PRAISE FOR *YOUR METABOLIC SHIFT*

Professor Robert Lustig

Dr Sharief Ibrahim is both a physician and a patient, which makes him doubly qualified to present and explain the complex topic of metabolic syndrome. You can't solve a problem if you don't know what the problem is. Dr Ibrahim's erudite explanation of these pathologies will help you tackle this modern scourge.

Robert Lustig, MD, MSL

Author of *Fat Chance: The Hacking of the American Mind,* and *Metabolical*

Dr. David Perlmutter

Dr Sharief Ibrahim transforms the complexities of metabolic dysfunction into a clear, empowering, and deeply human journey of renewal. Drawing on decades of clinical experience and personal transformation, he breaks down the science of metabolism into practical, actionable steps anyone can follow, providing an action plan for reclaiming vitality and guiding readers from confusion to confidence with clarity, compassion, and hope. Turns the science of metabolism into a roadmap for transformation.

Dr. David Perlmutter, MD

New York Times bestselling author of *Grain Brain,* and *Brain Defenders*

Professor Stuart Pringle

This book has something for everyone, from medical students to practising doctors, and Healthcare professionals to anyone interested in their own or their family's health and well-being.

Dr Sharief Ibrahim writes in a clear and engaging style. Each chapter is well-structured, featuring practical recommendations and concise summaries that make it easy to follow. It is an encyclopaedic tour de force on the history, science, and consequences of metabolic syndrome.

Drawing on a varied and successful career across multiple disciplines and regions, Dr Ibrahim distils his expertise into a work that will benefit readers, patients, and professionals alike. This valuable book deserves a place in healthcare institutions, personal libraries, and wellness centres as a trusted guide to health promotion and disease prevention.

Stuart D Pringle, MD FRCP

Honorary Professor & Consultant Cardiologist (retired)

Ninewells Hospital and Dundee Medical School

Michael Ash

Bridging the gap between traditional and functional medicine, *Your Metabolic Shift* reframes chronic disease through a metabolic lens.

Dr Sharief Ibrahim FRCP IFMCP, a consultant physician with decades on the NHS front line, reveals the biochemical mechanisms linking insulin resistance, visceral adiposity, inflammation, and neurodegeneration. Each chapter translates complex science into clinically actionable strategies for reversing metabolic syndrome through nutrition, movement, stress recalibration, and sleep optimisation.

A must-read for clinicians seeking a systems-based, patient-centred approach to chronic disease prevention and reversal.

Michael Ash DO, ND, BSc (Hons), RNT, FRSM,

Co-Founder & Chief Medical Strategy & Education Officer

Dr Christos Demetriou

I've had the privilege of working with Dr Sharief Ibrahim for nearly a decade and consider him both a mentor and a friend. His personal journey and professional expertise make him a rare voice in medicine, a doctor who can honestly say, "I've tried it, and it works." With over 45 years of frontline experience, he is the most seasoned Functional Medicine doctor in the United Kingdom.

This book is essential reading for anyone seeking to improve their health and vitality. Metabolic syndrome now affects roughly one in three adults, dramatically increasing the risk of heart disease, Type 2 diabetes, and stroke. **Your Metabolic Shift** arrives at a crucial time, offering a clear, practical path to reclaiming metabolic health. It empowers readers to take ownership of their well-being, sustain energy as they age, and live the vibrant life they were meant to enjoy.
Dr Christos Demetriou
Songwriter, record producer, and television host, is the author of *The Voice*.

Richard Abrahams

Four years ago, my wife and I visited Dr Ibrahim for a consultation that changed our lives. *Your Metabolic Shift* captures the essence of that experience, combining personal stories with precise, evidence-based science.

Dr Ibrahim explains how the human machine truly works and how simple, practical changes can transform health. This book offers both academic depth and human warmth, an inspiring guide for anyone ready to understand their body and take charge of their well-being.
Richard G. Abrahams
Science Fiction author of *The Chronicles of the Mediocrats*.

Steve Till

In Your Metabolic Shift, Dr Sharief Ibrahim, who has personally experienced many of the challenges he now helps others overcome, combines his personal experience with decades of clinical practice to guide his patients toward lasting well-being. With clarity, compassion, and scientific insight, he shows how simple lifestyle changes can prevent and reverse metabolic illness. His passion for helping others is evident throughout, and his work represents a valuable service not only to individuals but also to the NHS, which faces an ever-growing burden from obesity, diabetes, and related diseases.

Steve Till

Author of *The Run of Life, How any runner can reach their mountain top*

Professor Sam Lingam

As a healthcare professional, I found Your Metabolic Shift to be an outstanding bridge between clinical knowledge and real-world application. The book doesn't just discuss disease; it goes directly to the metabolic root causes and explains how lifestyle and nutrition can both prevent and reverse chronic conditions. The real-life case studies and the straightforward functional medicine approach make this a resource I would confidently recommend to patients and practitioners alike. It offers a holistic, effective framework for those seeking to take control of their health.

Professor Sam Lingam, MD (Hons), FRCPCH, FRCP, DCH, DRCOG

Author of *Appraisals in Medicine*

Your Metabolic Shift

by Dr. Sharief Ibrahim FRCP IFMCP

Published by Vitality Publishing

Paperback ISBN: 978-1-9192769-0-8
Harback ISBN: 978-1-9192769-2-2
eBook ISBN: 978-1-9192769-1-5

Copyright © 2025 Sharief Ibrahim

All rights reserved. No part of this book may be reproduced, stored in a retrieval system, or transmitted in any form or by any means, electronic, mechanical, photocopying, recording, or otherwise, without the prior written permission of the publisher, except in the case of brief quotations embodied in critical articles or reviews.

The moral right of the author has been asserted.

This book is intended solely for educational and informational purposes. The content of Your Metabolic Shift does not constitute medical advice and should not be used as a substitute for professional diagnosis or treatment. Readers are strongly advised to consult a qualified healthcare provider before making any changes to their diet, lifestyle, exercise routine, or medication.Although every effort has been made to ensure the accuracy of the information presented, the author and publisher disclaim any liability for loss, injury, or adverse effects that may result, directly or indirectly, from the use or application of the material in this book.

YOUR METABOLIC SHIFT

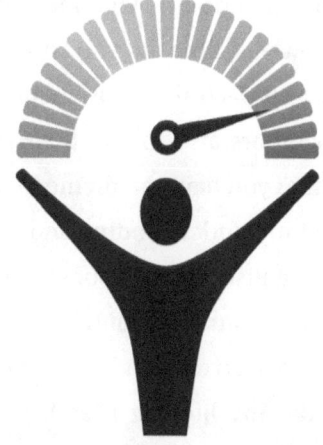

Dr Sharief Ibrahim
FRCP IFMCP

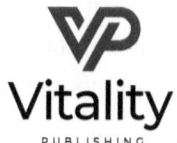

ACKNOWLEDGEMENTS

To my patients: Many of you sought comfort in my support during challenging periods of your life, and you entrusted me with your health. However, little did you know that your openness to exploring a new approach through functional medicine could open the doors for others also to end their suffering. This book brings together all that you have taught me in my clinical practice. You have sharpened my understanding and transformed my skill in crafting truly personalised plans. Your stories bring my teaching alive, and in respect of your contributions, I recall them here. Of course, all names have been changed, but the truth remains intact.

To my wife, **Hala**, my lifelong friend, personal doctor, and saviour. You stood beside me through illness and nurtured me back with love, one day at a time: from small steps to over 120 marathons completed now. Your consistency and resolve showed me the path to a lasting recovery. All that I have gained since then stems from your support.

My children, **Nada and Yasir**, your belief in me has been unshakable from day one. Despite neither of you being in the medical field, your interest and endless questioning developed my ability to explain functional medicine. The story of Your Metabolic Shift began in our kitchen on Saturday mornings and evolved into an ongoing narrative. Thank you for your patience, endurance and support in completing this project.

To my grandchildren, **Omnia and Amin**, your active lives have taught me the importance of teaching a healthy lifestyle from an early age. Of course, it is never too late, but since you were raised on a "rainbow" of fruit and veg and park races from infancy, I hope you find a special appreciation for this book as a directory of all the teachings I have tried to instil in you.

A few close friends have also shaped my work, including **Pastor Chris Demetriou** of Cornerstone Church, my first patient who followed the programme thoroughly and achieved life-changing results. Your step in the right direction proliferated my teachings and opened the path to a series of highly successful courses with your congregation. Thank you. To my lifelong friend, **Professor Ahmed Yagi**, for broadening my scope in molecular biology and subcellular metabolism through regular discussions of patient cases and Laboratory results. To my closest friend, **Richard Swift**, you championed my transition into Functional Medicine and guided me in refining my vision to focus on metabolic health. Thank you. To my dear friend **Pavlos Papanicolaou**, who continually provided current thinking that shaped my teachings over the years and was pivotal in laying the foundations of this book, thank you. Heartfelt thanks also to **Chris and Elisabeth Scappatura (Canada)** for shaping the plans of this book and for our ongoing collaboration, which now includes over 70 YouTube videos on metabolic health.

My path to disease prevention has also been profoundly shaped by some of the great minds in the field, both in the UK and the US. In the 90s, **Professor Pringles** in Dundee, Scotland, ignited my interest in community cardiology. Sincere thanks to **Professor Robert Lustig**, whose groundbreaking work on sugar and its detrimental effects on metabolism has significantly transformed public and scientific understanding of metabolic health. **Professor Roy Taylor (Newcastle University)** changed the narrative by demonstrating to the world how a simple dietary change can lead to long-term remission of type 2 diabetes. I want to express my deep appreciation to **Dr David Perlmutter**, whose pioneering work established uric acid as a key driver of insulin resistance. His insights into the roots of disease and the brain–body connection have significantly influenced my understanding and approach to metabolic health. **Dr Jason Fung (Canada)** inspired me with his work on diet and fasting, and most notably, **Dr Bob Rountree**, who makes the complex simple and unforgettable. Thank you.

Gratitude to my London and Surrey colleagues, **Professor Sam Lingam, Dr John Moran, and Pete Williams,** for the inspiring presentations we built together; to **Andrea Lecky** and colleagues in natural therapy in Weybridge for their regular local support and encouragement and to **Dr Shabir Pandor** for thoughtful case discussions and exemplary biological dentistry for my patients. Thanks to **Chris Moore** at Nordic VMS (Denmark) for his support of my patients over the years and for his steady interest and encouragement throughout every stage of this book's development.

To the incredible team who brought this book together: Special thanks to **Jenny Hasan**, a leading UK nutritionist, thank you for building most of Section 4 (Recipes) from the ground up. Your flavour-forward, whole-food dishes make metabolic health practical, delicious and convenient. Much gratitude also to **Steve Till**, my editor and fellow marathon runner, for meticulous planning and clarity; **Jonathan Howkins**, my outstanding social media strategist; **Flossie Burch**, my thorough research and marketing backbone; and my PA, **Shakira Elliott**, for coordinating the many moving parts. And to **Spiffing Publishing**, for the dedication that brought this book to life.

May these pages serve you well: read them, use them, and let Your Metabolic Shift begin.

CONTENTS

Introduction: A Personal Invitation 1
Note on the Author 13
History of Metabolic Syndrome 18

Section 1: Metabolic syndrome components

1. Metabolic health screening 26
2. Metabolism: The Engine of Vitality 43
3. Insulin Resistance: The Hidden
   Spark Behind Metabolic Chaos 66
4. Central Obesity: The Core of the Metabolic Storm 94
5. The Hidden Pulse of Metabolic Syndrome:
   Understanding High Blood Pressure 108
6. The Sweet Danger: A Personal Reflection on
   High Blood Glucose 128
7. Cholesterol: Friend, Foe, or Misunderstood? 153

Section 2: Metabolic syndrome-related conditions

8. Fatty Liver Disease: The Silent Invasion 180
9. A Breath of Insight: Sleep Apnoea and the Metabolic Maze 191
10. Periodontal Disease: A Local Problem
    with Systemic Consequences 204
11. Benign Prostatic Hyperplasia: A Metabolic or
    Hydraulic Problem? 214

12. Polycystic Ovary Syndrome: A Metabolic
    Disorder with Far-Reaching Impact..................................226
13. Osteoarthritis: When Joints Reflect Metabolic Distress 237
14. Varicose Veins: Metabolic, Ubiquitous, and Unsightly........251

Section 3: The natural solution

15. Health Goal Setting: A Personal Turning Point....................264
16. The Metabolic Diet Prescription..275
17. The Metabolic Exercise Prescription.....................................294
18. The Metabolic Sleep Prescription 307
19. The Metabolic Stress and Relationship Prescription 317
20. Baby Boomers Got It Wrong: Blue Zoners Got It Right!.......332
The Final Word: Your Journey to Health and Vitality 342

Section 4: Natural recipes and meals

The Art of Clean Eating: Simple recipes, Big Flavour 349
Additional Reading...410
End Notes 418
Index 435

INTRODUCTION

A Personal Invitation

If you've ever struggled with your weight, blood pressure, blood sugar, energy levels - or just felt that your body was working against you - you're not alone. I know, because I've lived it. Not just as a doctor, but as a patient.

Metabolic syndrome isn't an abstract medical concept to me. It's personal. I've grappled with it for most of my life - quietly at first, then more openly, as I began to connect the dots between my own experience and what I was seeing in my patients.

For more than 45 years, I've worked on the front lines of chronic disease. I've seen the silent creep of high blood pressure, the daily burden of type 2 diabetes, the heartbreak of premature heart disease. I've walked with thousands of patients through their struggles.

And I've come to believe this: most chronic illnesses don't appear out of the blue. They build up, silently and steadily, over years - sometimes decades - until one day, your body raises the alarm. That alarm may sound like a diagnosis, a crisis, or simply a sense that something isn't right.

This book is my response to that alarm.

It's rooted in science but shaped by stories - my own and those of the many patients who've taught me what textbooks never could. It's a call to look beyond symptoms and surface-level fixes and to understand the deeper, interconnected nature of metabolic health.

Because here's the truth: with accurate knowledge, support, and a few powerful changes, metabolic syndrome doesn't have to define your future.

Let's begin with two stories that fuelled my passion for holistic medicine.

The First Case: Her Boyfriend Left Because of Her Snoring

One of the earliest patients I saw with classic signs of metabolic syndrome was a 35-year-old woman from Portugal who had recently arrived in London. She was morbidly obese, plagued by constant headaches, exhausted beyond reason, and struggling to stay awake during the day. Initially, we suspected a neurological cause - perhaps even a minor stroke - so we arranged a head scan. It came back clear.

She was admitted for observation, but by a stroke of fate, she was placed in the wrong bed, in the high-dependency unit.

It turned out to be a serendipitous mistake.

During the morning rounds, the nurses raised red flags: overnight emergencies, wildly erratic blood pressure, oxygen levels that plunged to dangerous lows, and snoring so thunderous that fellow patients couldn't sleep. What at first seemed like a mild mystery was now a critical concern.

The diagnosis: Obstructive sleep apnoea - a condition where

breathing repeatedly stops and starts during sleep, starving the body of oxygen.

She was offered a CPAP machine, a device that helps keep airways open by wearing a mask at night. But she was desperate to solve the problem naturally. With my holistic medical hat firmly on, I advised her to lose weight, and she did. The transformation was extraordinary. Not only did her symptoms resolve, but she avoided a lifelong dependency on a noisy, uncomfortable breathing machine.

Her story unfolds entirely in Chapter 9.

The Second Case: Understanding the Person Behind the Condition

About twenty years ago, an accountant came to see me. His diabetes was poorly controlled despite a battery of medications. His GP was ready to escalate things with insulin. But as we spoke, it became clear the issue wasn't just biochemical. It was human.

He was drowning in stress. Missed deadlines. Client complaints. A mountain of paperwork he could never conquer. The more he tried to cope, the worse his blood sugars became.

As I listened, I saw something the numbers didn't reveal: he was a classic "golden retriever" - loyal, warm, people-oriented. He wasn't built to crunch numbers all day; he came alive when guiding others.

So, I offered him a radical suggestion: change your job. At first, he was stunned. "But I've been an accountant for 25 years," he protested. I wasn't asking him to quit, just to restructure - or at least, change how he does it. He brought in a junior colleague to handle the routine tasks, freeing him to focus on what he loved -

advising clients and forming meaningful connections.

The results were remarkable. His blood sugar normalised, without insulin. And for the first time in decades, he *enjoyed* his job. Aligning his work with his natural strengths, the simple adjustment helped him restore his health and live a happier life.

This book is about those stories. It explores the hidden roots of modern diseases, many of which begin silently as a cluster of risk factors known collectively as **metabolic syndrome.** Left unchecked, this slow-burning storm can ignite more than 1,200 chronic conditions - from high blood pressure and type 2 diabetes to heart attacks, strokes, dementia, and even cancer.

The scale is staggering. In the UK alone, metabolic syndrome affects one in three adults - a number that soars to one in two among those with obesity and overweight.

Why Is It Called 'Metabolic' Syndrome?

To understand metabolic syndrome, we must first understand **metabolism** - the elegant, behind-the-scenes process that sustains every breath you take, every thought you form, every step you walk. Metabolism is your body's built-in engine room, converting the food you eat into usable energy. This energy fuels everything from heartbeats and digestion to brain function and muscle movement. It's not just a buzzword thrown around in diet ads; it's the currency of life.

Each of the trillions of cells in your body functions like a miniature powerhouse, complete with its energy factories known as the **mitochondria.** But these factories don't run on goodwill - they require a steady supply of fuel, primarily in the form of glucose, the simple sugar that comes from digesting carbohydrates.

When everything runs smoothly, glucose enters cells efficiently with the help of **insulin**, a hormone produced by the pancreas.

Think of insulin as the key that unlocks the door to each cell, allowing glucose to come in and power the cell's activities. But here's where things can go wrong.

In many people today - often without obvious warning - this system begins to falter. **Insulin resistance** develops, meaning the "lock" on the cell's door becomes stubborn or jammed. The key (insulin) still tries to do its job, but the door only opens a crack. Glucose can't enter the cells efficiently, leading to two major problems: the sugar builds up in the bloodstream (where it doesn't belong), and the cells are starved of the very fuel they need to function.

This slow but steady breakdown lies at the heart of a wide array of modern illnesses - often long before any formal diagnosis is made. The remarkable thing is that **addressing this one root issue - insulin resistance - can have a ripple effect, improving multiple chronic conditions simultaneously.** Whether it's high blood pressure, heart disease, or type 2 diabetes, fixing the sugar-delivery system often improves all of them, making it a more innovative and integrated approach than tackling each disease separately.

You'll find a deeper dive into insulin resistance in Chapter 3 - but for now, let's unpack what causes it and how we can intervene.

What Causes Insulin Resistance?

Insulin resistance doesn't suddenly appear out of nowhere - it's typically years in the making. And it often starts with the food on your plate.

Modern diets have undergone significant shifts in recent decades. Gone are the days of simple, whole ingredients cooked from scratch. In their place, we've welcomed ultra-processed, calorie-dense, nutrient-poor foods: sugary cereals, fizzy drinks, chips, convenience meals, and the ever-expanding fast-food menu.

These foods trigger **chronic, low-grade inflammation** within the body and disturb how we process sugars and fats.

Fortunately, the reverse is also true. **A diet rich in unprocessed, nutrient-dense foods - such as vegetables, healthy fats, nuts, fish, legumes, and unrefined grains - helps restore insulin sensitivity.** This isn't about dieting for short-term weight loss. It's about restoring your body's internal balance, calming inflammation, and giving your cells the fuel they need, delivered in the right way.

Lifestyle choices beyond food also play a vital role. **Movement, restful sleep, and stress management** each enhance how well your body responds to insulin. It's not about perfection but about building a daily rhythm that supports - not sabotages - your metabolism.

By targeting the root causes instead of merely chasing symptoms, we can reduce dependence on multiple medications. It's not just a dream - it's a reality that's achievable for many people through thoughtful, evidence-based lifestyle changes.

So, What Exactly Is Metabolic Syndrome?
Metabolic syndrome is not a disease in itself - it's a red flag, a signal that your body's engine is misfiring. A **cluster of five risk factors defines it**, and you only need **three** to meet the criteria[1]:

- **Central obesity:** excess fat around the abdomen (not just cosmetic—it's metabolically active and inflammatory).
- **High blood pressure:** 130/80 mmHg or higher.
- **Elevated fasting glucose:** above 6.0 mmol/L, suggesting impaired sugar metabolism.
- **High triglycerides:** over 1.7 mmol/L, indicating poor fat processing.
- **Low HDL cholesterol:** less than 1.0 mmol/L—the "good" cholesterol that helps protect arteries.

Each of these risk factors may seem small in isolation. Still, together, they set the stage for serious diseases like heart attacks, strokes, type 2 diabetes, fatty liver disease, and even certain cancers. As you'll discover in later chapters, inflammation from abdominal fat can directly damage blood vessels, accelerate plaque formation (atherosclerosis), and drive hormonal imbalances.

The Early Signs Are Often Missed
Here's the problem: **you can have metabolic dysfunction for years without a diagnosis.** You may not feel overly sick - but you're not well either. This "grey zone" encompasses symptoms that we often dismiss as part of modern life, such as persistent fatigue, brain fog, unpredictable energy fluctuations, frequent hunger, mood swings, or restless sleep.

Later, as insulin resistance worsens, signs of high blood sugar become more visible - blurred vision, increased thirst and urination, frequent infections (especially of the skin or urinary tract), and a weakened immune response. But by this stage, considerable damage may already be done. (See Chapter 6 for a fuller picture of early and advanced symptoms)

Who Is At Risk - And How Young Is Too Young?
Traditionally, metabolic syndrome was considered a midlife problem, often appearing around the age of 40, when metabolism naturally begins to slow and hormone balances shift. However, modern lifestyles have rewritten the timeline. **We're now seeing the early stages of metabolic disease in younger people.**

Childhood obesity rates have skyrocketed. Teenagers are being diagnosed with what was once called "adult-onset" diabetes. Twenty-somethings are turning up in coronary care units with heart attacks and strokes. This shift is not just alarming - it's preventable.

Men with insulin resistance may present with issues like **erectile dysfunction or prostate enlargement** (explored in Chapter 11). At the same time, women often notice irregular menstrual cycles, acne, or difficulty conceiving - key signs of **polycystic ovary syndrome (PCOS)**, which has strong ties to insulin resistance (see Chapter 12).

A Hidden Epidemic

Perhaps the most dangerous aspect of metabolic syndrome is how quietly it spreads. **Many people with high blood pressure, high cholesterol, or high blood sugar don't realise they are connected - because we've been trained to treat each one as a separate issue.** Even many healthcare providers miss the forest for the trees.

This book is here to shift the narrative from disease management to disease prevention and reversal. By understanding what metabolic syndrome truly is and recognising the power of lifestyle interventions, we can rewrite our health story. Not with a medicine cabinet full of pills, but with habits that nourish our cells, restore our metabolism, and give us back the energy and vitality that modern life quietly steals.

Type 3 Diabetes? Yes, It's A Thing

You might be surprised to learn that Alzheimer's disease - the most common cause of dementia in older adults - has increasingly been referred to by another, rather unsettling name: **Type 3 diabetes**. This isn't just a catchy label; it reflects a more profound truth that's been emerging from decades of research. Alzheimer's is not only a degenerative brain disorder; it is also fundamentally a **metabolic disease**.

In Alzheimer's, the brain's ability to process glucose - the primary fuel for brain cells - deteriorates. Imagine trying to power a city when the electricity grid is failing. Neurons begin to starve, communication breaks down, and over time, regions of the brain start to shrink.[2] This is no small insight: it means that many of the risk factors for type 2 diabetes - such as insulin resistance, inflammation, and poor diet - also lay the groundwork for cognitive decline.

Studies now show that increased abdominal fat - a hallmark of metabolic syndrome - is closely linked to reduced brain volume. To put it plainly, this means the wider your waistline, the smaller your brain will be.[3] This metabolic-cognitive connection highlights the profound impact that our daily lifestyle choices have on brain health.

Silent Casualties: The Liver And Kidneys

While the brain may be the most feared site of metabolic fallout, it's far from the only one. Let's talk about the liver.

Non-alcoholic fatty liver disease (NAFLD), a condition once considered rare, is now the most common reason people need a liver transplant. It has quietly eclipsed alcohol as the leading cause of liver failure in many parts of the world. NAFLD can progress stealthily from a fatty liver to inflammation, fibrosis, cirrhosis, and eventually liver cancer (explored more fully in Chapter 8).

And then there's the kidney - our unsung hero of a filtration system. Chronic high blood sugar and elevated blood pressure damage the delicate vessels within the kidneys, leading to **chronic kidney disease (CKD)**. For some, this condition quietly progresses until dialysis or a transplant becomes the only option. It's a slow and often silent decline - one that many people never see coming until it's too late.

Turning the Tide: Yes, You Can

So, where does that leave us? Thankfully, not in despair - but in **opportunity**. The scientific consensus is crystal clear: diets rich in ultra-processed carbohydrates and refined sugars, when combined with inactivity, are driving this global metabolic meltdown.

The good news is also powerful: **these can be changed**. And contrary to popular belief, reclaiming your metabolic health doesn't require superhuman effort. It starts with small, strategic steps. This book is here to guide you through those steps - armed with up-to-date science, practical tools, and deeply personal stories from my journey and those of my patients.

Over the years, I've observed a common and immediate reaction when I talk to patients about sugar: *"But I don't eat sugar."* The confusion here is understandable, but it is also dangerous. Most people think "sugar" refers only to the white granules they stir into coffee or the obvious sweets, such as cake, chocolate, or soda. However, biochemically speaking, **all carbohydrates ultimately break down into glucose**. That includes many foods people consider "healthy" or "innocent": bread, pasta, rice, cereals, and yes, even your beloved wholemeal toast.

Eating a bowl of cereal or a sandwich can be metabolically equivalent to dumping sugar straight into your bloodstream. These "fast carbs" spike your blood glucose just as quickly as a spoonful of sugar - if not faster. In contrast, unrefined whole foods, such as vegetables, legumes, and whole fruits, are digested more slowly, releasing glucose in a gentle, steady stream that your body can handle.

Short-Term Temptations vs. Long-Term Rewards

As a holistic doctor, I don't just treat lab values - I treat people, with all their hopes, fears, and cravings. I understand the emotional pull of chocolate cake or a glass of wine at the end of a long day. But I also know that true motivation comes from aligning our habits with something more profound.

So, I often ask my patients to picture something real and meaningful, such as *playing with their grandchildren, hiking in their seventies, or dancing at their granddaughter's wedding*. When your goals are vivid and emotionally compelling, they become powerful enough to outweigh fleeting temptations.

Why Health Matters More Than Ever
At first glance, it may seem evident that health is essential, but in the 21st century, **health has taken on a whole new dimension**. We are living longer than ever before, but we are not necessarily living **better**.

Consider this: in 1900, the average life expectancy in the UK was approximately 50 years. Today, it's over 80. That's a gift of more than three decades of extra life. But what are we doing with those years?

Here's the catch: many people now spend the last 12 to 15 years of life coping with multiple chronic conditions - diabetes, arthritis, frailty, memory loss, and heart disease.[4] We are not dying young anymore - we're living long and unwell.

To truly thrive in this new age of longevity, **we must extend not just lifespan, but health span** - the years during which we remain energetic, independent, and mentally sharp. And the key to this, you guessed it: **metabolic health**.

A Doctor's Wake-Up Call
Let me end this section with a story I know intimately - because it's mine. I was no different from the patients I now try to help. Long hours. Fast food. Stress. No exercise. Until one day, I collapsed at work. I nearly died.

That was my wake-up call.

Today, at 70, I have gone from a 40-inch waist (102 cm) to a 32-inch waist (81 cm). I've run over 120 marathons. I have more energy now than I did in my forties. I share this not to boast, but to show what's possible.

Please let me help you reclaim your health - not just for today, but for the decades ahead. You don't have to settle for decline. The future is still yours to shape.

A Note on the Author

As a child, I was lean - but not entirely healthy. Despite my slender frame, a small potbelly persisted like an unsolved riddle. No matter how active I was, that little protrusion never quite went away. Later, in early adulthood, I threw myself into diet and exercise in a bid to flatten it - but with little success. What I didn't know then was that this belly wasn't just fat. It was the outward sign of a deeper issue: fatty liver disease, one of the early red flags of metabolic syndrome.

At the time, I had no name for what I was experiencing. I simply knew that my energy would crash, especially after meals. I was often hungry, in a way that went beyond ordinary appetite - craving carbs with a kind of urgency I couldn't explain. In retrospect, those were early signs of blood sugar instability. Yet, growing up in a household where sweets were rare and snacks were forbidden, my hunger remained largely unacknowledged.

Our family meals followed a strict rhythm. My father, ever punctual, would return from work by 4:30 p.m., rest briefly, and rise just in time for dinner, synchronised with the 5 o'clock news. But for me, this was the day's most anxious moment. As the iconic chimes echoed from the radio, I would break into a sweat, my hands trembling, my heart racing. I was experiencing hypoglycaemia - low blood sugar - long before I had the language or training to recognise it. Only eating would bring relief, often just in the nick of time. I dreaded any delay in lunch, not because I was spoiled or impatient, but because my physiology demanded it.

That was my introduction to metabolic dysfunction - long before I studied medicine or stood in a clinic coat. And years later, it would return in a more dramatic form, completely changing my life.

I graduated from Khartoum Medical School in 1980, trained in the classical medical tradition - system by system, organ by organ. On ward rounds, we were expected to narrow our attention: the heart during cardiology, the brain during neurology. But even then, a quiet question stirred in me: how do all these parts work together? What is the body trying to achieve as a whole.

That Question has Guided my Entire Medical Career
In Saudi Arabia, I had the privilege of directing a primary health care program under the World Health Organisation's guidance. There, I saw a broader picture of health: not just the absence of disease, but the presence of energy, mental clarity, purpose, and connection. This wider definition inspired me, but I also began to see how rarely modern medicine allowed space for it.

Later, after moving to the United Kingdom in the early 1990s, I pursued postgraduate training and earned the MRCP (Membership of the Royal College of Physicians). Unlike many of my peers, I chose not to pursue a narrow subspecialty. I remained a generalist, deliberately so. I trained across Guy's, St Thomas's, and King's College Hospitals, earning dual accreditation in general and geriatric medicine. Eventually, I was awarded a Fellowship from the Royal College of Physicians and Surgeons of Glasgow.

I often joked with colleagues that I suffered from "professional claustrophobia" - I needed to roam across disciplines. Like a nomad at heart, I found it challenging to settle in a single silo of medicine. My curiosity about how systems interconnect never left me. And so, I embraced general medicine - its complexity, breadth, and humanity.

But Professional Success Came at a Steep Cost

Beneath the surface of achievement, I was burning out. Years of night shifts, mounting stress, poor sleep, and an increasingly processed diet began to take their toll on the body. My waistline expanded. My knees ached. My blood pressure climbed. My fitness vanished to the point where walking half a mile to the train station felt like a challenge. I relied on taxis for distances I once would've jogged.

Eventually, my Body Gave Out

One day, I collapsed in a hospital corridor - ironically, the same corridor where I'd once cared for patients. A bleeding cyst in my thyroid had compressed my windpipe, triggering a medical emergency. Surgery followed - then another, after a second bleed. This time, I remained unconscious for seven days in the intensive care unit.

When I finally awoke, I was no longer the doctor. I was the most critically ill patient in the very hospital where I had spent years treating others.

That was my Turning Point

Determined not only to recover but to reclaim true vitality, I embarked on a personal transformation. At 70, I now have a 32-inch waist (down from 40 inches), and I've completed over 120 marathons. My energy and health today far surpass what I had decades earlier. This book is the story of that transformation - and what I've learned from both sides of the consultation table.

The Inevitable Shift

The effects of metabolic disease didn't just touch my patients - they shook the foundation of my own life. It became clear to me: I could no longer practise medicine the same way.

And so, I made the hardest decision of my life. I left my secure role as a senior consultant in the NHS. No salary. No pension. Just conviction. I wanted to pursue a field of medicine that treated the whole person, not just parts in isolation.

The Path Ahead was Uncertain

Then, a simple conversation changed everything. My son Yasir, an architect, mentioned a doctor he'd heard on a podcast who spoke in a language that sounded uncannily like mine. That doctor was Dr. Mark Hyman. He indirectly introduced me to the field of functional medicine.

Within weeks, I was on a flight to Chicago for my first module. What followed was a deep immersion in this systems-based approach to health. I met Dr. Jeffrey Bland, the father of functional medicine, and discovered a community that finally reflected my long-standing philosophy. This was more than a new career direction - it was a homecoming.

That decision - risky, unconventional, and wildly uncertain - became the most rewarding of my life.

"I Feel 30 Years Younger"

Eager to bring this new paradigm into the community, I approached Pastor Chris Demetriou, a well-respected local church leader, and offered to run a free health course for his congregation. Cautious but curious, he decided to try it himself first.

Eight weeks later, the results spoke for themselves. He lost 8 kilograms, eliminated chronic back pain, came off all medications, and told me, grinning, "I feel 30 years younger."

Word spread. The program took off. One woman, who had depended on insulin for three decades, was able - for the first time - to stabilise her blood sugars naturally. Her consultant at the hospital was so astonished, he reportedly "almost fell off his chair."

Looking back, I now realise that I was practising functional medicine long before I had a name for it. Even within the constraints of hospital wards, I had always viewed the patient as a whole person, shaped by biology, behaviour, environment, and belief.

Functional medicine didn't just confirm what I believed - it gave me the tools to act on it.

This book is the result of everything I've lived, studied, endured, and overcome. If something in my story echoes with yours, know this: it's never too late to take your health - and your future - into your own hands.

The History of Metabolic Syndrome

Metabolic syndrome is as ancient as humankind itself. Our distant hunter-gatherer ancestors may not have experienced the full range of effects that we do today, but biological vulnerabilities have always been present. What has changed dramatically is our environment - especially our diet, activity levels, and stress levels. It wasn't until relatively recently that metabolic syndrome was formally recognised and named. The journey to that recognition is a fascinating tale of medical discovery, social transformation, and industrial impact.

Medical Milestones

The formal story of metabolic syndrome dates to the early 20th century. In 1921, Elliot P. Joslin - one of the pioneers in diabetes research - first reported a striking connection between diabetes, hypertension, and elevated uric acid levels.[1] Just two years later, Swedish physician Eskil Kylin expanded on these findings, conducting additional studies on what was then an emerging clinical pattern.[2]

Fast forward to 1947: French physician Jean Vague observed that obesity concentrated in the upper body (particularly the abdomen) was closely linked with chronic conditions such as diabetes, atherosclerosis, kidney stones, and gout. Her insights were more than observational - she and her colleagues demonstrated that dietary interventions, particularly low-calorie and low-carbohydrate regimens, could lead to significant improvements in triglyceride levels, blood sugar, and cholesterol.[3]

By 1967, researchers such as Piero Avogadro, Gaetano Crepaldi, Giuliano Enzi, and Antonio Tiengo formally diagnosed patients with obesity who also exhibited diabetes, elevated cholesterol, and high triglycerides.[4] Their findings revealed that these metabolic issues could improve substantially on calorie-restricted, low-carb diets. Around this time, P. Singer introduced the term *metabolic syndrome* to describe a constellation of conditions: obesity, gout, diabetes mellitus, hypertension, and elevated blood lipids.[5]

The momentum continued. In 1977, German internist Hermann Haller emphasised the *additive* nature of risk factors, suggesting that together they significantly increase the likelihood of atherosclerosis and heart disease.[6] His list included obesity, diabetes, high uric acid, elevated blood fats, and fatty liver.

One year later, Gerald Phillips further advanced the understanding. He highlighted that the risk of heart attack was linked to a combination of abnormalities: glucose intolerance, high insulin levels, dyslipidaemia, and hypertension.[7] He even speculated that hormonal changes - particularly those involving sex hormones - might be the unifying thread.

Then came a pivotal moment in 1988. Gerald Reaven introduced the term "Syndrome X," proposing that insulin resistance was the key underlying mechanism.[8] This was revolutionary: it shifted the conversation from treating symptoms to addressing root causes. According to Reaven, insulin resistance ties together many of the metabolic issues that precede type 2 diabetes and cardiovascular disease.[9]

Modern Definitions and Discoveries

As scientific consensus grew, organisations began standardising definitions. In 2005, the International Diabetes Federation (IDF), in collaboration with Japanese researchers, proposed that *abdominal obesity* be a core diagnostic criterion for metabolic syndrome.[10] This made intuitive sense: waist circumference often reflects the accumulation of visceral fat - the most metabolically harmful type.

But research continued to evolve. In 2008, animal studies highlighted that it's not just the fat that causes harm, but the *inflammation within fat tissue*. This insight helped shift attention from simple weight metrics to deeper biochemical processes.[11]

By 2009, several major health organisations - IDF, the American Heart Association, the World Heart Federation, and others - agreed on a revised set of diagnostic criteria. Crucially, this updated model no longer requires abdominal obesity to be present, acknowledging that metabolic dysfunction can also exist in lean individuals.[12]

In 2010, the World Health Organisation reinforced insulin resistance as the central factor. They recommended the oral glucose tolerance test and fasting insulin measurements as tools to assess risk. Their conclusions were clear: the interaction between insulin resistance and abdominal obesity is the driving force behind the development of metabolic syndrome.[13]

A Breakthrough in Reversal

In 2011, a groundbreaking study by Professor Roy Taylor of Newcastle University brought new hope. He demonstrated that type 2 diabetes could be reversed - yes, reversed - using a carefully controlled low-calorie diet. MRI scans confirmed that excess fat in the liver and pancreas vanished, and 11 out of 13 participants maintained normal blood sugar levels a year after the intervention. This wasn't just another weight loss study; it was a paradigm shift.[14]

Professor Taylor made the intervention accessible through a public website, and the impact was profound. Seventy per cent of participants lost approximately 4.5 kilograms (roughly 10 pounds) and remained in remission for over two years. These findings were so compelling that the NHS in the UK adopted the programme, and the American Diabetes Association acknowledged that long-term remission is a viable and desirable treatment goal.

Metabolic Syndrome: Upstream Causes, Downstream Effects
The timeline of discovery highlights a profound truth: metabolic syndrome is not a single disease, but rather a complex cascade of upstream risk factors that manifest as diverse downstream conditions. Where the symptoms emerge depends on your genetic and physiological vulnerabilities - your so-called "weak link."

For example:

- If your weak link lies in your arteries, metabolic syndrome may show up as high blood pressure, heart disease, stroke, or dementia.
- If it affects your joints or bones, it may lead to conditions such as gout, osteoarthritis, or osteoporosis.

Understanding this variability is essential. It reminds us that while metabolic syndrome affects everyone differently, its root causes are remarkably consistent - and often preventable.

What Causes Metabolic Syndrome?
Metabolic syndrome does not stem from a single cause, but rather from the convergence of multiple lifestyle and biological factors - poor diet, sedentary behaviour, chronic stress, sleep disruption, and underlying genetic susceptibilities. At its core, metabolic

syndrome is the body's reaction to an environment it was never designed for: one saturated with cheap, calorie-dense, nutrient-poor foods and opportunities for physical inactivity.

A major accelerant of this crisis came not from a medical breakthrough, but from the political arena. In the early 1970s, U.S. President Richard Nixon, facing inflation, a looming re-election campaign, and public unrest, set out to make food cheaper and more abundant. To do so, he appointed Earl Butz as Secretary of Agriculture. Butz dismantled traditional farming subsidies and encouraged the development of massive industrial-scale monoculture farming, particularly of corn. The result was an explosion in the production of high-fructose corn syrup (HFCS), a sweetener far cheaper and more potent than cane sugar.

HFCS quickly became a staple of the modern processed food industry. It found its way into soft drinks, cereals, condiments, and fast food. But unlike natural sugars, fructose does not stimulate insulin or leptin - the hormones that tell us we're full. This biochemical loophole encouraged overeating, promoted fat accumulation (especially visceral fat), and helped fuel an unprecedented rise in obesity.

To lower the cost of food, Butz also encouraged the production of corn oil to support the fast-food industry, which led to the emergence of companies such as McDonald's, Burger King, and KFC, which are now global brands.

The numbers tell the story starkly: in the early 1970s, only about 15% of Americans were classified as obese. By 2022, that figure had nearly tripled to 42.4%.[15] Between 1970 and 1990, consumption of HFCS increased by more than 1,000%.[16]

Then came the COVID-19 pandemic, which acted like fuel to a fire already burning. Lockdowns, remote work, disrupted routines, and emotional stress created the perfect conditions for metabolic deterioration. Physical activity plummeted, snacking and comfort eating soared, and sleep quality declined. Studies across various populations have shown consistent weight gain and worsening of metabolic markers during lockdown periods.[17,18]

In essence, the pandemic didn't just expose our vulnerabilities - it magnified them. And nowhere was this more evident than in the dramatic rise in conditions linked to metabolic syndrome: obesity, insulin resistance, fatty liver disease, and type 2 diabetes.

Looking Forward: Screening the Modern Metabolism

The story of metabolic syndrome - spanning nearly a century of clinical observation, scientific discovery, and societal transformation - has brought us to a crucial turning point. We now understand that metabolic syndrome is not merely a coincidence of symptoms, but a predictable, preventable, and often reversible progression of biological dysfunction driven by modern lifestyles. It begins subtly, usually decades before disease manifests, with silent shifts in blood sugar, cholesterol, blood pressure, and body fat distribution.

This raises an essential question: how can we detect metabolic risk early, before it develops into a disease? Fortunately, we now have powerful tools to do just that. Advances in blood testing, imaging, and risk scoring allow us to identify individuals at risk long before they develop diabetes, heart disease, or other complications.

In the next chapter, we will delve into the evolving science of **metabolic screening** - what it entails, who should undergo it, and how early detection can be a game-changer in preventing chronic illnesses. If history has taught us anything, it's that waiting for symptoms to appear is often too late. Prevention begins with awareness, and awareness starts with screening.

SECTION 1

METABOLIC SYNDROME COMPONENTS

CHAPTER 1

Metabolic health screening

A Time Bomb Ready to Explode

It was 2006, and I was working alongside Professor Pringle from the University of Dundee in a mobile cardiology clinic. Our mission was simple but urgent: to detect hidden heart disease early and reduce the toll of cardiac deaths. One day, we approached a cheerful man in his mid-30s, stepping out of a bingo hall. He looked fit, energetic, and in good spirits - hardly someone you'd suspect of harbouring a deadly condition.

But appearances can be deceiving.

When we measured his blood pressure, it registered an alarming 160/100 mmHg - well above the healthy average of 120/80 mmHg. Then came the real shock: his electrocardiogram (ECG) showed clear signs of ischemia - reduced blood flow to the heart. We immediately referred him for an urgent coronary angiogram.

What it revealed was chilling.

All three of his main coronary arteries were severely blocked. He was quite literally a walking heart attack, seconds away from catastrophe. The image on the screen wasn't just a clinical finding

- it was the portrait of a ticking time bomb.

Thankfully, the story didn't end there. He underwent emergency triple bypass surgery and began a lifelong regimen of medication to manage his condition.

That day, he may have been lucky at bingo, but his greatest stroke of luck was being in the right place at the right time, caught just before his silent killer struck.

A Missed Opportunity

Looking back, I can't help but think how different things might have been if we had met this gentleman just a few years earlier. With timely guidance, we could have addressed his risk factors and possibly prevented the need for major heart surgery. Unfortunately, his story is not unique.

Many people who suffer a heart attack never see it coming. They believe it struck without warning - an unfortunate twist of fate. What they don't realise is that their bodies were sending subtle signals for years, even decades. Underneath the surface, a condition known as metabolic syndrome had been quietly increasing their risk, unrecognised and unchecked.

In this book, you'll learn what metabolic syndrome is, how it silently drives serious conditions like heart disease, and - most importantly - what you can do about it. By understanding your body's warning signs and making simple, targeted changes, you can reduce your risk and take control of your health. Early intervention doesn't just change outcomes - it saves lives.

What Is Metabolic Syndrome?

Metabolic syndrome is not a single disease but a dangerous combination of risk factors that, when present together, significantly increase your chance of developing serious conditions like type 2 diabetes, heart disease, and stroke. These risk factors include:

- **Central obesity** – excess fat around the waist (commonly called abdominal fat)
- **High blood pressure**
- **Elevated blood sugar levels**
- **High triglycerides** - a common type of fat found in the blood
- **Low levels of HDL cholesterol** - the "good" cholesterol that helps clear the "bad" one from the bloodstream

To be diagnosed with metabolic syndrome, a person must have at least **three of the five** risk factors.

But here's the alarming part: metabolic syndrome affects **1 in 3 people in the United Kingdom** - many without even knowing it. It creeps in quietly, often without symptoms, until it manifests as a serious, sometimes life-threatening event such as a heart attack or stroke.

Think of metabolic syndrome as a warning sign - a red flag waving before the onset of multiple chronic diseases. It opens the gate to a cascade of health problems, including obesity, type 2 diabetes, high blood pressure, cardiovascular disease, arthritis, dementia, and even certain types of cancer.

That's why early identification is critical.

We urgently need simple, practical, and sensitive tools to detect those at risk before it's too late. While these tools do not replace proper medical evaluation, they can play a decisive role in **raising awareness and prompting action**. The goal isn't to encourage self-diagnosis or self-treatment but to **empower you** to take charge of your health and partner with your healthcare providers to protect and improve it.

Are You at Risk of Metabolic Syndrome?

Identifying your risk for metabolic syndrome early could be one of the most critical steps you take for your long-term health.

Start by asking yourself a few key questions:

- Do you have a family history of conditions like obesity, high blood pressure, type 2 diabetes, heart disease, stroke, dementia, or gout?
- Do you lead a sedentary lifestyle?
- Do you smoke or consume alcohol excessively?

If you answered "yes" to any of these, it's time to pay closer attention. These factors - especially in combination - can significantly increase your risk of developing metabolic syndrome. Fortunately, many of them are within your power to change. Quitting smoking, cutting back on alcohol, moving your body more, and improving your daily habits can dramatically lower your risk and enhance your overall well-being.

While your family history is something you can't change, it can serve as a powerful motivator. You may not be able to rewrite your genetics, but you can rewrite your lifestyle story. Factors like a poor diet, lack of sleep, high stress, inactivity, and strained relationships can all be modified to work in your favour.

At its core, metabolic syndrome often stems from the body's inability to process glucose effectively - the very fuel your body needs for energy (we explore this in depth in Chapter 3). When glucose can't enter your cells adequately, it's stored as fat instead, gradually altering your body's shape and undermining your health.

That's why measuring body fat - not just weight - can be a practical early warning sign. It offers insights into how well your metabolism is functioning, even before a formal diagnosis is made.

Understanding Body Fat: A Key to Unlocking Metabolic Health

Body fat isn't just about appearance - it plays a central role in your risk of developing metabolic syndrome and related diseases. Accurately measuring body fat helps us assess that risk. But with so many tools available - from simple tape measures to advanced scanning technologies - which methods truly matter?

Let's explore how body fat is measured, starting with the basics and progressing to more sophisticated techniques, and examine how each method relates to disease risk.

Body Weight: A Starting Point, Not the Full Picture

Your total body weight includes fat, muscle, bones, organs, and water. While it's easy to track, weight alone doesn't reflect body fat. However, comparing your current weight to when you were in your physical prime (typically around age 20-25) can be helpful. If you weighed 60 kg back then and now weigh 90 kg, you've gained 30 kg - likely fat. That realisation can be a powerful motivator to make changes that improve health and lower disease risk.

Body Mass Index (BMI): Popular but Imperfect

BMI, calculated as weight (in kilograms) divided by height squared (in meters), is a widely used measure of health. It categorises individuals into weight status groups based on population averages.

BMI Categories for Caucasians (UK):
- Underweight: <18.5 kg/m^2
- Normal: 18.5-24.9 kg/m^2
- Overweight: 25-29.9 kg/m^2
- Obese: 30-39.9 kg/m^2
- Morbidly Obese: ≥40 kg/m^2

For Asian populations, the risk thresholds are lower:
- Underweight: <18.5 kg/m^2
- Normal: 18.5–22.9 kg/m^2
- Overweight: 23–27.4 kg/m^2
- Obese: ≥27.5 kg/m^2

However, BMI has limitations. It does not account for fat distribution or muscle mass. An athlete with high muscle mass may have a "high" BMI but low fat. Likewise, many people with a "normal" BMI may carry excessive body fat, particularly around the abdomen - a key risk factor for metabolic syndrome. Studies show that **33% of men and 52% of women with a normal BMI still have excess body fat**.

Waist Circumference (WC): A Window into Belly Fat

Unlike BMI, waist circumference (WC) specifically targets **central obesity**, which is fat stored around the abdominal organs. This type of fat, known as **visceral fat**, is strongly linked to metabolic diseases such as type 2 diabetes, heart disease, and dementia.

To measure your waist circumference (WC), wrap the tape measure around your torso midway between your lower ribs and the top of your hip bone, near your belly button.

Risk thresholds:
- **Men:** ≥94 cm increases risk; ≥102 cm significantly increases risk
- **Women:** ≥80 cm increases risk; ≥88 cm significantly increases risk

Waist-to-Hip Ratio (WHR) and Hip Circumference (HC)

WHR compares the waist circumference to the hip circumference to estimate fat distribution. It's informative but can be misleading due to hormonal and muscular variations. For example, oestrogen encourages fat storage around the hips (beneficial in childbearing years), which may skew the ratio in women. Similarly, athletes may have larger hip muscles, which can influence the measurement.

Hip circumference (HC) is taken at the widest point of the hips (greater trochanter). While HC can help calculate ratios, it's rarely used on its own for disease risk assessment.

Waist-to-Height Ratio (WHtR): Simple and Effective

To overcome the limitations of WHR, experts in the UK's National Institute for Health and Care Excellence (NICE) recommend using the **waist-to-height ratio**. It's easy to calculate and highly predictive of abdominal fat and disease risk.[1]

Interpretation:
- **Healthy:** 0.4–0.49
- **At risk:** 0.5–0.59
- **High risk:** ≥0.6

Put simply, your waist should be **less than half your height**. If it's more, your risk of metabolic syndrome rises sharply.

Neck Circumference (NC): A Simple, Telling Indicator

Neck circumference (NC) is emerging as a practical alternative to waist measurement for assessing obesity and the risk of metabolic syndrome. Quick and non-invasive, NC is measured just below Adam's apple, with the individual standing upright, shoulders relaxed, and looking straight ahead.

Research suggests that an NC greater than 34 centimetres (13.4 inches) in women and 37 centimetres (14.5 inches) in men is associated with central obesity, a key metabolic risk factor. Because it reflects upper-body fat accumulation, NC may offer a more consistent marker, especially in populations where standardising waist measurements is challenging.

Body Roundness Index (BRI): Looking Beyond the Scale

The Body Roundness Index (BRI) provides a more comprehensive understanding of body fat distribution and visceral fat - the hidden fat that surrounds internal organs. Unlike BMI, BRI incorporates height, weight, waist circumference, and hip circumference into a single formula that estimates both total and central adiposity.

A healthy BRI falls below 10 on a scale of 0 to 20. Higher scores reflect increased roundness of the body, signalling a greater risk for obesity-related conditions, including metabolic syndrome. As a visual and numerical indicator, BRI helps clinicians and patients better understand how fat is distributed in the body and why it matters.

Measuring Body Fat and Composition: Tools for Understanding Metabolic Health

In the next section, we'll examine modern technologies - such as bioelectrical impedance and DEXA scans - that provide a deeper and more precise understanding of your body fat and its impact on your health.

Bioelectrical Impedance Analysis (BIA)

Bioelectrical impedance is a modern, non-invasive method for estimating body composition. It works by measuring how easily a mild electrical current passes through the body. Since fat and bone resist electrical flow more than muscle or water-rich tissues, these differences help estimate body fat percentage.

You can find basic BIA devices that resemble regular bathroom scales - some even feature handgrips for enhanced accuracy. While these consumer versions offer useful insights, more advanced and precise machines are often available in gyms, wellness centres, and medical clinics.

DEXA Scan: A Comprehensive Body Composition Tool

Originally developed to evaluate bone density in osteoporosis, dual-energy X-ray absorptiometry (DEXA) scans have become a gold standard for body composition analysis. In addition to measuring bone health, DEXA accurately quantifies fat mass, lean tissue, and visceral fat - the fat stored deep around your internal organs.

Healthy total body fat ranges vary:

- **Men:** ideally 12%–20%, acceptable up to 25%
- **Women:** ideally 20%–30%, acceptable up to 35%

Visceral Fat: The Hidden Threat

Visceral fat is more than just a cosmetic concern - it surrounds vital organs and plays a significant role in metabolic syndrome. High levels are associated with an increased risk of inflammation, insulin resistance and cardiovascular disease.

While CT and MRI scans offer the most precise measurements of visceral fat, they are costly and often impractical for routine screening. The DEXA scan, by contrast, provides a reliable and more accessible alternative. For optimal metabolic health, visceral fat should account for **no more than 12%** of your total body fat. Anything above that threshold significantly raises the risk for metabolic disorders.

High Blood Pressure: The Silent Driver of Risk

High blood pressure - also known as hypertension - is a key component of metabolic syndrome and a major contributor to life-threatening events like heart attacks and strokes. Often symptomless, it's sometimes called "the silent killer" because it can quietly damage blood vessels and vital organs over time.

Fortunately, thanks to the widespread availability of digital home blood pressure monitors, keeping track of your blood pressure has never been easier. Regular self-checks can help detect elevated readings early, enabling timely intervention and improved long-term outcomes.

A blood pressure measurement includes two values:

- **Systolic pressure:** the peak pressure when your heart beats.
- **Diastolic pressure:** the lowest pressure when your heart rests between beats.

These numbers are written as a ratio - **systolic over diastolic** (e.g., 120/80 mmHg). Here's how to interpret your readings:

- **Optimal:** below 120/80 mmHg
- **Normal:** below 130/85 mmHg
- **Pre-hypertension:** 130–139 / 85–89 mmHg—warning signs of metabolic syndrome.
- **Grade 1 hypertension:** 140–159 / 90–99 mmHg
- **Grade 2 hypertension:** 160–179 / 100–109 mmHg
- **Grade 3 hypertension:** 180+/110+ mmHg

Knowing where your numbers fall is the first step in preventing the cascade of problems associated with high blood pressure. For an in-depth look at hypertension - its causes, consequences, and treatments - turn to Chapter 5.

Monitoring Your Blood Glucose at Home

Keeping track of your blood glucose levels is a powerful way to understand how your body responds to food, activity, and stress - key factors in managing metabolic syndrome.

Traditionally, this has meant using a glucose meter, which requires a small drop of blood obtained through a finger prick. While effective, this method can be inconvenient and uncomfortable for regular use.

Fortunately, technology now offers a more user-friendly alternative: **Continuous Glucose Monitoring (CGM)**. With CGM, a small sensor inserted just under your skin continuously tracks your blood sugar levels throughout the day and night - no finger pricks required. Download the companion app, follow the instructions to insert the sensor, and let the system handle the rest. Most continuous glucose monitors (CGMs) can provide data for up to 14 days, offering a detailed picture of how your glucose levels fluctuate in response to meals, exercise, and sleep.

This real-time feedback empowers you to make smarter lifestyle choices - adjusting your diet, tweaking your activity level, or identifying hidden triggers that cause glucose spikes.

As a general guideline:

- **Fasting glucose** should ideally be below **5.5 mmol/L (100 mg/dL)**
- **Two hours after eating**, it should remain under **7.8 mmol/L (140 mg/dL)**

We'll take a deeper dive into interpreting CGM data and maximising your results in **Chapter 6**.

Metabolic Risk Factors: What Your Lab Results Reveal

When it comes to evaluating your metabolic health, your blood doesn't lie. A routine blood test at your doctor's office can reveal early signs of metabolic imbalance - often before symptoms appear. Understanding what these lab markers mean empowers you to take control of your health. Here are two of the most telling indicators:

Fasting Insulin: Your Early Warning System

Before blood sugar levels rise, your body sends out a quieter signal: elevated insulin. Insulin resistance, where your cells fail to respond appropriately to insulin, is the first step toward developing metabolic syndrome. In response, your pancreas works overtime, producing more insulin to regulate blood sugar levels.

That's why **fasting insulin** is such a powerful early marker. Even if your blood sugar still looks "normal," a fasting insulin level of **10 µU/mL or higher** suggests your metabolism is already struggling. Catching this early gives you a crucial head start in reversing the process.

Blood Glucose: The Later Stage Marker

Fasting insulin levels rise early, while **elevated blood glucose** tends to show up later in the development of metabolic syndrome. A key early indicator? Blood glucose is measured **two hours after a meal,** specifically after a **glucose tolerance test (GTT)**. If your level is **7.8 mmol/L (140 mg/dL)** or more two hours after consuming 75 grams of glucose, it's a sign your body is having trouble managing sugar.

As metabolic dysfunction progresses, fasting blood glucose levels also begin to rise. Levels between **6.0 mmol/L (108 mg/dL)** and **6.9 mmol/L (124 mg/dL)** indicate metabolic syndrome and are considered **prediabetic**, increasing your risk of serious complications like heart disease and stroke. A fasting glucose of

7.0 mmol/L (126 mg/dL) or more crosses the threshold of **type 2 diabetes.**

Glycated Haemoglobin: A Hidden Clue to Metabolic Risk

While glycated haemoglobin (HbA1c) isn't officially listed among the diagnostic criteria for metabolic syndrome, it offers powerful insight into who might be heading in that direction.

HbA1C reflects the average blood glucose level over the past three months - the typical lifespan of a red blood cell. During this time, excess glucose binds to haemoglobin in a process called glycation, similar to how iron rusts when exposed to moisture. The more sugar in the bloodstream, the more haemoglobin gets "rusted."

This marker is reported as a number and a percentage of total haemoglobin and can serve as an early warning sign for metabolic dysfunction:

- **Below 5.5% (42 mmol/mol)**: Normal range, low risk.
- **5.5% to 6.4% (42–48 mmol/mol)**: Suggestive of insulin resistance or prediabetes - warning signs of metabolic syndrome.
- **6.5% and above**: Diagnostic of diabetes.

Monitoring HbA1C can help catch metabolic issues before they escalate into full-blown diabetes, offering a crucial opportunity for early intervention.

Triglycerides and HDL Cholesterol: Silent Signals of Risk

The two markers, often overlooked yet powerful indicators of metabolic syndrome, are **high triglycerides (TG)** and **low high-density lipoprotein (HDL) cholesterol levels.** These lipid markers aren't just lab numbers - they're silent signals that your metabolism may be off balance.

A triglyceride level of **1.7 mmol/L (150 mg/dL) or higher** is considered elevated. While often called the "forgotten" risk factor for heart disease, high triglycerides play a critical role in cardiovascular health and should not be ignored.

Equally important is your HDL cholesterol - often referred to as the "good" cholesterol. HDL acts like a metabolic cleanser, helping to remove damaged LDL, or "bad" cholesterol, from the bloodstream. Low levels of HDL (less than **1.0 mmol/L or 40 mg/dL**) are among the strongest predictors of heart attack.

The good news? **Regular exercise and a diet rich in healthy fats** - such as those found in avocados, nuts, seeds, olive oil, and fatty fish - can help boost your HDL levels and lower your triglycerides, thereby improving your overall metabolic profile.

Other Metabolic Risk Factors

Beyond the well-known contributors to metabolic syndrome, several other biomarkers can reveal hidden risks, often quietly at work long before symptoms appear.

Chronic Inflammation: The Silent Instigator

At the root of insulin resistance lies chronic, low-grade inflammation - a key disruptor of how the body handles glucose (see Chapter 3). One of the best tools for detecting this is the high-sensitivity C-reactive protein (hs-CRP) test. Even a modest elevation - above 1.0 mg/L - indicates an increased risk of metabolic syndrome and cardiovascular complications. While not specific to any one disease, a high hs-CRP should prompt closer attention to overall metabolic health.

Uric Acid: More Than Just Gout

You might associate uric acid with gout, where it crystallises painfully in the joints. However, high uric acid is also a broader marker of metabolic dysfunction. Elevated levels often result from diets rich in purines (found in red meat and beer) and consumption of high-fructose corn syrup (HFCS), a common ingredient in soft drinks and processed foods. A level of 0.41 mmol/L (7 mg/dL) or more, particularly in men, is a red flag for insulin resistance. (For more on high-fructose corn syrup and its metabolic impact, see Chapters 2 and 3.)

Leptin: The Hunger Regulator Gone Rogue

Leptin, a hormone secreted by adipose (fat) cells, plays a crucial role in regulating hunger and energy balance. As we eat, leptin levels rise, signalling us to stop. But when levels climb above 10.0 ng/mL, the signal no longer works, and leptin resistance sets in - another hallmark of metabolic disruption.

Adiponectin: The Protector

Adiponectin is a beneficial hormone that enhances insulin sensitivity and supports vascular health. Unlike leptin, *low* levels of adiponectin are cause for concern. A deficiency in this anti-inflammatory marker suggests rising insulin resistance and a growing risk of full-blown metabolic syndrome.

HOMA-IR: A Window into Insulin Resistance

The Homeostatic Model Assessment of Insulin Resistance (HOMA-IR) is a scientific tool that calculates insulin resistance using fasting glucose and insulin levels. While primarily used in research, some clinical laboratories offer this test to patients who require a more comprehensive understanding of their metabolism.

Homocysteine: A Hidden Threat to Arteries

Homocysteine is a naturally occurring amino acid, but when its levels rise above 8 μmol/L, it becomes dangerous, damaging artery walls and promoting blood clots. Elevated homocysteine is a well-established, independent risk factor for cardiovascular disease and stroke.

Markers of Fatty Liver: Early Clues to a Silent Threat
Elevated liver enzymes - such as alanine aminotransferase (ALT), aspartate aminotransferase (AST), and gamma-glutamyl transferase (GGT) - serve as red flags for non-alcoholic steatohepatitis (NASH), a more advanced and potentially dangerous form of non-alcoholic fatty liver disease (NAFLD). These enzymes are often the first biochemical hints that the liver is under metabolic stress.

In addition to blood tests, imaging tools such as ultrasound can detect fatty changes in the liver, providing visual confirmation of metabolic liver disease, often before symptoms appear.

Alarmingly, sugar has emerged as a modern-day toxin for the liver, rivalling alcohol in its potential to cause lasting damage. Excessive sugar intake can lead to the same end-stage outcomes as alcohol abuse: cirrhosis, liver failure, and liver cancer. NAFLD is now the leading indication for liver transplantation worldwide.

The good news: Early detection and intervention can halt or even reverse this process. Spotting the signs of fatty liver disease early isn't just about preventing complications - it's about saving lives.

Final Thoughts
Taking charge of your metabolic health early can lead to surprising and rewarding results. Even modest changes - such as losing just 10% of your body weight - can dramatically improve your health. This small but powerful step can reduce inflammation, stabilise blood pressure and blood sugar, and lower triglyceride levels. Most importantly, it significantly cuts your risk of a heart attack and sets

the stage for a future of vitality and well-being.

The key is early detection. When metabolic risk factors are identified in their early stages, they are often much easier to reverse. That's why it's essential to be proactive. Partner with trusted healthcare professionals - your doctor, dietitian, or wellness coach - who can guide you, support your progress, and help you stay on the right path.

Start now. Your future self will thank you.

CHAPTER 2

Metabolism: The Engine of Vitality

To begin our exploration of metabolic health, let's consider the contrasting post-retirement journeys of two football legends: Brazil's Pelé and Argentina's Diego Maradona. Both retired at 37 after illustrious careers that captivated millions. Yet, their lives took strikingly different turns. Pelé remained active in the sport, coaching teams and promoting fitness, while Maradona battled obesity and related health issues, ultimately unable to continue in the sport he once dominated. What caused such a stark divergence?

The answer lies in **metabolism** - the body's engine for converting food into energy. A healthy metabolism fuels vitality, performance, and resilience. When it falters, the consequences ripple through every aspect of health.

Though metabolism may sound like a technical concept, at its core, it's simple: it's how your body transforms what you eat into the energy that powers everything you do. But here's the critical question: **Are the foods you eat fuelling wellness, or feeding disease?**

Since the 1970s, the rise of the Western diet - characterised by high sugar and processed carbohydrate consumption - has disrupted our metabolic flexibility, the natural ability to switch between burning sugar and fat. This metabolic adaptability was once essential to the survival of our hunter-gatherer ancestors. Without it, many modern bodies are locked in sugar-burning mode, leading to fatigue, weight gain, and chronic illness.

In this chapter, we'll demystify how the body generates energy, define what a truly healthy metabolism looks like, and explain how imbalances develop. You'll learn how to spot the early signs of metabolic dysfunction - and, most importantly, how to reclaim your metabolic health.

By the end, you'll discover your **metabolic type**, a powerful key to understanding your body's weight, shape, and energy patterns. Because your metabolism isn't just about burning calories - it's the foundation of a thriving, energised life.

Understanding Metabolism: Your Body's Hidden Power Plant

Let's take a closer look at metabolism - the intricate, behind-the-scenes system that keeps your body running.

At its core, metabolism is a series of processes that convert the food you eat into usable energy. This journey begins with digestion and absorption, followed by the transport of nutrients to your cells. Once there, these nutrients are transformed into the energy needed to power your body's daily activities, remove metabolic waste, and provide the building blocks that support growth, repair, and maintain the body's structures.

But where exactly does this energy go?

You might be surprised to learn that about **70%** of your daily energy is spent on basic life-sustaining activities - things your body does automatically and continuously, like keeping your heart beating, your lungs breathing, and your blood circulating - even when you're at rest. This is called your **basal metabolic rate (BMR)**.

Another **20%** of your energy is used for your everyday physical activities, including walking, working, cleaning, gardening, and even recreational pursuits. Interestingly, intense exercise and vigorous tasks rarely make up more than **5%** of this total.

The final **10%** is used to process the food you eat - a process known as the **thermic effect of food**.

Many people imagine metabolism as a single "furnace" buried somewhere in the abdomen, where food is burned to release energy. But this isn't how it works. There's no central engine. Instead, every one of your **trillions of cells** functions like its own miniature furnace. Energy isn't created in one place and sent out; it's generated at the cellular level, everywhere in your body, all at once, working tirelessly to fuel your every move, thought, and breath.

Healthy, Fast, and Poor Metabolism: What They Mean

Metabolism is the process by which your body converts the food you eat into energy. When metabolism is functioning optimally, calories from food are efficiently delivered to your cells, fuelling your body for everything. This is what we refer to as a **healthy** metabolism - one that supports consistent energy, ideal body weight, and protection against chronic disease.

In everyday conversation, people often refer to a "fast metabolism" as the ability to overeat without gaining weight. While partly true, this oversimplification overlooks the broader context. A truly healthy metabolism isn't just about burning calories quickly - it's about using those calories effectively to power your body's systems.

In contrast, a **poor** or "slow" metabolism means that the calories you consume aren't being properly used for energy. Instead, they're diverted and stored as fat. Over time, this can lead to fatigue, weight gain and increased risk of metabolic disorders - even in people of normal weight.

Here's a sobering reality: research shows that **88% of U.S. adults** have signs of metabolic dysfunction. This includes **90% of those who are overweight**, **95% of those with obesity**, and even **65% of adults at a normal weight**.[1] This means that a "healthy weight" doesn't always equate to a healthy metabolism.

Understanding the difference between a fast metabolism, a healthy one, and a poor one is crucial. It's not just about how much you eat or how quickly you burn calories - it's about how well your body uses food to keep you vibrant, active, and well.

How Does Poor Metabolism Lead to Disease?

When your metabolism slows, your body becomes less efficient at utilising calories for energy. Instead of fuelling your cells, those calories are increasingly stored as fat, particularly around your waist. This buildup of abdominal fat, known as central obesity, is not just a cosmetic concern. It's the defining and most dangerous hallmark of metabolic syndrome.

As fat accumulates, a chain reaction begins. Blood pressure gradually increases due to several factors. At the same time, a slower metabolism allows excess sugar to circulate in the bloodstream. This not only spikes blood glucose levels but also drives the liver to convert surplus sugar into triglycerides - unhealthy fats and lower levels of protective HDL "good" cholesterol (covered in detail in Chapter 7).

This scenario brings together all five markers of metabolic syndrome: central obesity, high blood pressure, elevated blood sugar, high triglycerides, and low HDL cholesterol. But you only need three of these to receive a diagnosis.

Today, one in three adults in the UK has metabolic syndrome. It's not just a warning sign - it's a launchpad for over 1,200 related conditions that dominate the global burden of non-communicable diseases. These range from diabetes, heart disease, and stroke to conditions like dementia, non-alcoholic fatty liver disease, erectile dysfunction, PCOS, and even some cancers. Many of these are explored in Section 2 of this book.

Metabolic syndrome is more than a collection of risk factors - it's the root system of the most significant public health crisis of our time.

Living Longer, but Not Healthier: The Hidden Cost of Modern Life
As mentioned earlier, life expectancy in the United Kingdom has increased significantly over the past century, with a gain of over 30 years. On the surface, this appears to be a triumph of modern medicine and science. But there's a catch: while we may be living longer, we're not necessarily living better.

A growing number of those extra years are spent in poor health. According to official UK statistics, the average man will spend 16 of his final years battling chronic illness. For women, it's 19 years.[2] This decline in quality of life is primarily driven by metabolic diseases, like type 2 diabetes and cardiovascular diseases. These diseases not only shorten our health span but also strip away independence, leaving many older adults reliant on nursing and care homes.

This wasn't always the case.

Our hunter-gatherer ancestors followed a natural rhythm of feast and famine. During times of abundance - typically in summer - they ate generously. Raising their insulin levels and encouraging their bodies to store fat. This stored energy was vital for surviving leaner months when food was scarce, and fasting was often unavoidable. During these periods, the body switches to burning fat, showcasing remarkable metabolic flexibility: it burns sugar in times of plenty and fat in times of scarcity.

Today, that balance has vanished. We live in a perpetual state of feast. Additionally, ultra-processed foods, high in sugar and refined carbohydrates, have replaced the natural, seasonal diet our biology evolved to thrive on. The famine never comes, and with it, our ability to switch metabolic gears fades away, paving the way for chronic illness.

The result: A longer life, perhaps, but one too often overshadowed by disease.

Changing the Fuel: How Our Diet Went Off the Rails

The roots of our modern metabolic crisis can be traced back to a pivotal moment in the early 1970s. In 1971, facing mounting unpopularity due to the Vietnam War and desperate for re-election, President Richard Nixon turned his attention to a growing domestic concern: the soaring cost of food.

To ease inflation and appeal to struggling Americans, Nixon's administration introduced sweeping changes to the U.S. food system. Central to this effort was the subsidisation of corn production, leading to the mass manufacturing of cheap, calorie-dense ingredients like high-fructose corn syrup (HFCS) and corn oil. This marked a dramatic shift in how food was produced, moving away from farms and into factories.

The outcome: Processed foods packed with sugar and unhealthy fats flooded the market. HFCS-laced soft drinks and fast food cooked in corn oil became staples of the American diet. Nixon's strategy worked politically - he won re-election - but the long-term health consequences were profound.

This dietary revolution ignited a cascade of global effects. Grocery store shelves became dominated by highly processed products, with roughly 90% of offerings coming in boxes and cans. These foods weren't just high in sugar; they were stripped of fibre and essential nutrients, leaving only empty calories behind.

Contrast this with the diet of our hunter-gatherer ancestors, which was rich in whole foods, fibre, and nutrients, and contained only 75–125 grams of carbohydrates per day. Today's Western diet often delivers more than 300 grams of mostly refined carbs daily. The result is a metabolic slowdown. Where the original human diet energised the body and supported efficient metabolism, our modern fare overwhelms it, contributing to the rise of obesity, insulin resistance, and metabolic syndrome.

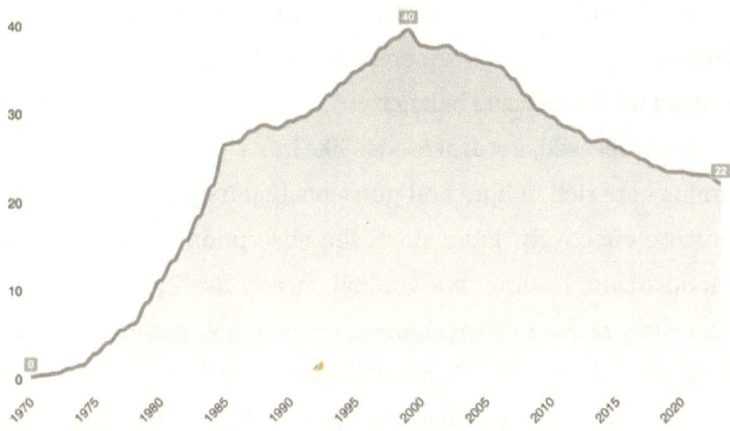

U.S. per capita annual consumption of high-fructose corn syrup (lbs) (1970 - 2023)

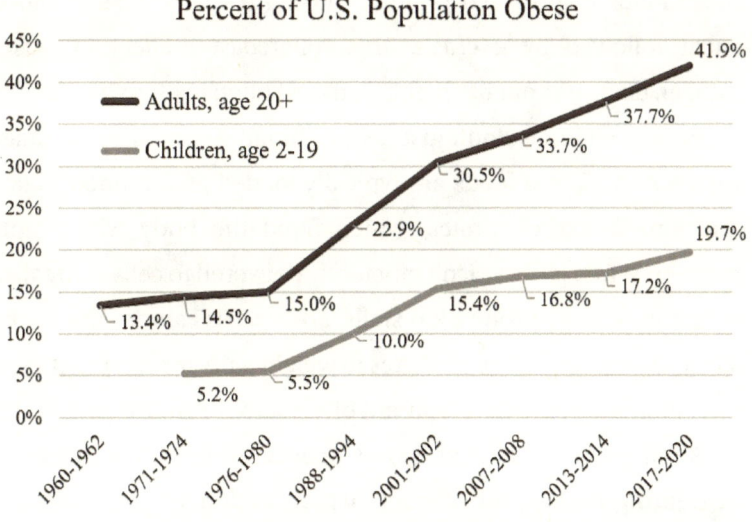

Obesity in the US population

The sharp rise in obesity after 1990 in the US reflects the delayed effects of the sugar calories consumed by children in the 1970s and 1980s, as well as a repeated pattern.

Western Diet

Glucose is the body's primary source of energy, and maintaining steady blood glucose levels is essential for metabolic health. However, not all foods are created equal when it comes to their impact on this delicate balance.

Unprocessed, natural foods - like fruits, vegetables, and whole grains - are rich in fibre and nutrients that help the body manage glucose effectively. Fibre slows the absorption of sugar into the bloodstream, leading to a gradual, steady rise in blood glucose. This slow release provides sustained energy, minimises insulin spikes, and helps cells absorb glucose efficiently.

In contrast, **ultra-processed foods** - a hallmark of the modern Western diet - strip away fibre and essential nutrients to maximise shelf life and consumer convenience. Without fibre, glucose from these foods is absorbed rapidly, causing a sharp spike in blood sugar followed by a crash. This rollercoaster effect increases hunger, disrupts appetite regulation, and often leads to overeating.

Processed foods don't just disrupt blood sugar - they sabotage metabolism. These foods are typically loaded with refined sugars and simple carbohydrates, which flood the body with empty calories. When glucose isn't efficiently delivered to cells along with nutrients, energy production stalls, and excess calories are stored as fat. Over time, this contributes to weight gain, insulin resistance, and, ultimately, the development of metabolic syndrome.

Adding to the problem is how **processed food has reshaped our eating habits.** The average person no longer sticks to three meals a day. Instead, we consume up to six eating occasions, fuelled by the easy availability and low cost of snack foods. Since the 1970s, daily calorie intake in the U.S. has increased by 24%, and obesity rates have skyrocketed from 15% to 42%.[3]

This dramatic shift in what - and how - we eat is a major driver of the metabolic crisis we now face.

The Cuban Case Study:
When Sanctions Sparked a Health Revolution

What happens when the Western diet is suddenly stripped away? An unexpected and compelling natural experiment occurred in Cuba in the early 1990s. Following the collapse of the Soviet Union, the United States tightened its economic sanctions, drastically reducing Cuba's access to imported processed foods. As a result, Cubans were forced to rely primarily on locally grown staples, including fruits, vegetables, legumes, nuts, and seeds.

The health effects were nothing short of remarkable. On average, Cubans lost about 12 pounds (5.5 kilograms), and rates of diabetes, cardiovascular disease, and even cancer dropped dramatically, reaching their lowest recorded levels.[4]

This real-world, population-wide shift in dietary patterns offers robust evidence: it's not just how much we eat, but what we eat that shapes our metabolic health.

The Thyroid: Your Body's Metabolic Accelerator

Think of your thyroid gland as the gas pedal of your metabolism. Nestled in your neck, this small but mighty gland orchestrates the pace at which your body converts food into energy. When functioning properly, it maintains balance throughout. But when it's out of sync - either too fast or too slow - every system in your body feels the impact.

An **overactive thyroid** (hyperthyroidism) revs the metabolic engine. Your heart races, body temperature rises, sweat increases, and you may feel jittery or anxious. Despite having a healthy appetite, you may still experience rapid weight loss. It's as if your body is stuck in overdrive.

Conversely, an **underactive thyroid** (hypothyroidism) puts the brakes on metabolism. You feel sluggish, your heart rate slows, you become cold intolerant, and you may experience constipation or excessive weight gain. Even your mood and mental clarity can suffer.

So, what causes thyroid function to falter?

One common culprit is **Hashimoto's thyroiditis**, an autoimmune condition often triggered by gluten sensitivity. But sometimes, the problem lies in something far simpler: missing nutrients. Your thyroid depends on a team of **10 essential nutrients** to produce and activate its hormones. These include:

- **Iodine** and **tyrosine** (an amino acid from protein) are used to build thyroid hormones.
- **Vitamins A, B, C, D, and E**, **zinc**, and **iron** to support hormone production and function.
- **Selenium** (200 µg daily, or just 2-3 Brazil nuts) to convert the prohormone T4 into the active form, T3.

Here's a fascinating fact: only **20% of T4 is converted to T3 inside the thyroid**. The rest happens mainly in the **liver and gut**. That means **your digestive health and liver function are critical** to maintaining an optimal thyroid function and a healthy metabolism.

How Does the Body Make Energy?

Ever wonder how your body powers everything from a heartbeat to a sprint? The answer lies in a fascinating, three-stage process that transforms glucose - the sugar in your blood - into energy your body can use. Don't worry if the science sounds intense; I'll break it down clearly and summarise at the end.

Stage 1: Glycolysis – The Quick Start

This first step takes place in the cytoplasm, the fluid inside your cells, and doesn't require oxygen. It's your body's go to basic method for a quick energy boost, especially when oxygen is in short supply, like during high-intensity exercise or poor breathing.

In glycolysis, one six-carbon glucose molecule is broken down into two three-carbon molecules of pyruvate. This process produces four ATP molecules - the body's energy currency - but two are used up in the process, leaving a net gain of **two ATP**. It also generates two molecules of **NADH**, which will be useful later.

If oxygen isn't readily available, pyruvate is converted into **lactate**. You've probably felt this as the burn or soreness in your muscles after a challenging workout. Thankfully, lactic acid clears up quickly, especially with light movement, such as walking or swimming.

Stage 2: The Krebs Cycle – Powering Up

When oxygen is available, pyruvate enters the **mitochondria**, the cell's powerhouse. Aided by factors - vitamins B1, B2, B3, and **alpha-lipoic acid** - all of which are found in whole foods. Inside the mitochondria, pyruvate loses one carbon atom and is converted into **acetyl-CoA**, releasing **two additional NADH** molecules.

Now comes the **Krebs cycle** (also called the citric acid or TCA cycle), a ten-step sequence that spins like a wheel to extract more energy. It starts when acetyl-CoA combines with oxaloacetate to form **citric acid** - hence the name. This cycle produces **two ATP**, six more **NADH**, and two **FADH2**, which are also electron carriers.

Fun fact: The cycle was discovered by Sir Hans Krebs, who received a Nobel Prize in 1953 for this groundbreaking work.

Stage 3: Oxidative Phosphorylation – The Energy Jackpot

Here's where the big payoff happens. In the **electron transport chain**, located within the mitochondria, the NADH and FADH2 molecules deliver their electrons. With the help of oxygen - the final electron acceptor - a powerful electrical gradient forms. This drives the production of ATP by converting **ADP** into **ATP**, your body's primary usable energy unit.

The results: One glucose molecule can produce up to **32 ATP molecules**:

- **2 ATP** from glycolysis
- **2 ATP** from the Krebs cycle
- **28 ATP** from oxidative phosphorylation (25 from NADH and 3 from FADH2)

Stages of cellular energy production and approximate ATP yield from one molecule of glucose

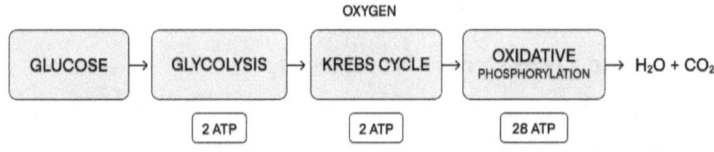

A diagram illustrating the stages of cellular energy production from a single glucose molecule, showing the ATP (energy units) yield at each step. Glycolysis generates 2 ATP, and the Krebs cycle produces another 2 ATP. Most energy is generated in the final stage (oxidative phosphorylation), when oxygen is incorporated to yield 28 ATP, along with the by-products water and carbon dioxide.

The Vital Role of Oxygen in Energy Production

Oxygen is the game-changer. Without it, your body can only settle for just 2 ATP from glycolysis. However, with a steady oxygen supply, it unlocks the full 32 ATP from a single glucose molecule. The difference is staggering and underscores a vital truth: **oxygen**

is the limiting factor in efficient energy metabolism. That's why **breathing efficiently and deeply isn't just for relaxation - it's essential for energy production.**

Think of a peacefully sleeping baby - the gentle rise and fall of their belly with each breath. This is the body's natural, optimal way to breathe - deep, diaphragmatic, and efficient. Yet, as we grow older, stress and lifestyle changes often cause our breathing to shift into a shallow, rapid pattern, which starves our cells of oxygen.

Restoring your natural breathing rhythm can powerfully support your metabolism. One time-honoured method is **Pranayama**, the traditional Indian practice of controlled, abdominal breathing. By practising deep, mindful breathing, you not only improve oxygen delivery to your cells but also awaken the full potential of your body's energy systems.

The Powerhouse
Mitochondria, often called the cell's powerhouses, generate a staggering 90% of the body's energy. When their numbers dwindle or they lack the essential nutrients needed to function, energy levels drop sharply. This energy shortfall hits the body's most demanding organs first, especially the brain and muscles.

The effects can be profound: persistent fatigue, mental fog, difficulty concentrating, muscle cramps, anxiety, and even depression. Meanwhile, with less energy being used, surplus calories are stashed away as fat, paving the way for unwanted weight gain.

Other Essential Nutrients: Powering Up Your Mitochondria
To keep our cellular engines - our mitochondria - running efficiently, a host of essential nutrients play a crucial role.

Iron, for instance, is indispensable for energy production. It acts as both an electron donor and acceptor in the electron transport chain, the final step of cellular respiration, where most of our body's energy (ATP) is made. Unsurprisingly, iron deficiency is a common underlying factor in chronic fatigue.

A suite of other nutrients - including the **B vitamins**, **coenzyme Q10 (CoQ10)**, **alpha-lipoic acid**, and **L-carnitine** - are also vital for mitochondrial health. These compounds support the production of energy within cells. However, deficiencies are widespread, particularly among individuals who consume nutrient-poor, processed diets.

Worryingly, some medications can also deplete these crucial nutrients. For example, **statins**, widely prescribed to lower cholesterol, are known to reduce CoQ10 levels. Similarly, **oral contraceptives** may interfere with CoQ10 metabolism, compromising mitochondrial function in women who use them long-term.

Environmental toxins further complicate the picture. **Pesticides**, **herbicides**, and **heavy metals** - such as **cadmium** in cigarette smoke and **mercury** from large fish like tuna or dental amalgams - can disrupt mitochondrial activity, impairing your body's ability to produce energy efficiently.

In short, maintaining robust mitochondrial function - and preventing fatigue and metabolic dysfunction - requires not only a clean diet but also avoidance of certain medications and environmental exposures that may deplete essential nutrients or disrupt energy production.

Age-Related Metabolic Decline:
Why Midlife Demands a Shift in Strategy

By our mid-30s, the body begins to slow down in subtle but meaningful ways. This is around the age when most professional athletes retire, not just due to external competition, but also because of internal, biological shifts. From that point onward, our metabolic efficiency gradually declines. However, the rate and impact vary from person to person - compare the diverging paths of sports legends like Pelé and Maradona.

One of the earliest and most noticeable changes is in body composition. Starting in our 40s, we begin to lose muscle mass - about 5% every decade - and simultaneously, our ability to process glucose diminishes. These two factors combine to lower your basal metabolic rate (BMR), the number of calories your body burns at rest. As BMR drops, unused glucose is more likely to be stored as fat, leading to gradual but persistent weight gain.

The math is unforgiving yet straightforward: less muscle equals lower calorie burn, and poor glucose handling means more fat storage. By midlife, many people are dealing with both excess body fat and a reduction in muscle mass. If you're still eating like you're 25 - mainly processed foods high in sugar and starch - your body will quietly rebel, storing those extra calories as fat.

However, there's good news: while metabolic decline is a natural process, it's not irreversible. The key lies in adapting your lifestyle to this new biological reality. Building or preserving muscle through resistance training, incorporating intermittent fasting, and consuming whole, nutrient-dense foods can all help restore metabolic balance.

For context, a 70-year-old requires roughly 400 fewer calories per day than they did at 30 years old to maintain an ideal weight. That doesn't mean drastically reducing your food intake - it means eating smarter and moving with purpose.

The lives of Pelé and Maradona remind us that ageing is inevitable, but how we age is not. Metabolic health in your 40s and beyond is about making intentional choices - trading fat for muscle, optimising your diet, and tuning into your body's changing needs. With the right approach, your metabolism can remain a powerful ally well into the later chapters of life.

The Impact of Oestrogen and Menopause on Metabolic Health

Hormones are potent regulators of health, particularly in relation to metabolism and bodily functions. Among them, oestrogen plays a crucial role in maintaining metabolic balance in women. The transition into menopause, marked by a dramatic decline in oestrogen levels, often brings significant metabolic changes. To better understand this, let's examine a real-life example.

Jane, a 59-year-old woman, came to see me with a troubling cluster of symptoms: constant fatigue, unexpected weight gain, irritability, forgetfulness, and unpredictable mood swings. Most distressing for her were the hot flushes, excessive sweating at night, and frequent nighttime trips to the toilet that disrupted her sleep.

She'd visited her GP, where she was found to have gained nearly two stone (28 pounds). Her blood pressure was elevated at 145/90 mmHg - well above the ideal of 120/80 mmHg. Blood tests revealed that her fasting glucose was 6.6 mmol/L, placing her in the prediabetic range. Her lipid profile was also concerning, with high levels of total cholesterol and triglycerides, and low levels of protective HDL cholesterol.

Jane exemplifies a pattern seen in up to 60% of postmenopausal women: metabolic syndrome linked to hormonal changes. Her symptoms began about three years earlier, during the transition to menopause. With no periods for over 12 months, her menopause was confirmed. During this time, she entered a state of energy imbalance, as her appetite increased, her physical activity declined, and her diet shifted toward high-calorie foods, such as pizza, pasta, and crisps.

Most of her weight gain settled around her abdomen. Her waist measured 39 inches, and her hips measured 41 inches, giving her a waist-to-hip ratio of 0.95 (the ideal ratio for women is typically under 0.85; see Chapter 6). This abdominal, or visceral, fat is especially harmful because it drives chronic low-grade inflammation, a process we'll explore in detail in Chapter 3. Compounding the problem, the natural decline in oestradiol - an anti-inflammatory sex hormone produced by the ovaries - left her more vulnerable to these metabolic disruptions.

The turning point came with a tailored intervention: bioidentical oestrogen replacement combined with strategic lifestyle changes. Over time, Jane lost weight, improved her metabolic markers, and regained control of her health.

Her story highlights an essential truth: before menopause, oestrogen offers a protective metabolic buffer. After menopause, its loss can open the door to weight gain, inflammation, and disease. But with awareness and early action, women can navigate this transition with confidence and resilience. Understanding the role of oestrogen in metabolism empowers women to take practical, lasting steps toward better health.

Rethinking Conventional Weight Loss Advice

For decades, the standard advice for losing weight has been simple: eat less and move more. But this oversimplified mantra has led many to obsess over calorie counting while overlooking a critical truth: **not all calories are created equal**.

Focusing solely on calorie quantity can backfire. When you drastically cut calories, your body slows its metabolism to conserve energy, making it even harder to shed weight. Meanwhile, pushing yourself to exercise more without changing your diet can increase stress, heighten hunger, and fuel cravings for high-calorie, ultra-processed foods.

Scientific research now paints a clearer picture: **what you eat matters more than how much you eat**. As we have seen, Western diets high in sugar, refined carbs, and unhealthy fats can impair your metabolism. In contrast, whole, natural foods such as fruits, vegetables, legumes, nuts, and seeds support metabolic health. Even reducing the number of times we eat or taking dinner 2 to 4 hours before bedtime can have a positive influence on metabolism.

Another long-held myth that's been debunked is the fear of fat. **Healthy fats** - found in foods like avocados, nuts, seeds, coconut, and olive oil - can boost metabolism and support weight loss. In contrast, excess sugar has the opposite effect, promoting fat storage and metabolic slowdown.[5]

Protein is another key player. High-quality protein not only helps control your appetite - keeping you satisfied longer and reducing the urge to overeat - but also helps preserve and build muscle. Since muscle mass is a major driver of your metabolic rate (which declines with age), maintaining it is crucial. Protein has a higher thermic effect, meaning your body uses more energy to digest and process it compared to carbohydrates or fats.

Excellent protein sources include organic eggs, pasture-raised chicken, grass-fed beef, and wild-caught fish, such as salmon. Incorporating these foods into your diet can help stabilise hunger, encourage fat loss, and rev up your metabolism - all while promoting long-term health.

Simple Ways to Fire Up Your Metabolism
Think of your metabolism as your body's internal engine - it runs faster when you're active and idles when you're not. The good news: You can take charge and keep that engine revving.

Regular physical activity is one of the most effective ways to boost your metabolism. Whether it's brisk walking, high-intensity interval training (HIIT), strength training, or even standing while working, movement of any kind triggers your body to burn more energy. (For a full workout plan, see Chapter 17.)

Hydration is another key. Drinking enough water helps your cells function efficiently and supports a faster metabolic rate. Likewise, quality sleep is crucial - your metabolism doesn't just rest while you do; it resets and recharges.

Even the foods you eat can make a difference. Spices, especially chilli peppers, have a thermogenic effect, slightly increasing your metabolic rate. Caffeine gives a temporary boost, though it's short-lived. Green tea, however, offers a gentler lift, thanks to its combination of caffeine and metabolism-supporting antioxidants.

Small changes add up. When combined, these habits can help shift your body out of metabolic stagnation and into a more energised, fat-burning mode.

Become Metabolically Flexible
Your body is a "hybrid" designed to run on two fuel sources: glucose and fat. **Metabolic flexibility** refers to your body's ability to switch effortlessly between different fuels based on their availability and needs. When glucose is abundant - either from the food you've just eaten or glycogen stored in your liver and muscles - your body prioritises it for energy. The liver can store up to 2,000 calories worth of glycogen, enough to fuel your body for about a day without eating.

After an overnight fast, your body naturally shifts gears, switching from burning glucose to tapping into fat stores. When you eat again, it returns to glucose. This seamless transition is a hallmark of metabolic health.

In ancient times, this adaptability was essential for survival during periods of feast and famine. Today, it's no less important. Being metabolically flexible gives you steady energy, helps maintain a healthy weight, and supports overall well-being. It also reduces your risk of metabolic disease and may even slow the ageing process.

But here's the catch: **you can't burn fat efficiently if your insulin levels are constantly high.** Insulin is the hormone that helps glucose enter your cells, but when it's chronically elevated, it promotes fat storage and blocks fat burning. A poor diet and lack of physical activity can lead to insulin resistance, where your cells fail to respond adequately to insulin. This leads to more glucose being stored as fat instead of being used for energy, contributing to weight gain and increasing your risk for obesity.

The good news: Metabolic flexibility can be restored. The first step is addressing insulin resistance - a critical topic we'll explore in depth in **Chapter 3**.

Know Your Metabolic Type
Have you ever followed a strict diet or reduced your calorie intake, only to see little or no change in your weight? That's because metabolism isn't one-size-fits-all.[6] It plays a crucial role in shaping your body weight, size, and composition. While diet and lifestyle are essential, understanding your unique metabolic type can be the missing piece of the puzzle.

Researchers have identified four distinct metabolic types. Each one processes calories differently, and knowing yours can help you make smarter, more effective decisions about your health.

1. Stable Metabolism
Individuals with a stable metabolism tend to experience predictable fluctuations in their weight. They can gain or lose weight relatively easily by adjusting their calorie intake. Their metabolic response is steady and responsive to lifestyle changes.

2. Efficient Metabolism
This type tends to conserve energy and store excess calories as

fat. People with an efficient metabolism extract more energy from fewer calories, storing the rest as fat, making it difficult to lose weight. They often require significant calorie reduction to see results, and even then, progress can be slow.

3. Inefficient Metabolism

In contrast, people with an inefficient metabolism burn through calories rapidly. Their bodies expend more energy on passive movements, such as fidgeting, and burn more calories per activity. For example, a 30-minute walk might burn 75 calories for them, while it burns only 50 calories for someone else. Gaining weight can be challenging - they struggle to maintain their body mass.

4. Adaptable Metabolism

Individuals with an adaptable metabolism tend to maintain a stable weight regardless of their calorie intake. Their metabolism becomes efficient during calorie restriction but inefficient with overfeeding. This adaptability helps keep their weight fluctuations to a minimum.

Discover Your Metabolic Body Type

One evening, while I was explaining metabolic body types to my family, my son jumped in mid-sentence: "I'm a mesomorph! That means I need to cut back on carbs and stay consistent with my workouts to keep my weight in check." His quick insight surprised me, but he was right.

Understanding your metabolic body type can empower you to make smarter decisions about nutrition, exercise, and overall health. Just like my son, you too can identify your type and tailor your lifestyle for optimal results.

Here are the three primary metabolic body types:[7]

- **Ectomorph**
  Characterised by a slim build, narrow shoulders, and a small frame, ectomorphs have a fast but often inefficient metabolism. They tend to fidget, are naturally hyperactive, and may struggle to gain weight or muscle mass.

- **Mesomorph**
  With a naturally athletic and muscular physique, mesomorphs tend to gain muscle and fat more easily than other body types. They respond quickly to training but should be cautious with carbohydrate intake and maintain a regular exercise routine to stay lean and healthy.

- **Endomorph**
  Endomorphs typically have a rounder body and thicker limbs. They conserve energy efficiently, which often results in a slower metabolism. As a result, they may feel tired easily and struggle to maintain a healthy weight. Achieving and maintaining a healthy weight typically requires a significant reduction in calories and a well-planned fitness regimen.

By identifying your metabolic body type, you can begin to personalise your approach to health, making your goals more achievable and sustainable.

BODY TYPES

Ectomorph　　　Mesomorph　　　Endomorph

Find the body type that looks like you. Then read the relevant section in the book to learn the specific features of each body type.

Final Thoughts

Metabolism is the body's way of turning food into energy, fuelling every cell and function in the body. At the heart of this process is glucose, our primary source of energy. Under normal conditions, glucose travels from the bloodstream into cells, where it's used to generate power. But when metabolism falters, this system breaks down. Instead of being used to feed our cells, glucose is redirected and stored as fat. This shift is primarily due to insulin resistance - a condition in which the body struggles to effectively move glucose into cells. We'll explore this critical process in more detail in Chapter 3.

CHAPTER 3

Insulin Resistance: The Hidden Spark Behind Metabolic Chaos

Insulin resistance is the silent warning sign - an early and invisible shift that signals trouble ahead. It's the starting point of a cascade. This small snowball can rapidly grow into an avalanche of metabolic diseases such as type 2 diabetes, heart disease, dementia, and even cancer.

In this chapter, we'll explore how insulin - a hormone crucial for delivering glucose, the body's primary energy source - can lose its effectiveness. What causes our cells to stop responding to insulin's signal? What damage follows? And most importantly, how can we restore our body's sensitivity to this vital hormone?

Understanding insulin resistance isn't just a scientific pursuit for me - it's personal. A severe bout of insulin resistance nearly cost me my life. That experience fuels my passion to uncover its dangers and, more critically, how we can fight back against it.

Lucky To Be In A Hospital, Fortunate To Be Alive
When I moved to the United Kingdom more than 30 years ago, I was in peak condition - fit, energetic, and full of life. But within

just two years, everything changed. I became chronically fatigued and often struggled with debilitating episodes of "brain fog." My work as a doctor began to suffer. My thoughts were consumed by food, and I convinced myself that more calories might give me the energy I lacked. I was in and out of the doctors' mess for buttered toast and biscuits. I found comfort - and a false sense of vitality - in crisps, chocolate bars, and fizzy drinks from the hospital shop. My weight ballooned from 67 to 97 kilograms.

Despite my growing concern, medical support was disappointingly absent. Normal blood tests reassured my general practitioner, and even a hospital consultant couldn't identify anything wrong. The downward spiral continued - until one night when everything changed. In minutes, I went from a busy, responsible doctor to the most critical patient in the same hospital.

It was a cold December night. I was on duty covering medical emergencies, and the hospital was under pressure. We had just responded to our third cardiac arrest call when a junior colleague turned to me and said, "Dr Ibrahim, do you want to use your inhaler? You're very wheezy." It was the first clue that something was seriously wrong.

Within minutes, my breathing became laboured. My colleagues rushed me to radiology, where an X-ray revealed a shocking discovery: my windpipe was kinked like a "starter handle," compressed by a massive swelling in my neck.

I was lucky to be in the right place. I had suffered a ruptured thyroid cyst that triggered heavy bleeding, pressing against my windpipe and bringing me to the edge of suffocation. Emergency surgery was performed immediately. Half of my thyroid gland was removed, and the relief was almost instant. My family came to visit that evening, grateful and shaken.

But the crisis was far from over.

At midnight, I deteriorated again - this time with severe, asthma-like symptoms. Fearing a rebleed, I urgently asked the surgical house officer to remove my surgical stitches before getting help. Those were my final words before I slipped into a deep coma.

Seven days later, I awoke in the intensive care unit, a ventilator tube still in my throat. I remember thinking, *'This isn't right.' I'm supposed to be helping patients get better, not lying here as the sickest one in the hospital.*

A second haemorrhage had filled my surgical wound. More surgery followed. I was placed on a ventilator and kept in the ICU. When I finally regained consciousness, my vital signs were dangerously low - my heart rate was just 30 beats per minute, and my blood pressure was 70/30 mmHg (normal is around 120/80). It took several days before these readings stabilised.

Later, I came to understand the underlying cause: insulin resistance. It had contributed to the thyroid cyst, which ruptured and set in motion the cascade that nearly killed me. I have battled sugar and insulin issues my entire life - a struggle I first described in the "Note on the Author." Though I've won some battles and lost others, I've never given up. Over time, I've learned to live with my condition and manage it better, but the journey has never been easy.

Why Is Insulin So Important?

Every moment of every day, your body demands energy. Whether you're thinking, walking, or simply breathing, your trillions of cells need a steady fuel supply to keep you going. That fuel is glucose, a type of sugar carried in your bloodstream. But glucose can't get into your cells on its own. It needs a key to unlock the door. That key is insulin.

Produced by the pancreas, insulin is a hormone that acts as the gatekeeper for glucose. Every time you eat, your blood sugar rises, and your pancreas responds by releasing insulin. This hormone travels through your bloodstream, knocking on the doors of your cells. When insulin binds to receptors on the cell surface, it signals the arrival of a special transporter called **GLUT4**, which opens the door and allows glucose to flow into the cell.

Think of it this way: insulin knocks, GLUT4 opens, and your cells receive the energy they need. This elegant process happens every time you eat.

But what if the door doesn't open?

That's the problem with **insulin resistance**. Over time, your cells may become less responsive to insulin's signal. Insulin keeps knocking, but the door barely budges. Less glucose enters the cells, leaving them hungry for energy. The body reacts by asking the pancreas to release even more insulin to force the glucose in. This leads to a state of **hyperinsulinemia** - too much insulin circulating in your blood.

Insulin resistance creates a **triple threat** to your health:

1. **Excess insulin** floods the body, affecting everything from blood vessels to fat storage.
2. **Glucose fails to reach your cells**, causing fatigue and persistent low energy.
3. **Sugar remains in the bloodstream**, where it can damage tissues and organs over time.

Understanding insulin's role is crucial to grasping metabolic syndrome and reclaiming control over your energy, health, and longevity.

Do All Types of Sugar Have the Same Effect?
When it comes to sugar and its impact on your body, not all types

are created equal, but they often end up in the same place: glucose.

Glucose is the body's primary source of fuel. However, the foods we eat rarely contain pure glucose. Instead, sugar usually arrives in more complex forms - either as **disaccharides** (two sugar units) or **polysaccharides** (long chains of sugar units, commonly known as starches).

Once ingested, your body breaks these larger sugar molecules into **monosaccharides**, or simple sugars. For example, **sucrose** (table sugar, made from sugarcane or sugar beets) is a disaccharide composed of glucose and fructose. After you eat it, the glucose quickly triggers the pancreas to release insulin. Fructose, on the other hand, does not directly stimulate insulin production. Another common sugar, **lactose** (found in milk), is composed of glucose and **galactose**, which is converted into glucose before absorption and thus impacts blood sugar levels.

But sugar doesn't just hide in sweet foods.

Many people proudly claim they "don't eat sugar," unaware that many carbohydrates - like those in white bread, potatoes, or pasta - are essentially sugar in disguise. Starches are simply long chains of glucose molecules. When you chew a starchy food, enzymes in your saliva begin breaking it down, and if you hold it in your mouth, you might notice a sweet taste emerging - that's glucose being released.

And when starches like white pasta or refined flour are fully digested, they flood your bloodstream with glucose, much like eating spoonfuls of sugar would. In fact, a plate of refined pasta can act much like a bag of sugar once your digestive system has done its work.

Understanding this hidden sugar effect is crucial when managing or preventing metabolic syndrome. It's not just about avoiding dessert - it's about recognising all the ways sugar enters your system.

Food Processing: The Carbohydrate Trap and the Power of Fibre

Modern food processing has significantly altered the way our bodies metabolise sugar and carbohydrates. Ultra-processed foods - think biscuits, crisps, sugary cereals, and the endless snack options on supermarket shelves - now dominate many people's daily diets. But this convenience comes at a cost. The rise in processed food consumption has paralleled a surge in obesity, insulin resistance, and metabolic diseases. Let's unpack why.

When we eat carbohydrates like wheat, oats, or rice, our digestive system breaks them down into glucose - the body's primary energy source. Whole grains, when left largely intact, are packed with nutrients and soluble fibre that help regulate blood sugar and improve insulin sensitivity. But once these grains are processed - stripped of their fibre and nutrients - they're transformed into rapidly digestible starches found in foods like white bread, pasta, pizza, and pastries.

The result: A sudden spike in blood sugar followed by an equally rapid crash. You feel hungry again soon after eating, and over time, your cells become less responsive to insulin. This sets the stage for persistent high blood sugar levels, weight gain, and eventually, metabolic syndrome.

Fibre is a critical - yet often overlooked - part of this equation. It's essential for healthy digestion and a robust gut, but our modern diet contains only about 15 grams of fibre daily. Contrast that with our ancestors, who consumed up to 100 grams per day. Fibre exists in two forms, both vital:

- **Soluble fibre**, found in foods such as oats, apples, lentils, and berries, slows the absorption of sugar and fat, helping to prevent blood sugar spikes. It also feeds beneficial gut bacteria, which produce compounds like butyrate that reduce inflammation and support colon health.

- **Insoluble fibre**, found in whole grains, nuts, carrots, and leafy greens, doesn't dissolve in water. Instead, it adds bulk to stool and helps food move smoothly through the gut, promoting regularity.

Together, these fibres improve digestion, protect against disease, and support metabolic health. You need both for maximum benefit.

Fibre also plays a crucial role in determining how a food affects your blood sugar, measured by its **glycaemic index (GI) and glycaemic load (GL):**

- **Glycaemic index** measures how quickly a food raises your blood sugar.
- **Glycaemic load** considers both the speed and the amount of sugar in a typical serving.

Foods high in fibre usually have a low GI and GL, meaning they cause slower, more gradual increases in blood sugar, a key factor in managing insulin sensitivity. For example:

- A medium apple has a GI of 35 and a GL of 5.
- A doughnut GI of 75, GL of 20.
- A green salad GI of 15, GL of 5.
- French fries GI of 75, GL of 25.

In short, more fibre = better blood sugar control. So next time you're deciding between fries or a salad, remember: the green stuff is not just lower in calories - it's actively protecting your metabolism.

The Sweet Poison in Our Diet:
Fructose and High-Fructose Corn Syrup

The explosion of food processing in the 1970s introduced a deceptively sweet villain into our diets: **high-fructose corn syrup (HFCS)**. As discussed in Chapter 2, HFCS is not only the cheapest but also one of the sweetest forms of sugar available. It quickly became the darling of the food industry, fuelling the meteoric rise of soft drink giants like Coca-Cola and Pepsi, and sneaking its way into cookies, sweets, bread, ketchup, and countless processed foods.

But HFCS's sweetness hides a darker truth.

A single can of HFCS-sweetened soda can deliver **30–40 grams of fructose,** far more than the **less than 10 grams** found in an apple, and without any of the fibre or nutrients that nature includes as a buffer. Unlike glucose, **fructose doesn't trigger insulin release** from the pancreas. Instead, it bypasses this system entirely, heading straight to the liver. There, about 30% is converted into glucose, while the rest is used to produce **fat (triglycerides)**, with **uric acid** as a toxic byproduct.

Over time, this turns the liver into a **fat-producing factory**. As fat accumulates, the liver becomes resistant to insulin, laying the groundwork for **non-alcoholic fatty liver disease**. Fructose also **blocks leptin**, the hormone that tells your brain you're full. The result: You stay hungry, overeat, and gain more weight.

But the impact doesn't stop at weight gain.

HFCS consumption significantly increases **uric acid levels** - a hidden metabolic saboteur. Elevated uric acid, or **hyperuricaemia**, is linked not just to **gout**, where crystals inflame the joints, but also to a **reduction in nitric oxide**, the molecule that helps keep blood vessels relaxed and blood pressure low. Uric acid also suppresses **adiponectin**, a hormone that improves insulin sensitivity. [1] Together, these changes promote **high blood pressure, insulin** resistance, and metabolic dysfunction.

In fact, a uric acid level above **420 µmol/L in men** and **360 µmol/L in women** is associated with **higher risks of cardiovascular disease and stroke**.[2]

Yet not all fructose is equal. **Whole fruits**, despite containing fructose, are not harmful. Their **high fibre content** slows down absorption, and their **abundant nutrients** support energy production rather than fat storage. In contrast, HFCS delivers a concentrated, nutrient-devoid hit of fructose that the body is not equipped to handle in large amounts.

While medications like **allopurinol** can help lower uric acid and relieve gout symptoms, **dietary changes** are your most powerful tool. Reducing or eliminating foods high in fructose - especially those containing high-fructose corn syrup (HFCS) - and avoiding purine-rich foods like **beer and organ meats** can naturally lower uric acid levels and support better metabolic health.

The Inflammatory Path to Insulin Resistance

If we had to identify one primary cause of insulin resistance, inflammation would top the list. Without it, insulin resistance wouldn't even exist. Inflammation disrupts the normal delivery of glucose to your cells, laying the foundation for metabolic syndrome. But before you jump to the conclusion that all inflammation is harmful, let's take a closer look.

Not All Inflammation Is Bad

Inflammation comes in two forms: **acute** and **chronic**.

Acute inflammation is your body's rapid response to injury or infection. If you cut your finger, it swells, reddens, and becomes painful - classic signs of acute inflammation, first described by the Roman writer Aulus Celsus. Later, Galen, a Roman physician, added a fifth sign: loss of function. This short-term response is your body's way of boosting circulation and sending immune cells to the site of injury. Once the threat is neutralised, your immune system cleans up the debris and starts repairing the tissue - a vital part of healing.

Acute inflammation is essential. It protects and heals. **Chronic inflammation, however, is a slow and silent destroyer.**

The Real Enemy: Chronic Inflammation

Chronic inflammation is the root cause of insulin resistance and metabolic syndrome. Unlike acute inflammation, this type lingers - low-grade, persistent, and without an obvious purpose. It quietly damages tissues and disrupts normal metabolic function.

One of the primary drivers is **your diet.** Consuming simple sugars and refined carbohydrates fuels this internal fire. These foods trigger an immune response even though there's no injury or infection - just a flood of harmful molecules overwhelming your system.

"But My Tests Came Back Normal…"

Many people are surprised to hear that inflammation is behind their metabolic issues, especially if their recent blood tests showed no signs of infection or inflammation. The catch: Most standard tests only detect inflammation caused by infections or injuries, not the low-grade, chronic inflammation linked to metabolic problems.

That's why more sensitive tools, like the **high-sensitivity C-reactive protein (hs-CRP)** test, are essential. They can pick up the subtle signs of inflammation that underlie insulin resistance and metabolic syndrome.

What's Causing the Inflammation?

Let's break down the usual suspects:

- **Simple sugars & refined carbs**: High-fructose corn syrup (HFCS) is one of the worst offenders. It makes your liver and muscles resistant to insulin, boosts your appetite, and raises uric acid - another marker of insulin resistance. Other culprits include white bread, pasta, rice, cereals, and processed snacks that spike blood sugar quickly.
- **Cheap cooking oils**: Corn, sunflower, and safflower oils are high in omega-6 fatty acids, which promote inflammation, especially when heated. Trans fats, found in fast food and fried restaurant fare, are equally harmful.
- **Food allergens**: Gluten is the leading inflammatory allergen for many, but dairy, soy, eggs, and peanuts can also provoke an immune response in sensitive individuals.

Belly Fat: The Hidden Engine of Chronic Inflammation

When it comes to chronic low-grade inflammation - a key player in metabolic syndrome - what we eat might light the match, but belly fat keeps the fire burning. Visceral fat, often referred to as belly fat, isn't just a passive energy store. It acts as a dynamic endocrine organ, constantly releasing hormones and inflammatory molecules that fuel inflammation and exacerbate insulin resistance.

This type of fat is especially potent because it releases inflammatory mediators, such as tumour necrosis factor-alpha (TNF-α) and interleukin-6 (IL-6). IL-6, in particular, travels through the bloodstream, influencing appetite, metabolism, and the body's energy balance. It also stimulates the liver to produce C-reactive protein (CRP), a key marker and driver of inflammation. Elevated CRP levels are closely tied to weight gain and serve as a significant indicator of increasing insulin resistance. Encouragingly, losing weight tends to lower CRP levels, restoring a healthier metabolic state.

On the flip side, not all fat-derived hormones are harmful. Adiponectin, another hormone secreted by fat cells, plays a protective role. It reduces inflammation, enhances insulin sensitivity, and supports cardiovascular health by increasing nitric oxide production and raising levels of "good" HDL cholesterol. High levels of adiponectin are associated with a healthier metabolic profile. However, low levels are commonly seen in people with excess abdominal fat, creating a dangerous link between belly fat, insulin resistance, and metabolic syndrome. [3]

How Ultra-Processed Foods Disrupt Your Gut—and Your Health
Ultra-processed foods do more than spike your blood sugar - they alter the very ecosystem of your gut. One of the most damaging features of these foods is their lack of dietary fibre. Fibre isn't just roughage; it's a vital prebiotic that nourishes beneficial gut bacteria. Without it, the balance tips toward harmful microbes - a condition known as gut dysbiosis.

This shift has serious consequences. Harmful bacteria produce a toxin called **lipopolysaccharide (LPS)**. When LPS breaches the gut lining, it creates microscopic holes that allow the toxin to enter the bloodstream. The result: A persistent, low-grade inflammation that plays a key role in the development of insulin resistance and other metabolic disorders.

LPS-driven inflammation is a hidden driver of obesity, type 2 diabetes, and many features of metabolic syndrome. By restoring a healthy gut microbiome - through reducing ultra-processed foods and increasing fibre intake - we can lower inflammation, improve insulin sensitivity, and reclaim metabolic health.

Emerging research is shedding light on the hidden dangers of ultra-processed foods. These industrially engineered products have been strongly linked to increased body fat and rising obesity rates.[4] One study revealed that children with obesity exhibit elevated levels of zonulin, a key marker of intestinal permeability, often referred to as "leaky gut." Even more concerning, a recent study found that ultra-processed foods can trigger widespread inflammation by activating multiple inflammatory pathways in older adults. This may help explain why chronic conditions and comorbidities are so prevalent in this age group.[5]

The Dangerous Duo: Fat and Sugar
That fast-food burger with a large cola may seem like a convenient indulgence, but it's also a metabolic trap. Initially, the sugar in the soda causes your blood glucose levels to surge. Then, the fat from the burger steps in - not to help, but to prolong the spike. Unlike carbohydrates, fat digests slowly, keeping your body in a heightened state of energy absorption for hours.

Here's where the trouble starts: as insulin arrives to shuttle glucose into your cells, the high fat load signals that your cells are already full. They resist the glucose, essentially saying, *"No thanks - we've got more than enough."* This traffic jam of nutrients can lead to insulin resistance, a key player in the development of metabolic syndrome.

But the damage doesn't stop there. Saturated fat from meat and dairy can trigger inflammation in the hypothalamus - the brain's command centre for hunger and energy balance. This inflammation dulls satiety signals, leading to increased appetite and overeating. Over time, this vicious cycle contributes to weight gain, insulin resistance, and the cascade of health issues that define metabolic syndrome.

What About Protein?

Protein plays a vital role in the body, but not all protein sources have the same impact on metabolic health. In the short term, consuming animal protein can stimulate insulin release and improve blood sugar control.[6] However, over time, the story changes. Long-term intake of animal protein - especially from red and processed meats - has been linked to insulin resistance and impaired blood glucose regulation.

Unlike carbohydrates, animal proteins can raise insulin levels without causing a corresponding spike in blood sugar. This stealthy effect may worsen insulin resistance, potentially fuelling the development of full-blown metabolic syndrome.

Multiple studies have found that excessive meat consumption increases inflammation, insulin resistance, and the risk of type 2 diabetes. Red meat is high in saturated fat and produces a compound called trimethylamine N-oxide (TMAO), both of which can trigger harmful metabolic changes. Swapping red meat for nuts, which are rich in polyunsaturated fats, or opting for fish and seafood - low in saturated fat and high in anti-inflammatory omega-3 fatty acids - can offer protective benefits.

To support muscle health while minimising risk, protein intake should be moderate. Young adults need about 60 grams of protein per day (roughly the size of your palm), while older adults should aim for around 75 grams.

Even dairy, another common protein source, comes with a caveat. Although milk, cheese, and other dairy products are protein-rich, research shows that high dairy consumption may reduce insulin sensitivity more than diets high in lean red meat.[7] Choosing your protein sources wisely can make a meaningful difference in preventing or managing metabolic syndrome.

Why Too Much Salt Can Sabotage Your Metabolism

We often hear about sugar and refined carbs being the culprits behind metabolic issues, but salt, especially in processed foods, plays a surprisingly similar role. Beyond their high glycaemic index, these foods can promote insulin resistance through a lesser-known mechanism: sodium overload.

When sodium levels in the blood rise, the body interprets it as a sign of dehydration. In response, the brain releases an antidiuretic hormone to help the body retain water. But here's the catch - this hormone also signals the liver to produce more glucose as part of an emergency response. Over time, this leads to chronically elevated blood glucose and insulin levels, essentially mimicking the effects of consuming excessive sugar.

So, it's not just sweets you need to watch out for. A salty diet can quietly undermine your metabolic health in ways that are easy to overlook but hard to undo.

Dehydration And Caffeine:
Hidden Drivers Of Metabolic Imbalance

In our modern lifestyle, dehydration has become the norm rather than the exception. We sip dehydrating beverages like coffee, tea, and soft drinks throughout the day, and often follow with alcohol at night - yet neglect the most essential drink of all: water. Most people in the United Kingdom fail to meet daily water intake recommendations, contributing to a chronic state of dehydration. This seemingly small habit can have profound consequences. Dehydration elevates blood sodium levels, which disrupts insulin sensitivity and impairs blood glucose regulation, both key factors in metabolic syndrome.

When we're dehydrated, our cells shrink and lose their ability to function optimally. This cellular stress interferes with insulin signalling and sets the stage for insulin resistance and type 2 diabetes.[8] Fortunately, adopting one simple habit can make a difference: drinking water before and after meals (but not during) helps rehydrate cells, reduces insulin resistance, and prevents post-meal blood sugar spikes. (See Chapter 16 for more guidance on hydration within the dietary plan.)

Alcohol, while socially accepted and calorically dense at 7 calories per gram, offers little nutritional value. It contains nearly twice the energy of carbohydrates or protein, and slightly less than fat, yet lacks vitamins, minerals, and fibre. More importantly, alcohol promotes dehydration and places stress on the liver - an organ vital to maintaining blood sugar balance. Excessive alcohol use is a well-established risk factor for insulin resistance, weight gain, and type 2 diabetes.

Caffeine, too, plays a more complex role than most realise. By blocking adenosine receptors in the brain, caffeine keeps us alert and energised. But this stimulation comes at a cost: studies show that even moderate caffeine intake can reduce insulin sensitivity by up to 15%.[9] The risk is higher in individuals with a genetic variation in the **CYP1A2** gene, which slows caffeine metabolism. For them, caffeine lingers longer in the system, amplifying its effects on blood sugar regulation.

Timing matters as well. Drinking coffee first thing in the morning on an empty stomach - especially after a poor night's sleep - can impair glucose metabolism. A small meal beforehand may help buffer this response. And with average caffeine consumption ranging from 200 to 400 mg daily, moderation is key. One 8-ounce cup of brewed coffee contains 80 - 100 mg of caffeine, but other sources, such as energy drinks, soft drinks, hot chocolate, and even some sports beverages, can significantly contribute to your daily total.

The Hidden Cost of Smoking:
Insulin Resistance and Diabetes Risk

While smoking is widely known for its impact on lung health and cardiovascular disease, its role in metabolic syndrome is often overlooked. Nicotine impairs your cells' ability to respond to insulin, promoting insulin resistance - a key feature of metabolic syndrome. It also elevates cortisol levels, a hormone that further disrupts insulin action and drives up triglycerides, another hallmark of the condition.

Research shows that smokers face up to twice the risk of developing type 2 diabetes compared to non-smokers.[9] The good news: This risk isn't permanent. Remarkably, just two years after quitting, the likelihood of developing diabetes begins to decline, eventually returning to the level of a non-smoker within a decade.[10]

Sitting is the New Smoking

Emerging evidence leaves little doubt: prolonged physical inactivity is a significant contributor to insulin resistance and adverse metabolic and cardiovascular changes. That's why I make it a point to ask every patient with metabolic issues about their daily activity levels.

Over the years, I've encountered surprising stories. Former athletes - once paragons of health - have slipped into sedentary habits after retiring from sports. (Remember Maradona from Chapter 2) Others gave up walking or using public transport in favour of driving - and paid a metabolic price. The most tragic case was an office worker whose inactivity led to end-stage kidney failure and regular dialysis.

Fortunately, physical activity remains one of the fastest, most effective ways to restore insulin sensitivity. Even without insulin, active muscles pull glucose from the bloodstream. It's no surprise, then, that a brisk 15-minute walk after lunch can dramatically flatten post-meal blood sugar spikes.

Exercise doesn't just burn calories - it builds muscle, which increases your body's demand for glucose. Aim for at least 60 minutes of moderate physical activity each day and adopt other healthy lifestyle habits to help ward off metabolic syndrome (see Chapter 17 for a comprehensive exercise plan).

The Hidden Role of the Thyroid

Metabolism doesn't run on willpower alone - it runs on hormones, especially thyroxine (see Chapter 2). When the thyroid underperforms, thyroxine levels drop, slowing metabolism to a crawl. This sluggish state fosters insulin resistance, weight gain, and higher levels of circulating fats - all key contributors to metabolic syndrome.

Frequent Meals and Snacks:
A Hidden Driver of Insulin Overload

It's not just *what* we eat that affects our insulin levels - *when* we eat matters as much. In the mid-20th century, most people followed a consistent pattern of three meals a day. However, by the 1980s, a significant cultural shift had occurred. The rise of ultra-processed convenience foods - such as crisps, crackers, chocolate bars, and numerous snack options - ushered in a new norm: eating six or more times a day.

This near-constant grazing has a significant metabolic cost. Every time we eat, regardless of the portion size, our body produces insulin. Over time, frequent eating leads to chronically elevated insulin levels. This persistent stimulation can desensitise the body's insulin receptors, paving the way for insulin resistance - a core feature of metabolic syndrome.

Simply put, our modern eating patterns keep insulin levels high, day in and day out - and that may be silently driving the epidemic of metabolic dysfunction.

Let Me Stress This

When you're under chronic stress, your body goes into survival mode, redirecting fat storage to the abdomen. This visceral fat becomes a standby energy reserve, preparing you for an imagined threat that never comes. The result: A hormonal cocktail that fosters insulin resistance and lays the groundwork for conditions like obesity, type 2 diabetes, and cardiovascular disease.

But that's not all. Stress also messes with your appetite. It drives cravings for high-calorie, ultra-palatable comfort foods - just the kind that worsen insulin resistance. It's a metabolic trap: stress makes you hungry for the very foods that make your body less responsive to insulin.

Insulin Resistance:
The Silent Trigger Behind a Cascade of Health Problems

Our ancient ancestors adapted to seasonal cycles of feast and famine. During times of abundance - typically summer - their bodies ramped up insulin production to help store nutrients for the leaner months ahead (see Chapter 2). Insulin is not just a blood sugar regulator; it's a powerful growth signal. It fuels cellular division, growth, and repair - processes that all require cholesterol, a vital building block of cell membranes (see Chapter 7).

To meet this demand, insulin activates an enzyme called **HMG-CoA reductase**, which instructs the liver to produce more cholesterol. As a result, blood cholesterol levels rise. But here's the kicker: when insulin levels remain high - due to modern eating habits that mimic constant "feasting" - cholesterol production stays elevated. In contrast, lowering insulin levels naturally curbs this overproduction.

But the effects of high insulin go far beyond cholesterol.

Chronic elevation of insulin stimulates cell growth in the walls of arteries, leading to their thickening and narrowing. It also encourages the buildup of cholesterol plaques and calcium deposits along artery walls. This causes the heart to work harder to pump blood through increasingly stiff and narrow vessels, thereby raising blood pressure (see Chapter 5).

Meanwhile, high blood glucose - the frequent partner of high insulin - damages the endothelium, the thin inner lining of blood vessels. The endothelium produces nitric oxide (NO), a compound that relaxes blood vessels and helps maintain healthy blood pressure. When glucose damages this lining, NO production drops, and blood pressure rises. High insulin also increases sodium reabsorption in the kidneys, raising blood volume - and with it, blood pressure.

Insulin doesn't stop there.

It can trigger the formation of cysts in various organs - a phenomenon doctors often dismiss as incidental findings during imaging. I used to think the same - until I experienced a thyroid cyst rupture, causing life-threatening internal bleeding.

Repeated spikes in blood sugar also "rust" the body from the inside. This process, known as **glycation**, generates toxic compounds called **advanced glycation end-products** (AGEs). These AGEs accelerate ageing and weaken the immune system, leaving the body more vulnerable to infections, including the seasonal flu (see Chapter 6).

Moreover, blood glucose fluctuations are a leading - but often overlooked - cause of persistent neck and lower back pain.

Am I Insulin-Resistant?

Insulin resistance is often called a **"silent threat"** because it creeps in without apparent symptoms. It can quietly wreak havoc on your metabolism long before any diagnosis is made. Unfortunately, this makes early detection difficult, and a critical window to prevent more serious metabolic conditions is often lost.

But who should be concerned?

You're at higher risk if you:

- Smoke
- Lead a sedentary lifestyle
- Are overweight or obese
- Have a family history of diabetes or high blood pressure

For women

- Experienced gestational diabetes during pregnancy
- Delivered a baby weighing more than 9 pounds (4.0 kilograms)
- Are going through menopause
- Have polycystic ovary syndrome (PCOS)

For men

- Diagnosed with **benign prostatic hyperplasia (BPH)**

These groups should stay especially vigilant, as they are more likely to develop insulin resistance.

Why does this matter?

As mentioned above, chronically high insulin levels - **hyperinsulinaemia** - can drive cell division and growth. In men, this may lead to **benign prostatic hyperplasia (BPH)**, an enlargement of the prostate linked to uncomfortable urinary symptoms (see Chapter 11). In women, insulin resistance plays a key role in **PCOS**, often accompanied by weight gain, excessive body hair, and fertility issues (see Chapter 12).

Understanding your risk is the first step toward action and potentially reversing this silent but dangerous condition.

Could You Be Living with Insulin Resistance?

Do you often feel drained, foggy-headed, or constantly hungry? Do you battle intense food cravings or experience a pronounced energy crash in the afternoon? If these symptoms sound familiar, you may be experiencing **insulin resistance** - a silent yet powerful driver of metabolic dysfunction.

People with insulin resistance often notice that their energy levels fluctuate significantly with meals. A typical pattern includes feeling alert after eating, followed by a deep slump later in the day. Nighttime can also be restless - they often find themselves wide awake between 1 and 2 a.m., struggling to fall back asleep.

You may also notice physical signs, such as dark, velvety patches of skin in the armpits, neck, or face (known as **acanthosis nigricans**), skin tags, or unusual scarring. A potbelly in men or excess facial hair in women - especially in the context of obesity - can also be red flags. These signs are your body's way of sounding the alarm, even if traditional medicine doesn't always recognise them.

Mainstream healthcare often overlooks insulin resistance. Since it creeps in silently and doesn't present as a clear-cut disease early on, many doctors rely on conventional tests, such as **fasting**

blood glucose and **HbA1c** - both of which typically remain within normal limits until the condition is well advanced. Meanwhile, the pancreas is working overtime to produce more insulin to compensate for the reduced sensitivity in the body's cells.

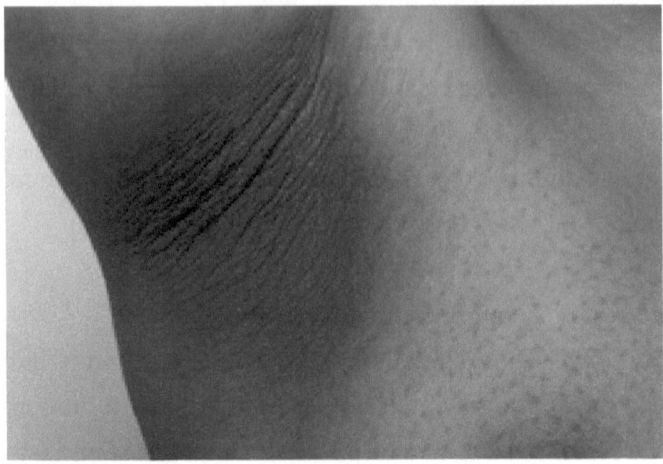

Acanthosis nigricans is characterised by patches of dark, thick skin, primarily on skin folds at the neck, armpit and groin or over skin scars. It is a sign of insulin resistance.

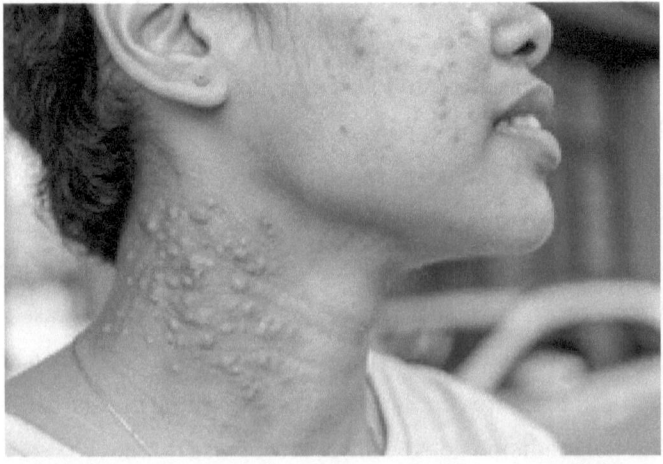

Skin Tags are painless, benign growths of skin that often appear in clusters, either the same colour as the skin or darker, and are frequently associated with insulin resistance.

Detecting the Early Warning Signs

Fortunately, there are better ways to catch insulin resistance before it spirals into something more serious:

- **Fasting insulin levels** above 10 mIU/L may be one of the earliest warning signs.
- **HOMA-IR (Homeostatic Model Assessment for Insulin Resistance)** is another early detection test, while primarily used in research, many labs now offer this test.
- **Triglyceride levels** over 1.7 mmol/L
- A **triglyceride-to-HDL cholesterol ratio** greater than 2.5 suggests a significantly higher cardiovascular risk.[11]

By tuning in to these early signals - both in how you feel and what your lab work reveals- you can take proactive steps to reclaim your metabolic health before more serious conditions, such as type 2 diabetes or heart disease, take root.

"It felt like my shoulders were touching my ears."

These were the exact words of a 72-year-old woman who came to see me not long after the loss of her husband. Grief had taken a toll on her, physically and emotionally. She complained of persistent neck and back pain and described a constant, almost comical sensation of tension, as if her shoulders were permanently hunched up near her ears.

I initially assumed this was purely stress-related. She was grieving, after all. I recommended a suite of stress-relieving practices: counselling, deep breathing, meditation, and gentle yoga. She promised to give them a try.

Six weeks later, she was back. Discouraged. The pain remained. The fatigue was worse. "I'm doing everything you said," she told me, "But nothing's changing."

That's when we dug deeper. She admitted that after her husband's death, she had stopped caring for herself. Cooking felt like a burden, so she lived on tea and biscuits, crackers, crisps - anything easy. Her sleep was poor, her energy flat, and the weight had crept on.

Routine blood tests, including blood glucose, all came back normal. But something wasn't adding up. I ordered more advanced metabolic tests. What we found stunned us both: her fasting insulin was 26 mIU/L - more than double the healthy upper limit of 10. She wasn't diabetic by conventional measures, but her body was struggling to process glucose. She was deep in the trenches of insulin resistance.

We tackled it together, changing her diet, gradually reintroducing whole, nourishing foods, and restoring a sense of routine and care to her day. As her insulin levels came down, something remarkable happened: her shoulders dropped quite literally. Her posture improved. The pain eased. Her energy returned. She even shed a few kilos.

But most importantly, she regained control of her health, her habits, and her hope.

This transformation was not just biochemical - it was deeply human. The shift from being a supported partner to a grieving widow had reshaped her body and biology in powerful, measurable ways. Her case was a striking reminder that metabolic health is not only about numbers on a lab report. It's about how we live, how we eat, and how we carry the weight of our lives - sometimes quite literally - in our bodies.

Reflection on My Own Experience

As a doctor, I was surprised - and humbled - to find myself struggling with insulin resistance. Despite my medical training, I lacked the knowledge and clinical guidance to manage it effectively. What followed was a long journey of trial and error before I discovered that the real solution lies not in complex treatments but in simple, powerful lifestyle changes: eating whole, high-fibre foods, practising intermittent fasting, and committing to regular exercise.

I remember feeling angry that my condition had gone unnoticed for so long, especially after it led to a burst thyroid cyst. But looking back, I also understand. Thirty years ago, insulin resistance was poorly understood, and my doctors were working with limited knowledge.

Still, I can't help but feel let down by the system. If my insulin resistance had been recognised earlier, I might have avoided two major surgeries and a series of life-threatening complications. Early diagnosis doesn't just benefit individuals - it could prevent prediabetes, diabetes, hypertension, and even cancer in countless others.

In my case, the roots of insulin resistance ran deep. It wasn't just the junk food from hospital canteens or sugary drinks from vending machines. It was the chronic stress, sleepless nights, sedentary routine, and relentless demands of hospital shift work that quietly set the stage.

My story isn't unique, and that's exactly why it needs to be told.

The Prognosis of Insulin Resistance

Insulin resistance is more than just a warning sign - it's a gateway to serious health complications. Around 60% of individuals with insulin resistance eventually develop one or more metabolic disorders, including type 2 diabetes, heart disease, stroke, or even dementia. The outlook becomes more concerning with prediabetes: up to half of those affected will progress to full-blown diabetes within 5 to 10 years if no intervention is made.[12] Understanding this progression is critical because early action can alter the path.

Managing your condition

You can manage insulin resistance naturally by eating a whole-food, nutrient-dense diet high in fibre but low in carbohydrates, following intermittent fasting, and losing 5% to 7% of your body weight.

A crucial step is to quell inflammation. In terms of food, you could summarise the remedy by going back to 'Mother Nature' - meaning whole natural food, which your great-grandmother would recognise as such. In practical terms, choose live food from the farm, not dead food from the factory. Adopt an anti-inflammatory lifestyle, including getting enough restful sleep, reducing stress levels, engaging in regular exercise, maintaining great and fulfilling relationships, enjoying the sunshine, sharing love, and finding purpose in life.

Final Thoughts

Insulin resistance doesn't appear overnight - it's driven by persistent, low-grade inflammation often fuelled by our modern diets. The regular intake of simple sugars and ultra-processed carbohydrates feeds harmful gut bacteria, which in turn release inflammatory molecules, such as LPS (lipopolysaccharides), into the bloodstream. This silent, chronic inflammation is a defining feature of insulin resistance.

A major contributor to this inflammatory state is abdominal fat, also known as central obesity. Far from being a passive store of energy, this type of fat actively promotes inflammation and plays a central role in the cascade of metabolic dysfunctions that follow.

Understanding central obesity is key to addressing the broader metabolic syndrome, and that's where we'll turn our focus in Chapter 4.

CHAPTER 4

Central Obesity: The Core of the Metabolic Storm

Why does fat accumulating around the waist - what we call **central obesity** - pose such a serious threat to our health? Is it simply a matter of appearance, or is this "belly fat" a powerful driver of disease? And more importantly, are there habits, dietary or lifestyle, that encourage this fat to settle in the abdomen? Most critically, what can we do to reduce it and safeguard ourselves from chronic illness?

"The Wider the Waist, the Smaller the Brain"
One of my patients once told me he was attending the clinic not just to prevent diabetes, but also to avoid **dementia**. I was intrigued - while the link between obesity and diabetes is well known, dementia seemed less obvious. When I asked what led him to that conclusion, he quoted a study: *"The wider your waist, the smaller your brain."*

That wasn't just a clever phrase. It was based on a remarkable study involving over 700 adults, which found that a higher volume of **visceral fat** - the deep fat surrounding internal organs - was associated with **smaller brain volume** and a greater risk of **dementia**, regardless of a person's overall weight. This was measured using detailed CT brain scans, reinforcing the fact that belly fat is far more than skin-deep.

From Survival Mechanism to Modern Risk
Fat storage has historically served an essential purpose. As described in Chapter 2, our ancestors evolved to store excess energy as fat during times of plenty - typically summer - to survive periods of scarcity, in winter. Women, in particular, stored fat around the hips to fuel the demanding processes of pregnancy and breastfeeding.

But today, we live in a world of constant abundance. We feast year-round without the corresponding famine. And the very mechanism that once protected us has turned against us. This overabundance leads to chronic fat accumulation, particularly in the abdomen, raising the risk of a condition we now call **metabolic syndrome** - a gateway to serious diseases like heart attack, stroke, diabetes, and more.

Why Belly Fat Is So Dangerous
Central or abdominal obesity isn't just a passive store of excess calories - it's biologically active. Visceral fat functions like an **endocrine organ**, releasing **hormones and inflammatory cytokines** that promote **low-grade chronic inflammation**. As you learned in Chapter 3, this inflammation drives **insulin resistance**, undermining the body's ability to use glucose efficiently. Over time, this disrupts metabolic function, opening the door to a range of diseases.

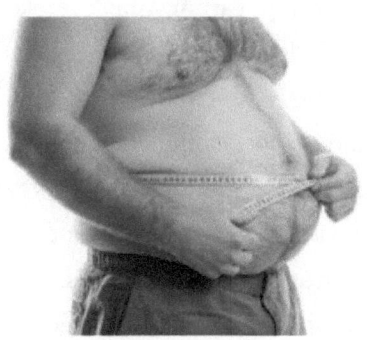

This is the critical difference between **physiological fat**, which supports us in times of need, and **pathological fat**, which silently contributes to the development of disease.

Abdominal fat accumulation (central obesity), particularly around the internal organs, is a risk factor for metabolic diseases, including high blood pressure, diabetes, heart disease and cancer.

The Hidden Epidemic: Normal-Weight Metabolic Syndrome

Here's a surprising fact: central obesity, rather than overall obesity, is the primary driver of metabolic syndrome. You don't have to be visibly overweight to be at risk. Studies show that up to **40% of people with a normal weight** have metabolic syndrome. Understanding and addressing central obesity is crucial because it's not just about the size of your waist. It's about the health of your **heart, liver, brain, metabolism, and future.**

Where Belly Fat Hides:
Understanding Abdominal Fat Distribution

Back in 1947, French physician Jean Vague made a striking observation: people with diabetes, heart disease, and gout often shared a common trait - excess belly fat. This insight shifted the medical community's focus from simply measuring body fat to understanding *where* it is stored. Vague and her colleagues discovered that lowering carbohydrate intake could improve diabetic control and reduce harmful triglycerides and cholesterol. More importantly, they realised that *body shape* - not just body size - holds the key to metabolic health.

Belly fat, also known as abdominal fat, plays a significant role in shaping our health risks. When fat accumulates around the waist, it creates what is known as android or "apple-shaped" obesity, which is more common in men. In contrast, fat stored around the hips and thighs results in a gynoid or "pear-shaped" body, which is typically associated with women. This pattern of fat distribution supports pregnancy and breastfeeding, serving a functional purpose. These "apple" and "pear" body types visually reflect two very different metabolic realities.

Thanks to modern imaging techniques like computed tomography (CT) and magnetic resonance imaging (MRI), we can now see that belly fat isn't just one type of fat. It falls into two major categories: **subcutaneous fat**, which lies just under the skin, and **intra-abdominal fat**, which surrounds and infiltrates internal organs. This distinction is crucial in understanding health risks associated with abdominal fat.

Subcutaneous fat is the layer that can be pinched, situated under the skin but above the abdominal muscles. It's a natural, physiological fat reserve found throughout the body. In healthy women, it often collects around the hips and thighs, creating a pear-shaped figure. This type of fat serves as a thermal insulator, an energy reserve, and a protective cushion for internal organs. It also has endocrine functions, producing hormones that support metabolic health. In moderation, subcutaneous fat is beneficial.

Intra-abdominal fat, however, is a different story. It includes **visceral fat** - the deep fat packed around abdominal organs, such as the intestines and kidneys - and **ectopic fat**, which accumulates *within* organs like the liver and pancreas. Visceral fat, especially in the omentum (a fat apron draped over the intestines), is closely linked to insulin resistance, inflammation, and cardiovascular disease. Ectopic fat can lead to fatty liver disease and impair organ function. Unlike subcutaneous fat, both visceral and ectopic fat are metabolically dangerous.

While not all fat is bad, **where** it is stored makes a world of difference. Subcutaneous fat may play protective roles, but excessive fat - especially when stored in the abdomen - can fuel the progression of metabolic disease.

How to Measure Your Body Fat and Risk of Disease

Understanding your body fat and where it's stored is key to assessing your risk of metabolic diseases - and you don't always need fancy tools to start. A quick self-check can be surprisingly revealing. Stand up and look down. If you can't see your feet, you likely have significant belly fat. If your waist circumference is more than half your height, that's another red flag. And yes, even a double chin can hint at dangerous visceral fat - the kind that surrounds your organs and raises your risk of metabolic conditions.

Measuring Methods: From Simple to Sophisticated

As introduced in Chapter 1, several methods exist for measuring body fat and central obesity. These include:

- **Body Mass Index (BMI)**
- **Waist Circumference**
- **Waist-to-Hip Ratio (WHR)**
- **Neck Circumference (NC)**
- **Waist-to-Height Ratio (WHtR)**

Let's take a closer look at how each of these can (or can't) help assess your health risks.

BMI: Misleading but Still Used

BMI is widely used, but it's not a reliable predictor of disease risk. It simply compares your weight to your height and categorises you accordingly. But here's the problem: BMI doesn't distinguish between fat and muscle. Athletes with high muscle mass or people with more subcutaneous (under-skin) fat may be wrongly labelled as unhealthy. Worse, it doesn't tell us where the fat is stored - information critical for assessing metabolic risk.

Why WHtR Outshines BMI

The **Waist-to-Height Ratio (WHtR)** offers a more accurate picture. Central obesity - fat around your waist - is more strongly linked to disease than fat elsewhere. WHtR highlights this better than BMI or WHR, and it works across genders and ages. If your waist is more than half your height, your risk is elevated - even if your weight is "normal."

Neck Circumference: An Underrated Indicator

Recent research suggests that **Neck Circumference (NC)** may be just as useful as waist measurements for identifying metabolic risk, and it's easier to measure, especially in people with obesity. Measure just below the Adam's apple, keeping your head level and shoulders relaxed.

- Over **12.5 inches (32 cm)** in women and
- Over **15 inches (38 cm)** in men
  Suggest an increased risk of central obesity and related diseases. NC is especially valuable when used in conjunction with BMI and WHtR.

Old-School Tools Still Matter - Skinfold Thickness

This tried-and-tested method has been used for decades. A simple calliper measures fat just under the skin, typically at the triceps, abdomen, hip, and thigh. These readings can be entered into apps or formulas to estimate total body fat percentage. While less high-tech, this method is effective and great for monitoring changes over time.

Modern Tech, Better Precision

Today's science brings precision tools for measuring fat and risk more accurately:

- **Bioelectric Impedance Analysis (BIA)**
  These devices measure how easily electricity flows through your body. Fat and bone resist electric flow more than muscle. You can get a simple scale-like device for home use or opt for more accurate versions in gyms. One caveat: results can be skewed by hydration levels - being dehydrated can falsely elevate your fat percentage.
- **DEXA Scan**
  The **Dual-Energy X-ray Absorptiometry (DEXA)** scan is the gold standard. It accurately measures fat mass, lean mass, and bone density - all in under five minutes. It's often used in hospitals to diagnose osteoporosis, but it's also an excellent tool for analysing body composition. The only downside is Cost. At around £100 per scan, it's not cheap, but its reliability and convenience make it a worthwhile investment.

In summary, no single measurement tells the whole story. Combining tools like WHtR, NC, and body composition scans can give a much clearer picture of your metabolic health. It's not just about how much fat you have - it's about where it's stored and what it means for your future well-being.

Outwardly Healthy, Yet Silently at Risk

At first glance, Andy appeared to be the picture of health. At 45 years old, he maintained a normal weight, didn't drink alcohol, and had no alarming symptoms beyond occasional indigestion.

But a routine check-up told a different story - one that revealed the hidden dangers of metabolic syndrome.

Andy's concern was sparked by unexpected blood test results: mildly elevated liver enzymes, borderline blood glucose, and rising cholesterol levels. What made this more worrisome was his family history. His father had died of a heart attack at just 46, and his mother succumbed to liver cirrhosis in her 50s, despite never drinking alcohol. This legacy of silent disease prompted his doctor to investigate further.

Although Andy's BMI was 24.5 kg/m^2 - technically within the normal range - this metric failed to tell the full story. As discussed in Chapter 1, BMI doesn't account for fat distribution, which can be a more crucial indicator of disease risk. When his waist was measured at 41 inches (105 cm) and his hips at 40 inches (102 cm), his waist-to-hip ratio (WHR) came out to 1.03 - well above the healthy limit of 0.9 for men. This pointed to significant abdominal fat accumulation, and an abdominal ultrasound confirmed the diagnosis: fatty liver disease.

Andy's lifestyle offered important clues. His diet was heavy in refined carbohydrates - cereals, oat porridge, pasta, bread, potatoes, and especially commercial fruit juices loaded with high-fructose corn syrup (HFCS). Though he didn't consume alcohol, he regularly snacked on crisps, chocolate bars, rice crackers, and cakes. Sedentary from working at home, he rarely exercised and struggled with chronic stress and sleep disruption - all of which compounded his risk.

The blood results painted a clear biochemical picture of metabolic dysfunction:

Liver enzymes: ALT was 73 U/L and GGT 99 U/L (both more than double the upper normal limit).

Glucose metabolism: Fasting blood glucose was 6.2 mmol/L (prediabetic), HbA1c was 5.9% (elevated), and fasting insulin was

21 mIU/L (more than double the normal).

Lipid profile: Total cholesterol was 5.5 mmol/L, LDL ("bad" cholesterol) was 3.5 mmol/L, HDL ("good" cholesterol) was a borderline 1.0 mmol/L, and triglycerides were alarmingly high at 3.3 mmol/L (nearly twice the upper normal limit).

Despite his "normal" BMI, Andy was metabolically unhealthy. His story is a powerful reminder that metabolic syndrome can lurk beneath the surface, even in those who appear healthy. Waist measurements, liver health, and lifestyle factors often reveal more about an individual's overall health than weight alone.

Causes of Central Obesity

Central obesity, or belly fat, is a key feature of metabolic syndrome, and it's on the rise. One of the primary culprit is the modern Western diet.

The Modern Diet and Belly Fat

Today's typical diet is rich in fat, sugar, and highly processed carbohydrates - think cereals, bread, rice, pasta, and pizza. These foods are energy-dense but low in fibre and essential nutrients, creating a perfect storm for fat accumulation, especially when combined with a sedentary lifestyle.

Sugary drinks and fruit juices, particularly those sweetened with high-fructose corn syrup (HFCS), are especially harmful. Studies consistently link HFCS and ultra-processed foods to central (abdominal) obesity more strongly than to general weight gain. In contrast, whole foods - such as unprocessed grains, lean proteins, and oily fish - are associated with reduced belly fat.

Alcohol: The Truth Behind the 'Beer Belly'

Alcohol is another well-known driver of abdominal fat. The term "beer belly" is not just colloquial - it's medically accurate. One study showed that consuming more than four litres of beer per week significantly increases abdominal fat, particularly in men. [1]

Stress, Cortisol, and Fat Storage

Modern life is stressful, and chronic stress triggers the body's appetite for comfort foods, which are typically high in sugar, fat, and calories. This stress-induced eating is driven by the hypothalamic–pituitary–adrenal (HPA) axis, which releases cortisol. Elevated cortisol promotes fat storage in the abdominal cavity.

High morning cortisol levels have been linked to abnormal metabolic markers, such as an increased BMI and waist-to-hip ratio, particularly in individuals who gain weight following stressful events.[3]

Hormones and Age: Why Fat Distribution Changes

Fat storage patterns shift with age, mainly due to changes in sex hormones. In women, oestrogen encourages fat storage in the hips, thighs, and buttocks - a healthy gynoid (pear-shaped) pattern that supports childbearing.

Men, on the other hand, benefit from testosterone, which promotes fat burning and prevents fat accumulation. As testosterone declines with age, men are more prone to central obesity.

After menopause, falling oestrogen levels cause women to adopt a more male-like (android) fat distribution. Fat shifts from the hips to the abdomen, increasing the risk of visceral fat accumulation and related metabolic diseases.

Genetics: The Role of Leptin

Leptin is the hormone that signals fullness. When leptin receptors are missing due to genetic mutations, the result is constant hunger and early-onset obesity. Affected individuals may exhibit extreme food-seeking behaviour - including hoarding or stealing food - due to their inability to feel full.

Environment Matters

Where you live can shape your waistline. Individuals who reside near supermarkets offering fresh, healthy food options are less likely to become obese.[1] In contrast, those surrounded by fast-food outlets, bars, and convenience stores are far more likely to accumulate belly fat.[2]

Why Belly Fat Is Especially Harmful:
The Hidden Risk Behind the Waistline

Not all body fat is created equal, and fat stored around your belly is particularly harmful. Unlike fat just beneath the skin (subcutaneous fat), abdominal fat - also called visceral fat- travels directly to the liver via the portal vein. This direct route floods the liver with fatty acids, overwhelming its ability to process them and triggering a cascade of metabolic dysfunction.

When the liver is overloaded with fat, it begins to store it, leading to **non-alcoholic fatty liver disease (NAFLD)**. As fat builds up, the liver becomes resistant to insulin, the hormone that helps regulate blood sugar. Meanwhile, excess fat also accumulates in the muscles, making them insulin resistant as well. Because the liver and muscles are the body's primary consumers of glucose, their dysfunction causes blood sugar to rise. Insulin levels increase to compensate, but the sugar has nowhere to go. Instead, the liver converts it into **triglycerides**, raising its blood levels - another risk factor for **metabolic syndrome**.

By contrast, subcutaneous fat (the type under your skin) enters the general circulation. In this case, fat becomes diluted and reaches the liver at a lower concentration. This fat is less likely to overwhelm the liver. It also adapts by creating new fat cells to store excess energy safely. Visceral fat, however, expands by enlarging existing fat cells. This unnatural growth stresses the cells, leading to damage and the release of **inflammatory chemicals** that disrupt insulin function and promote **low-grade chronic inflammation** - a hallmark of metabolic syndrome as discussed in Chapter 3.

Belly fat also acts like an endocrine organ, releasing **pro-inflammatory molecules** that further damage tissues and worsen insulin resistance over time. This slow-burning inflammation doesn't just raise blood sugar - it fuels the development of chronic illnesses such as diabetes and heart disease.[3]

In addition, excess fat around the midsection can restrict breathing. It limits lung expansion by flattening the diaphragm and putting pressure on the chest wall, which decreases **tidal volume** (the amount of air you can move in and out of your lungs). This is especially problematic for people with asthma. One study found that **75% of asthma patients in emergency departments were either overweight or obese.**[4] For these individuals, **weight loss isn't just cosmetic—it can significantly improve their breathing and overall asthma control.**

Central obesity also increases the risk of high blood pressure, high blood glucose, high cholesterol, gallbladder disease, gallstones, osteoarthritis, polycystic ovary syndrome (PCOS), and benign prostatic hyperplasia (BPH). One study also concluded that central obesity may impair the immune system, leading to a higher frequency of illnesses such as the flu and colds.

Risk of Thrombosis

People with central or general obesity are known to have a high risk of arterial and venous thrombosis due to their low ability to dissolve the clots that form. Obesity-associated chronic inflammation impairs fibrinolysis, the process by which clots are dissolved. Adipose (fat) tissue produces a plasminogen activator inhibitor (PAI-1), which prevents the dissolution of clots, thereby explaining the increased risk of thrombosis in individuals with obesity.

How to Reverse Central Obesity – Key Actions

- **Focus on food quality, not just calories**: Replace ultra-processed, factory-made foods with whole, nutrient-dense foods rich in fibre - fruits, vegetables, legumes, nuts, and seeds.
- **Reduce refined carbs**: Cut back on sugar, white bread, pasta, and other refined carbohydrates. These are primary drivers of belly fat and fatty liver.
- **Adopt a Mediterranean-style diet**: Prioritise olive oil, nuts, seeds, vegetables, and fish. This diet improves liver health and insulin sensitivity.
- **Embrace intermittent fasting**: Fasting for 16 hours daily encourages fat burning and mimics our natural evolutionary eating cycles.
- **Build and maintain muscle**: Engage in resistance training. More muscle raises your metabolic rate and helps burn fat even while resting.
- **Exercise regularly**: Both endurance (aerobic) and resistance training help reduce visceral fat and improve liver health.
- **Support your liver** by incorporating foods like citrus fruits, onions, and bitter melon, which promote liver detoxification and help reduce fat accumulation.
- **Boost your microbiome**: Eat more fibre and consider probiotics. A healthy gut supports appetite control, insulin sensitivity, and fat loss.

- **Try proven supplements**:
  - **Berberine**: Lowers blood sugar, insulin, and liver fat.
  - **Omega-3 fish oil**: Reduces liver fat and inflammation.
  - **Probiotics**: Restore gut balance, reduce appetite, and improve body composition.
- **Choose your proteins wisely**: opt for organic poultry and small, oily fish instead of red and processed meats, which are high in saturated fat.
- **Make small, sustainable changes**: You don't need to do everything at once. Choose progress over perfection.

Final Thoughts

Central obesity - commonly known as belly fat - is more than just a cosmetic concern; it's a major driver of metabolic syndrome. Surprisingly, this condition can affect not only individuals with obesity but also those who appear to have a normal weight. Its prevalence increases with age, making it a growing public health concern.

One of the primary culprits behind central obesity is the Western diet, rich in processed foods, sugars, and unhealthy fats. Coupled with sedentary habits and chronic stress, this lifestyle fosters fat accumulation around the abdomen. But the danger doesn't stop there. Belly fat is metabolically active, releasing inflammatory cytokines that trigger a state of chronic, low-grade inflammation. This persistent inflammation contributes to insulin resistance and elevated insulin levels, laying the groundwork for other metabolic complications.

As we will explore in Chapter 5, one of the most common consequences of this chain reaction is high blood pressure - a key component of metabolic syndrome.

CHAPTER 5

The Hidden Pulse of Metabolic Syndrome - Understanding High Blood Pressure

My first encounter with high blood pressure - also known as hypertension - was during an unforgettable medical school session. Our professor, known for his theatrics, called on an anxious student and began firing a series of tough questions. As the student struggled to respond, the professor's criticism intensified. Tension mounted. Sensing the pressure, the professor turned the moment into a teaching opportunity - he asked another student to measure the distressed student's blood pressure. As expected, it was sky-high. Without missing a beat, the professor carried on with the lesson. About fifteen minutes later, he asked for another reading. This time, the student's blood pressure had returned to normal.

The takeaway: **It's a grave mistake to diagnose hypertension based on a single blood pressure measurement.**

This lesson wasn't just about technique - it was about context, stress, and the body's dynamic nature. It's a perfect starting point for understanding why hypertension is more complex than it first appears.

The Scope of the Problem

In the United Kingdom, hypertension affects:

- **31% of men**
- **26% of women**
- **60% of individuals with overweight or obesity**

It's the **third leading cause of death.**[1] But what's more surprising - and dangerous - is that hypertension in **lean individuals** often goes unnoticed and untreated, making it potentially even more harmful.

"Is There a Natural Way Out?"

A question I frequently hear in the clinic is:
"I've been on blood pressure pills for years - can I come off them? Is there a natural therapy that works?"

The reality is sobering. A major study found that **only 30% of patients** on long-term antihypertensive medications achieve effective blood pressure control.[2] But here's the good news: **lifestyle changes can make a profound difference.**

For many, especially those who are overweight, losing even a modest amount of weight can significantly lower blood pressure, often reducing or even eliminating the need for medication. Achieving a normal Body Mass Index (BMI) through healthier eating and regular physical activity can help restore balance to the cardiovascular system and significantly reduce the risk of stroke and heart disease.

What This Chapter Will Cover

In the pages that follow, we'll uncover how **impaired glucose metabolism and insulin resistance** - key features of metabolic syndrome - can quietly contribute to the development of hypertension. You'll learn how this "silent disease" weaves itself into the fabric of our health, often without symptoms, and why early detection is crucial.

Most importantly, we'll explore a **natural, holistic approach to managing blood pressure**, focusing on diet, weight, and lifestyle - not just pills.

Why Does the Heart Have to Work Harder?

Think of blood as your body's delivery service - carrying oxygen and nutrients to every cell. At the centre of this system is the heart, the pump that keeps everything moving. Each heartbeat creates pressure in the arteries, allowing blood to flow efficiently. This pressure is what we refer to as **blood pressure**.

When everything is working well, your blood pressure stays below 120/80 mmHg. The top number (systolic) reflects the pressure when the heart contracts, while the bottom number (diastolic) reflects the pressure when the heart relaxes. These values aren't chosen at random. Decades of research have shown that the risk of heart disease, stroke, and death increases steadily once blood pressure begins to rise above this range - and skyrockets when it becomes very high.

We are born with arteries that are soft, flexible, and smooth inside. This allows the heart to pump with ease. But over time, our arteries can lose this natural elasticity. They become stiff, thickened, or even calcified. When this happens, the heart must pump harder to push blood through increasingly resistant vessels, raising blood pressure in the process.

You might wonder: What causes arteries to stiffen in the first place? That's a key question we'll explore later in this chapter.

The Silent Climb

Most people with high blood pressure, or **hypertension**, feel entirely normal. That's why it often goes unnoticed until it's discovered by chance - during a routine check-up, a pre-surgery screening, or an unrelated doctor's visit. Many are shocked by the diagnosis, simply because they didn't feel unwell.

Some individuals may experience symptoms such as fatigue, headaches, or dizziness. In rare cases, high blood pressure can cause tiny blood vessels in the nose to rupture, resulting in nosebleeds. But far too often, the first "symptom" of hypertension is a crisis: a heart attack, a stroke, or hospitalisation.

Studies show that about **one in three people** with high blood pressure don't even know they have it. You can live with it for years, unaware - until something serious happens. That's why hypertension is often called **"the silent killer."**

Classification of Hypertension
Understanding the different stages of hypertension is crucial for early intervention and long-term cardiovascular health. Blood pressure is considered **optimal** when it is below **120/80 mmHg**. As values rise above this threshold, the risk of cardiovascular complications increases significantly.

Pre-Hypertension (High-Normal Blood Pressure)

- **Systolic:** 120-139 mmHg
- **Diastolic:** 80-89 mmHg

This early stage of elevated blood pressure signals a need for preventive action. While not classified as full hypertension, pre-hypertension is a warning sign. Adopting a healthy lifestyle at this stage - through improved diet, physical activity, stress management, and weight control - can often prevent progression to full-blown hypertension.

Grade 1 Hypertension (Mild)

- **Systolic:** 140-159 mmHg
- **Diastolic:** 90-99 mmHg

Grade 1 hypertension typically responds well to a combination of lifestyle changes and prescribed medication. Early treatment can reduce the risk of heart attack, stroke, and kidney damage.

Grade 2 Hypertension (Moderate to Severe)
- **Systolic:** 160–179 mmHg
- **Diastolic:** 100–109 mmHg

At this stage, blood pressure is significantly elevated and requires close medical supervision. Medications are essential, often in combination, along with sustained lifestyle interventions.

Malignant (Accelerated) Hypertension
- **Blood Pressure:** ≥180/120 mmHg

This is a medical emergency. Malignant hypertension dramatically increases the risk of life-threatening complications such as stroke, heart failure, kidney failure, or cerebral haemorrhage. Without immediate treatment, survival rates are dismal - historically, fewer than 25% of patients survived one year, and only 1% survived five years. Prompt and aggressive intervention is critical.

Causes of Hypertension: A Dual Perspective
Traditionally, only about **10% of hypertension cases** are linked to an identifiable medical cause - termed **secondary hypertension**. Known causes include:

- **Chronic kidney disease**
- **Adrenal tumours** or **adrenal overactivity**
- **Coarctation of the aorta** (a congenital narrowing of the main artery)
- **Obstructive sleep apnoea**
- **Certain medications** (e.g., NSAIDs, contraceptive pills, cold remedies)
- **Illicit drugs** (e.g., amphetamines, cocaine)

The remaining **90% of cases** fall under **primary (essential) hypertension**, where no clear medical cause is identified. However, the absence of a cause does not mean it's untreatable.

A Functional Medicine View: Hypertension as a Lifestyle Disease
Functional medicine offers a fresh lens: it regards up to **80% of primary hypertension cases** as **lifestyle-related**. Rather than seeing the condition as permanent, this approach empowers patients. It emphasises root-cause resolution through:

- Dietary improvements
- Regular physical activity
- Weight management
- Stress reduction
- Sleep optimisation

This view gives patients hope and agency - encouraging them to take control of their health and, in many cases, reduce or eliminate the need for long-term medication.

A Case in Point: Turning the Tide on Metabolic Syndrome
Meet John, a 45-year-old man who visited his general practitioner complaining of a painful big toe. Blood tests revealed a high uric acid level, confirming a diagnosis of **gout** - a form of arthritis often linked to poor metabolic health. His blood pressure was elevated at **150/92 mmHg**, classifying as **grade 1 hypertension**, and routine bloodwork showed **high cholesterol levels at 6.6 mmol/L** (normal: <5 mmol/L). Although prescribed **allopurinol**, a standard treatment for gout, John was hesitant to start medication.

Until a few years ago, John had been in generally good health. However, a gradual shift in lifestyle had taken its toll. He began consuming a typical **Western diet** - rich in processed foods and low in nutrients - accompanied by a few glasses of wine each evening. His sleep was poor, limited to **six hours of interrupted rest**, and he often woke feeling unrefreshed. With a **BMI of 26 kg/m²** and a **waist-to-hip ratio of 0.99**, his body showed signs of **visceral fat accumulation**, a key indicator of metabolic dysfunction.

John's energy was consistently low - **just 5 out of 10 on most days**. Based on these findings, he was diagnosed with **metabolic syndrome**: a cluster of conditions that include **abdominal obesity, hypertension, high cholesterol**, and often, **gout**. Left unmanaged, this syndrome dramatically increases the risk of heart disease, stroke, and type 2 diabetes.

But John chose to reclaim his health. He adopted a diet rich in **whole, unprocessed foods** and incorporated **intermittent fasting** into his routine. Over time, he lost **28 pounds (12.7 kg)**. His sleep improved to a consistent **7-8 hours per night**, and he now wakes feeling refreshed. His daytime energy has surged to an **8/10**, and most importantly, his **blood pressure has stabilised under 120/80 mmHg** - without medication.

This case is a powerful example of how **lifestyle changes**, not just prescriptions, can reverse the course of metabolic syndrome.

Why Does Metabolic Syndrome Cause High Blood Pressure?
Metabolic syndrome doesn't just increase your risk of diabetes - it also has a powerful influence on blood pressure. When metabolism slows down, blood pressure tends to rise, setting the stage for a cascade of other health issues. But what's behind this connection?

As discussed in earlier chapters, metabolic diseases are often marked by elevated insulin and blood glucose levels. Together, these changes drive up blood pressure through several interconnected mechanisms:

- **Arterial thickening and narrowing**: Elevated insulin levels stimulate the growth of cells within the arterial walls. As the walls thicken and the vessels narrow, the heart is forced to work harder to push blood through, increasing pressure throughout the system.
- **Endothelial damage**: High blood glucose harms the endothelium - the thin, protective lining of blood vessels. This lining produces nitric oxide (NO), a molecule that helps blood vessels relax and stay flexible. When damaged, NO production drops, and blood pressure rises as vessels lose their ability to relax and remain flexible.
- **Cholesterol buildup and artery calcification**: High insulin boosts total and LDL ("bad") cholesterol. At the same time, elevated glucose oxidises LDL particles, triggering inflammation and plaque buildup along the artery walls. These plaques can harden into calcified deposits (as explored in Chapter 7), making arteries even more rigid. The result: The heart must pump with greater force to push blood through these stiffened, narrow vessels.
- **Fluid retention in the kidneys**: Insulin also increases the reabsorption of sodium and water in the kidneys, expanding blood volume and further elevating blood pressure.

In older adults, these effects are often compounded by **arterial calcification,** which can occur either as a natural part of ageing or because of atherosclerosis. When arteries become stiff and inflexible, the pressure inside them increases. Fortunately, modern diagnostic tools such as **coronary calcium scoring** allow doctors to detect calcified plaques early. This scan quantifies calcium buildup in the arteries and provides a reliable prediction of heart disease risk, including life-threatening events such as heart attacks.

How does Hypertension Damage the Body?

Hypertension is often called the "silent killer" for a reason - it quietly wreaks havoc on your body for years before any symptoms arise. Although it may seem harmless at first, persistently high blood pressure can gradually injure critical organs and systems. Left unchecked, it can lead to blindness, stroke, kidney failure, heart attacks, and even limb amputations.

Let's explore how this slow-moving threat affects the body:

A Hidden Threat to Vision

High blood pressure can damage the tiny blood vessels in the retina, the light-sensitive tissue at the back of your eye. This condition, called hypertensive retinopathy, may cause bleeding or blockages that result in blurred vision or complete vision loss. In severe cases, hypertension can lead to permanent blindness.

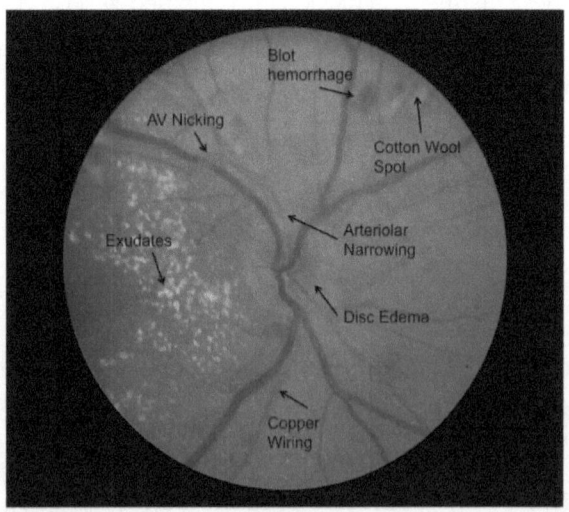

Hypertensive retinopathy: high blood pressure damages the retina at the back of the eye. The changes observed with the ophthalmoscope include flame-shaped haemorrhages (bleeding), blockage of the arterioles, which can cause infarcts (damage due to a lack of blood supply) known as cotton-wool spots and leakage of fluids and fat, leading to exudate formation.

Kidneys: Silent Organ Damage

Your kidneys filter waste from the blood, but hypertension damages the delicate blood vessels and filtering units (nephrons), causing scarring. This condition, known as hypertensive nephropathy, can eventually progress to end-stage renal failure, often requiring dialysis or kidney transplantation.

Brain: Stroke and Vascular Dementia

Hypertension increases the risk of both mini-strokes (transient ischaemic attacks or TIAs) and full-blown strokes by narrowing or blocking blood vessels in the brain. Over time, it can also lead to vascular dementia, a form of cognitive decline caused by reduced blood flow to the brain's tiny vessels. The result: Memory loss, impaired thinking, and diminished quality of life.

Arteries, Limbs, and Nerves

High blood pressure contributes to atherosclerosis, the hardening and narrowing of arteries, which affects not only the heart and brain but also peripheral circulation. Reduced blood flow to the legs and feet can lead to painful ulcers, slow-healing wounds, and, in severe cases, gangrene requiring amputation. Hypertension can also damage peripheral nerves, causing numbness, tingling, or burning sensations in the feet and legs (neuropathy).

When the Heart Can't Keep Up: Heart Failure

Initially, the heart compensates for high blood pressure by pumping more forcefully. Over time, this relentless strain causes the heart muscle - especially the left ventricle - to weaken, leading to **left-sided heart failure**. A hallmark symptom is breathlessness, particularly after exertion or when lying down, due to fluid accumulation in the lungs. Many sufferers sleep propped up with pillows to breathe more easily at night.

Eventually, this burden spills over to the right side of the heart.

Right-sided heart failure occurs when the right ventricle fails to pump blood efficiently into the lungs, leading to fluid buildup in the veins. This manifests as swollen ankles, a bloated abdomen (ascites), and even swelling of the genitals. Decreased blood flow to the pelvic region can also contribute to sexual dysfunction in both men and women.

The Hidden Link: Sleep Apnoea and Hypertension

Roughly 40% of people with high blood pressure also suffer from **obstructive sleep apnoea (OSA)**, a condition in which breathing repeatedly stops during sleep. Each time the airway collapses, oxygen levels drop, triggering a stress response that floods the body with cortisol, a hormone that raises blood pressure. In those with OSA, blood pressure often fails to drop at night, making it harder to control with medication.

Real-Life Stories: How Hypertension and Metabolic Syndrome Can Take Their Toll

The following two cases offer compelling insights into the hidden dangers of uncontrolled high blood pressure and its connection to metabolic syndrome. These stories underscore how seemingly minor symptoms can mask severe underlying conditions.

Case 1: The Burning Leg That Wouldn't Let Her Sleep

A woman I met had worn a 24-hour blood pressure monitor two decades earlier, which showed slightly elevated readings - but no treatment followed. Ten years later, she suffered a stroke, resulting in weakness on her right side. Thankfully, after three months of physiotherapy, her strength returned.

Two years after her stroke, she began to feel an unpleasant burning sensation in her lower legs. She no longer felt steady on her feet, dragging her right leg and struggling with balance.

Her lifestyle had changed significantly. She had stopped cooking and adopted a typical Western diet - low in fruits and vegetables - and slept poorly, averaging just six hours of broken sleep per night. She also developed a fatty liver, and doctors heard an abnormal abdominal bruit, hinting at possible kidney artery narrowing. A scan ruled out renal artery stenosis, but her high blood pressure persisted.

Her main issues included:

- **Chronic hypertension**
- **Peripheral neuropathy** (causing burning and heat sensations)
- **Impaired balance** from a prior cerebellar stroke

She would often wake at night just to uncover her hot leg - an overlooked symptom of nerve dysfunction.

Medical Insight: Chronic hypertension can silently damage blood vessels. Over time, it may dilate and thin the aorta (the main artery), increasing the risk of a life-threatening rupture or aneurysm—often with no warning signs.

Case 2: The Man Who Loved Sweets - and Paid the Price

I also treated a 60-year-old man who had undergone emergency surgery for a massive aortic dissection - a tear in the main artery. He also suffered a stroke, likely triggered by dangerously high blood pressure.

His health profile painted a familiar picture:

- He smoked hand-rolled cigarettes.
- He consumed a lot of sweets, cakes, and chocolate, but avoided healthy foods.
- He had 10 silver dental fillings, revealing a long-standing sugar habit.

Despite having an ideal weight (BMI 22.7), his waist-to-hip ratio (0.97) revealed dangerous central fat accumulation - a hallmark of **metabolic syndrome**. A scan also confirmed he had a fatty liver.

Neurologically, he exhibited signs of a stroke on his left side. Initially, he could manage a few steps with the aid of a stick and his wife's help. But over time, even walking short distances became difficult. He developed intermittent claudication - painful leg cramps due to poor blood supply and lactic acid buildup in the muscles.

Hidden Risks: Worse Outcomes in Lean Individuals

It's a common misconception that high blood pressure primarily affects people who are overweight or obese. However, research shows that hypertension is also surprisingly prevalent among individuals with a normal weight. In a U.S. study, 20.5% of adults with a BMI under 25 kg/m² were found to have hypertension between 2003 and 2004.[3]

Because hypertension is not typically expected in lean individuals, it often goes undiagnosed in this group. Unfortunately, this delayed detection can lead to more severe health consequences compared to those who are diagnosed earlier due to visible risk factors like obesity. This underlines the need for improved diagnostic strategies, including moving away from relying on a single blood pressure reading in favour of more accurate, consistent monitoring methods.

Medical Insight: High blood pressure doesn't just damage arteries - it reshapes the heart itself. Left ventricular hypertrophy (thickened heart muscle) increases the risk of sudden death due to fatal arrhythmias like ventricular fibrillation. Untreated, this condition can evolve into full-blown heart failure.

Lesson to learn
These stories highlight how metabolic syndrome and uncontrolled hypertension don't always announce themselves dramatically at first. Yet, their cumulative damage can be life-altering - or even fatal. The key lies in early detection, lifestyle changes, and consistent medical care.

Smarter Screening Strategies
Due to limited healthcare resources, not everyone can be screened for hypertension. Therefore, it's critical to prioritise high-risk groups. These include not only sedentary individuals with overweight or obesity, but also normal-weight people with central obesity (belly fat), or those with related metabolic conditions such as high cholesterol, type 2 diabetes, and gout.

Menopausal women should also be a key focus. Until age 65, men are more likely than women to develop high blood pressure. After menopause, however, the decline in protective oestrogen puts women at greater risk. The associated metabolic slowdown and weight gain make them more vulnerable to hypertension and related conditions.

Another overlooked group includes people living in socioeconomically deprived areas. These communities often face a higher burden of lifestyle-related risk factors - smoking, excessive alcohol and caffeine intake, and poor diets high in processed, salty foods and low in fresh produce - all of which contribute to elevated blood pressure.

Home Blood Pressure Monitoring: Empowers Patients

Thanks to affordable and accurate digital monitors, checking your blood pressure at home has never been easier. Home monitoring eliminates the anxiety often experienced during doctor visits - what's known as "white coat hypertension" - which can skew readings and mask the true nature of your condition.

Regular home readings, taken in a relaxed state over time, provide a clearer picture and help healthcare providers make informed treatment decisions. The American Heart Association recommends the following steps for accurate measurements:[4]

- Measure at the same time each day.
- Wait at least 30 minutes after consuming caffeine or engaging in exercise.
- Empty your bladder and rest quietly for five minutes before taking the measurement.
- Sit upright with your arm supported and the cuff at heart level.
- Take measurements on bare skin, not over clothing.
- Record 2–3 readings per session, spaced one minute apart.
- Remain still and silent during the readings.

Historically, clinics relied on single measurements, which often led to unreliable results, especially in anxious patients. Studies have shown that white coat hypertension is not harmless- it has been linked to increased risks of stroke, heart attack, heart failure, and other cardiovascular complications.[5]

To counter this, many Western healthcare systems have embraced 24-hour ambulatory blood pressure monitoring. This approach, which tracks readings continuously over a day and night, offers a much more accurate and comprehensive profile. It should be considered a cornerstone of hypertension diagnosis and management.

The Hidden Danger: Falls and Fractures in Older Adults

Managing high blood pressure in older adults requires more than a one-size-fits-all prescription. Without a thorough diagnosis, antihypertensive medications can do more harm than good, primarily by increasing the risk of falls and fractures. An extensive U.S. study found that older adults taking these medications had a significantly higher risk of serious fall-related injuries.[6] This is especially concerning for those with multiple chronic conditions.

Hip fractures, for instance, are not just painful - they're potentially fatal. In adults aged 65 to 69, a hip fracture increases the risk of death fivefold within the first year.[7] The lesson: Physicians must carefully weigh the benefits and risks before initiating treatment in elderly patients.

Salt: A Salty Issue with Blood Pressure

High salt intake and a sedentary lifestyle are well-known contributors to hypertension. However, interestingly, people who consume less than 50 mEq of salt per day and stay physically active are far less likely to develop high blood pressure. Even more fascinating, studies show that individuals who maintain a lean body and engage in regular exercise can effectively manage their blood pressure despite consuming relatively high amounts of salt.[8]

Genes Matter: The Role of Inherited Hypertension

Hypertension isn't just about diet and lifestyle - it's also in your DNA. Many individuals carry genetic variations that predispose them to high blood pressure, especially when combined with a high-salt diet. Three genes in particular stand out:

- **AGT**: Encodes angiotensinogen, a protein that plays a key role in raising blood pressure.
- **ACE**: Produces the angiotensin-converting enzyme, which amplifies this effect.
- **NOS3**: Encodes endothelial nitric oxide synthase (eNOS), crucial for relaxing blood vessels.

eNOS plays a vital role by producing Nitric Oxide from L-arginine (an amino acid), which relaxes arterial walls and controls blood pressure. In carriers of *NO3* variants, smoking and excess alcohol damage the endothelium (arterial lining) and often lead to severe hypertension.

Carriers of **AGT variants** may see a 45% higher risk of hypertension due to increased angiotensinogen levels. In these individuals, high sodium intake has a pronounced effect—making sodium reduction an essential strategy.

While **ACE variants** also raise blood pressure, their effects are milder. Still, lowering salt intake remains beneficial for these individuals as well.

Understanding the Renin-Angiotensin System

At the heart of blood pressure regulation lies a cascade known as the **renin-angiotensin system**:

1. The liver produces angiotensinogen.
2. The **kidneys** release **renin**, which converts angiotensinogen into angiotensin I.
3. The **lungs and kidneys** house **ACE**, which converts angiotensin I into angiotensin II, a potent vasoconstrictor that raises blood pressure.

This system is so critical that a significant class of blood pressure medications - **ACE inhibitors** - work specifically to block this pathway. These drugs are often the first line of treatment in managing hypertension.

Takeaway: Personalised Prevention and Care
Understanding your genetic background, lifestyle habits, and physiological responses can dramatically improve your blood pressure management. Whether it's avoiding falls through thoughtful prescribing, cutting back on salt, or identifying genetic risk factors, a personalised approach to hypertension is essential - especially for those navigating the complexities of metabolic syndrome.

Summary: Managing High Blood Pressure
– Essential Strategies & Skills

- **Seek immediate medical care** if blood pressure is very high before beginning lifestyle changes.
- **Achieve and maintain a healthy body weight**, especially for individuals with obesity.
  - Target: 5-10% body weight reduction for measurable improvement.

- **Adopt a heart-healthy diet**, especially the **DASH (Dietary Approaches to Stop Hypertension)** diet:
  - High in fruits, vegetables, potassium, fiber, and magnesium.
  - Low in sodium, caffeine, processed foods, and alcohol.
  - Includes healthy fats from oily fish and seeds.
- **Increase intake of specific nutrients**:
  - **Potassium** (green bananas, avocados, leafy greens)
  - **Magnesium** (nuts, seeds, dark chocolate)
  - **Vitamin D** (sunlight, supplements if needed)
  - **Vitamin K2** (egg yolks, butter, cheese)
- **Limit sodium intake**, especially from processed foods and all types of salt.
- **Incorporate physical activity**:
  - Start with walking; aim for 30–60 minutes brisk walking, 5 days/week.
  - Gradually add strength or interval training to build muscle.
- **Improve sleep hygiene**:
  - Prioritise restful sleep in a dark room; maintain a good circadian rhythm.
- **Practice stress reduction techniques**:
  - Meditation, deep breathing, music, laughter, nature walks, and Epsom salt baths.
- **Drink hibiscus tea** (2–3 cups daily) for natural support of your blood pressure.
- **Consider pet ownership** as a lifestyle enhancer; Studies show that pet owners tend to have lower blood pressure and are less likely to develop hypertension compared to those without pets. The calming presence of a furry companion may be more powerful than we realise.[9]

I have seen patients make simple lifestyle changes - like the ones listed above - and successfully manage their blood pressure enough to stop taking medication. Be sure to work closely with your doctor to make informed choices and prioritise your safety.

Final Thoughts

High blood pressure isn't just a cardiovascular issue - it's deeply rooted in metabolism. One of the earliest signs of trouble is your body's declining ability to process sugar, its primary source of energy. As glucose and insulin levels rise, they set off a cascade of effects that elevate blood pressure.

High insulin levels cause your arteries to stiffen and thicken, while also prompting your kidneys to retain salt and water - both of which increase blood volume and pressure. Meanwhile, elevated blood glucose inflicts silent damage on your blood vessels. It disrupts the production of nitric oxide, a critical molecule that helps vessels relax. At the same time, sugar reacts with proteins and fats through a process known as glycation - a biological "rusting" - that leads to plaque buildup and atherosclerosis, a defining feature of vascular disease.

Understanding this connection between blood sugar, insulin, and blood pressure is essential. In the next chapter, we'll explore the full impact of high blood glucose on your health - and most importantly, how you can restore your metabolic balance and protect your blood vessels from harm.

CHAPTER 6

The Sweet Danger - A Personal Reflection on High Blood Glucose

In 1979, I found myself navigating the grey drizzle and timeless rituals of London as a final-year medical student. Margaret Thatcher had just begun her first term as Prime Minister, and I was staying in a modest hotel in Sussex Gardens. Each morning, I strolled over to a mobile café parked in Hyde Park - one of those charming, steaming havens on wheels where tea was served with a side of British banter.

"With or without?" the lady behind the counter asked. I paused, clueless.

"With," I said, assuming she meant milk. But she meant sugar.

"One or two?"

"Two," I replied. But after that first cup, I quickly realised: I needed more. The next day, I asked for five teaspoons.

The look on her face was one of barely restrained horror. I could see her struggling - torn between polite service and the sense that she had some civic duty to save me from my sweet impulses. Each morning after, she delivered my tea with five teaspoons of sugar and a silent plea in her eyes: *Please stop doing this to yourself.*

Looking back, I realise she was right.

That moment has stayed with me - not just because it was slightly embarrassing, but because it was a perfect microcosm of the crisis I would come to understand in far greater depth: our global epidemic of high blood sugar.

Sugar: The Silent Spark of Metabolic Chaos

The story of high blood glucose is not just the story of diabetes. It's the origin myth of a vast constellation of modern illnesses - obesity, cardiovascular disease, dementia, cancer, and, of course, type 2 diabetes. At the centre of this lies a simple biochemical truth: our bodies were never designed to handle the sheer volume and frequency of sugar we consume today.

When blood glucose levels rise and remain elevated - what we refer to as **hyperglycaemia** - the body begins to falter. It starts subtly: fatigue that no coffee can fix, poor sleep despite exhaustion, dips in mental clarity, and cravings that feel more like compulsions. Then, more alarming signs emerge - abdominal fat accumulation, insulin resistance, and the early stages of metabolic syndrome.

This is the gateway. And for many, it remains unnoticed until complications arrive.

Prediabetes: The Misleading Middle Ground

High blood glucose often lurks in the shadows, unnoticed until the damage is well underway. Many people are shocked to discover they are "prediabetic," assuming this is a harmless prelude. However, the truth is that even mildly elevated glucose levels can wreak havoc.

Retinal damage. Kidney strain. Nerve deterioration. Poor circulation. These aren't future possibilities - they are realities unfolding quietly in millions of people whose blood sugar levels are just above normal. In clinical terms, this is not a waiting room.

It's the start of the fire.

In some cases, nerve damage becomes so severe that people lose sensation in their feet, leading to unnoticed injuries, infections, and – tragically - amputations. This is not rare. This is happening daily.

The Ripple Effects: Mind, Mood, Metabolism

High blood glucose doesn't stop at physical health. It affects:

- **Energy**: Glucose fluctuations drain the body's vitality, creating a cycle of crashes and cravings.
- **Brain Function**: Cognitive fog, mood swings, and even depression have been linked to poor glucose regulation.
- **Productivity**: You can't be your best self—at work or home—when your body is struggling to maintain basic metabolic balance.
- **Sleep**: Blood sugar instability can disrupt the hormonal patterns that regulate sleep, resulting in shallow and incomplete rest and recovery.

Over time, these disruptions accumulate. The body shape changes: visceral fat increases, muscle mass may decline, and ageing accelerates. The mirror becomes an uncomfortable truth-teller.

Why This Chapter Matters

In this chapter, I want to do what that kind woman at the tea truck tried to do for me. I want to offer a nudge - a pause - a moment of reflection. You may already know the dangers of sugar. Perhaps you've read about them earlier in this book. But this is not about repetition. This is about recognition.

Every moment of indulgence, every teaspoon of sugar added mindlessly, is not a harmless pleasure - it is a choice with consequences. But here's the good news: it's also reversible. If we detect the problem early, we can stop the chain reaction. We can maintain steady blood glucose, protect the body from damage, and restore metabolic resilience.

This chapter is not just a warning. It's an invitation to awareness, action, and health.

A Sweet Seduction — The Sugar Family Revisited
Sugar is the Jekyll and Hyde of nutrition. On one hand, it's a life-sustaining molecule - the simplest form of energy that powers every cell in our body, particularly our hungry brains. On the other hand, it is a ubiquitous villain in the modern diet, implicated in the growing epidemics of obesity, diabetes, and metabolic syndrome. Whether sugar is a necessary ally or a subtle saboteur depends not only on how much we consume, but also on the type, frequency, and form.

The Sugars We Know—and Those We Don't
What most people refer to as "sugar" is only the tip of a much larger biochemical iceberg. Nutritionally, sugars fall under the broader umbrella of carbohydrates. The simplest among them are *monosaccharides* - single-unit sugars like glucose (the bloodstream's primary fuel), fructose (found naturally in fruit and honey), and galactose (a component of milk sugar). When two monosaccharides link up, they form *disaccharides* - like sucrose (table sugar, made of glucose and fructose), lactose (milk sugar, composed of glucose and galactose), and maltose (often called malt sugar, a pair of glucose units).

Though many might proudly declare, "I don't eat sugar," they often overlook the invisible sugars hidden in plain sight. A slice of bread, a bowl of pasta, or a serving of rice may not taste sweet, but these complex carbohydrates are rapidly broken down into glucose during digestion. From the body's perspective, eating a bagel isn't much different from sipping a sugary soda - the resulting sugar flood is the same.

Sugar Consumption in the Modern Diet
The Western diet, particularly the standard American dietary pattern, is saturated with sugar in overt and covert forms. Average daily sugar consumption hovers around 85 grams - approximately 17% of total caloric intake. This is far above the World Health Organization's recommended ceiling of 10%. Alarmingly, sugar is not just in desserts and drinks but also hidden in sauces, processed meats, salad dressings, and even so-called "health" bars. It's woven into the very fabric of modern convenience food.

Glucose vs. Fructose: A Tale of Two Sugars
Once carbohydrates are digested, the resulting glucose and fructose molecules take very different metabolic paths. Glucose is the body's go-to energy source, stimulating the pancreas to secrete insulin, which helps ferry it into cells. Any surplus glucose is stored as glycogen in the liver and muscles or converted into fat when storage capacity is exceeded.

Fructose, though chemically similar, plays by different rules. It is metabolised almost exclusively in the liver, bypassing insulin's usual pathways. While this might sound advantageous, it's a metabolic sleight of hand with a dark side. Fructose is rapidly converted into fat through a process called *de novo lipogenesis*, which increases triglyceride levels in the blood and promotes fat storage, particularly in the liver. This paves the way for non-alcoholic fatty liver disease and contributes to insulin resistance. Adding to the problem, fructose also boosts uric acid production, which has been linked to inflammation and metabolic disturbances.

The Rise of High-Fructose Corn Syrup

No discussion of sugar in the modern diet is complete without addressing the phenomenon of high-fructose corn syrup (HFCS). Since its industrial debut in the 1970s, HFCS has become the sweetener of choice for processed food manufacturers: cheap, stable, and exceedingly sweet. Unlike sucrose, which has a 50:50 glucose-to-fructose ratio, HFCS often contains a higher percentage of fructose, sometimes as high as 55%. This subtle difference has outsized metabolic consequences. When glucose and fructose are consumed together in high amounts, especially in liquid form, they can overwhelm the liver's processing ability, resulting in a metabolic cascade that favours fat storage over energy utilisation.

HFCS isn't just a sweeter sugar; it's a molecular double whammy - fuelling appetite, feeding fat cells, and fostering insulin resistance in a way that ordinary sugar doesn't quite match. It's no coincidence that the rise of HFCS paralleled the surge in obesity and type 2 diabetes across the globe.

Sugar Alcohols: The Misunderstood Sweeteners

In the quest for "guilt-free" sweetness, sugar alcohols have gained popularity - sorbitol, xylitol, erythritol, and mannitol among them. These compounds resemble both sugar and alcohol in structure but are neither intoxicating nor calorie-free. Found in "sugar-free" chewing gums, candies, and health bars, they offer fewer calories and a lower glycaemic impact. But they are not entirely innocent. In sensitive individuals, they can cause digestive upset - bloating, gas, and diarrhoea - due to incomplete absorption in the gut. Moreover, the term "sugar-free" on products containing sugar alcohols is somewhat misleading; they still fall under the broader umbrella of carbohydrates and may affect blood sugar to varying degrees.

The Silent Siege — How High Blood Glucose Damages Your Body
In earlier chapters, we've followed the journey of glucose through the bloodstream, from its dietary origins to its storage in the liver, muscles, and fat. You've seen how insulin resistance gradually exhausts the pancreas, pushing it into overdrive until it can no longer cope. When insulin production finally falters, glucose levels spiral out of control - marking the onset of diabetes (see Chapter 3). But elevated blood sugar isn't just a number on a lab test. It is a relentless saboteur, gradually and silently dismantling the body's most vital systems.

Let's now delve into the myriad ways that chronically high blood glucose levels damage the body - first subtly, then catastrophically.

Glycation: When Sugar Becomes a Weapon
One of the most insidious effects of high glucose levels is **glycation** - a non-enzymatic process in which excess glucose binds to proteins or fats in the body, forming compounds known as **Advanced Glycation End-products (AGEs)**. These AGEs behave like biological rust. They weaken the structure of blood vessels, accelerate inflammation in organs such as the lungs and kidneys, and impair immune defences. Even food preparation can contribute to the fact that grilled, fried, and processed foods are rich in AGEs, compounding the internal damage from the outside in.

Glycation doesn't limit itself to major organs. It infiltrates the skin and hair, speeding up the ageing process with wrinkles, sagging, and premature greying. It targets immune proteins and white blood cells, dulling your body's defences and leaving you prone to recurring infections.

You've already met **glycated haemoglobin (HbA1C)** in earlier chapters - a clinical marker that reflects your average blood sugar over three months. But behind that tidy percentage is a grim tally of cellular wreckage.

Retina, Kidneys, and Limbs: Sugar's Favourite Targets

Eyesight: The Window Clouded

Chronic hyperglycaemia clouds the eye's lens proteins, triggering early onset cataracts. Deeper still, the fragile blood vessels in the retina become warped or burst, leading to **diabetic retinopathy** - a leading cause of blindness. White spots (areas of cell death) and red patches (microbleeds) are often visible in eye scans, even before symptoms appear.

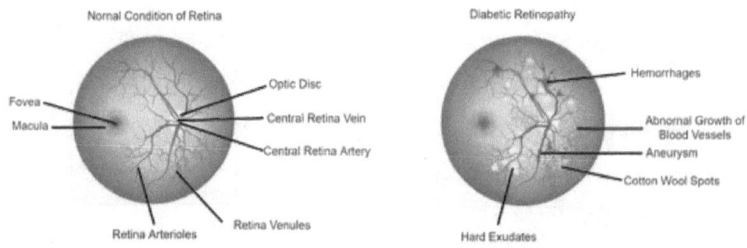

Diabetic retinopathy: diabetes damages the retina at the back of the eye. The changes observed with the ophthalmoscope include haemorrhages (bleeding), blockage of the arterioles, which can cause infarcts (damage due to a lack of blood supply) known as cotton-wool spots, dilatation of arterioles, leading to aneurysms, and leakage of fluids and fat, resulting in hard exudate formation.

Kidneys: The Silent Filter

Your kidneys act as vigilant gatekeepers, filtering blood to retain vital nutrients and eliminate waste. But there's a threshold. Once blood sugar levels cross this threshold, glucose spills into the urine, dragging along damage to the kidneys' delicate blood vessels. Over time, this wears down their filtering units, resulting in protein loss, declining function, and ultimately, **chronic kidney failure**. Many patients reach a point where dialysis becomes essential for survival.

Limbs: Numbness and Necrosis

Glucose also has a predilection for the limbs. Nerve endings are among its earliest victims, leading to **peripheral neuropathy** - a loss of sensation that may seem trivial until unnoticed injuries turn into **ulcers**, **gangrene**, or even **limb amputation**. Reduced blood supply only hastens the damage. A stubbed toe or minor blister can quickly escalate into a serious emergency.

Bones, Pain, and Premature Wear

Few associate blood sugar with back pain, but the link is very real. Fluctuating glucose levels cause muscular tension and spasms in the back and neck - initially presenting as unexplained aches, as described in Chapter 3. Over time, **oxidative stress** - akin to biological rusting - sets into spinal joints, fuelling early-onset **osteoarthritis**.

The Brain on Sugar: Depression and ADHD

Mood and Mental Health

The brain is particularly vulnerable to fluctuations in glucose levels. As blood sugar levels fluctuate, the stress hormone **cortisol** rises to compensate; however, this constant hormonal fluctuation undermines neurotransmitters such as **serotonin** and **BDNF**, which regulate mood. The result: Emotional exhaustion, low energy, and a higher risk of **depression**.

Attention Deficit Hyperactivity Disorder (ADHD)

Emerging research suggests a powerful link between **maternal insulin resistance** and the development of **ADHD** in children. The altered brain chemistry associated with ADHD not only impairs focus but also fuels **impulsive behaviour**, emotional dysregulation, and **poor dietary choices**. The result is a troubling cycle - ADHD begets weight gain, which worsens insulin resistance, increasing the risk of metabolic syndrome and cardiovascular disease. Adults with ADHD are 75% more likely to develop obesity and hypertension than their neurotypical peers.

Hormonal Havoc: The Glandular Fallout

Most people think of cortisol as a stress hormone, but its real name – **glucocorticoid** - reveals its deeper role in regulating blood sugar. Persistently high glucose levels overstimulate the adrenal glands, leading to **adrenal fatigue**. Symptoms include persistent tiredness, especially in the mornings, cravings for sugar or salt, and an unhealthy reliance on caffeine to "feel alive."

If left unchecked, adrenal fatigue devolves into **adrenal exhaustion** - a clinical burnout marked by apathy, depression, dizziness, and dangerously low blood pressure.

High cortisol levels also disrupt the **pituitary gland**, which regulates the **thyroid** and **reproductive organs**. This domino effect can manifest as an **underactive thyroid** (slowed metabolism, cold intolerance, weight gain) or **reproductive dysfunction** (missed periods in women, impotence in men).

A Cumulative Cascade

High blood glucose is not just a number - it's a complex cascade. One that begins with subtle insulin resistance and ends with widespread organ failure, cognitive decline, and chronic pain. By understanding the biological mayhem unleashed by excess glucose, we arm ourselves not only with knowledge - but with urgency.

The body speaks softly at first. A headache. A blurry vision. A stubbed toe that won't heal. But when glucose runs amok, these whispers can quickly turn into screams.

Do You Have a Blood Glucose Problem?

Imagine your body as a finely tuned orchestra, where each instrument plays in harmony to maintain balance within your systems. Now, picture sugar - sweet, seemingly innocent, as a disruptive force that throws the whole performance off rhythm. At first, the change is barely noticeable. A missed beat here, a slowed tempo there. However, left unchecked, sugar begins to dominate the entire composition.

So, how do you know if sugar is out of tune in your body? That's where careful observation - detective work comes in.

The Usual Suspects

While many people dismiss sugar problems as something that only happens to those with diagnosed diabetes, the truth is more complex - and far more common.

You might be at risk of **hyperglycaemia** (high blood glucose) if:

- You carry excess weight, especially around the waist
- You live a sedentary life or juggle chronic stress
- You smoke or drink heavily
- You struggle with high cholesterol or sleep apnoea
- Diabetes runs in your family
- You're a woman who's had gestational diabetes, delivered a baby weighing over 9 pounds (4 kg), or faced fertility challenges

Even those with an undeniable sweet tooth - who crave dessert or soda more than real meals - might unknowingly be living with constant blood sugar swings. For some, this preference is genetic and can be confirmed with specific tests. However, for many, it has become the norm.

Sugar's Subtle Whisper

Blood sugar problems don't announce themselves with blaring alarms. They sneak in with subtle hints:

- That foggy feeling after lunch that makes you stare blankly at your screen
- The desperate need for a nap at 3 p.m.
- Hunger pangs that hit even after a full meal
- Midnight wakeups with a racing heart or sweaty sheets

You might find yourself becoming a "grazer" - snacking constantly to avoid that hollow, shaky feeling. Or you may notice emotional eating patterns: stress leads to chocolate, boredom to biscuits, sadness to sweets. These behaviours aren't just psychological - they're biochemical.

When your blood sugar crashes after a spike, your brain rings the alarm bell. It pushes you to eat more sugar quickly. The problem is that the "quick fix" only fuels the next crash. You're not weak; you're trapped in what I call the **sugar rollercoaster**.

Why You Might Be Waking Up at 2 A.M.

One often-overlooked sign of blood sugar dysregulation is sleep disturbances. If you often wake up between 1 and 3 a.m., sugar could be the culprit.

Here's what happens: you eat a carb-heavy dinner, your blood sugar soars, then drops. In response, your body releases **cortisol** - a stress hormone meant to keep you alive by raising your blood sugar. However, cortisol also suppresses **melatonin**, a hormone that regulates the sleep cycle. And just like that, you're wide awake in the middle of the night.

This hormone tug-of-war disrupts your circadian rhythm, leaving you tired but wired. Over time, it depletes adrenal function, elevates insulin levels, and locks you into a cycle of poor sleep and worsening glucose control.

Physical Signs: Sugar Leaves Clues on the Outside Too
Sometimes, you don't even need a blood test to suspect a sugar issue. Just look in the mirror - or at the people around you.

As a clinician, I've learned to spot sugar problems by sight. Puffy faces, **central obesity** (also known as a "pot belly"), **skin tags**, **acanthosis nigricans** (dark, velvety patches in skin folds), and, in men, **gynecomastia** (breast development) are visual red flags.

How does gynaecomastia occur?

When insulin levels are chronically high:

- Testosterone gets bound up by **SHBG** (sex hormone-binding globulin), reducing its availability
- **Aromatase**, an enzyme made by fat cells, converts what little testosterone remains into oestrogen
- A fatty liver slows down oestrogen detoxification, compounding the effect

The resulting high oestrogen promotes gynaecomastia (breast development) in men. In general, hormonal imbalance, alters fat distribution, and for men, causes symptoms like prostate enlargement (explored in Chapter 11). For women, this can trigger polycystic ovary syndrome (see Chapter 12).

The Body Shape Shift: Apple vs. Pear
Think of your body shape as a reflection of your inner metabolic state.

The **apple shape** - characterised by fat around the waist is strongly linked to insulin resistance and an increased risk of heart disease and diabetes. This is no cosmetic concern; this type of fat surrounds organs and interferes with their function.

In contrast, **pear-shaped bodies** (fat stored in the hips and thighs) are less dangerous from a metabolic standpoint. The difference lies in how and where your body stores energy.

When insulin is high, fat burning halts. Your body starts breaking down muscle for energy while packing fat into your midsection. Cortisol - the stress hormone - amplifies this pattern. You may look soft and bloated despite a reasonable weight.

Earlier chapters (1 and 4) explored measurement tools like:

- Waist circumference
- Waist-to-hip or waist-to-height ratios
- Neck circumference
- Bioelectrical impedance analysis

These provide more insight than BMI alone and help identify **central obesity**, even in people who appear "normal" by weight.

The Truth in Your Blood

Blood tests offer clarity when symptoms are vague. If you suspect a sugar issue, these are the markers to watch:

- **Fasting insulin**: Elevated (>10 µU/mL) is often the first red flag—even when glucose appears normal
- **Fasting glucose**: Optimal is <4.7 mmol/L (85 mg/dL); over 6.0 mmol/L (108 mg/dL) suggests prediabetes
- **2-hour post-meal glucose / GTT**: Should stay under 7.8 mmol/L (140 mg/dL)
- **Haemoglobin A1C**: Reflects average blood sugar over 3 months, should stay under 42 or 5.5%.
- **Triglyceride:** Should stay under 1.7 mmol/L (150 mg/dL)
- **hs-CRP and homocysteine**: Indicate inflammation and vascular risk

Here's a crucial detail: your blood glucose may return to normal within two hours after a meal, but fats take longer to process. Elevated glucose **levels 3-5 hours** post-meal often point to a fat-processing issue, not just a sugar issue. This distinction helps avoid misdiagnosis and unnecessary panic.

Technology That Tells the Truth

You no longer need to guess what your body is doing. As discussed in Chapter 1, **Continuous Glucose Monitoring (CGM)** is a revolutionary tool. With a small wearable sensor and a phone app, you can see your real-time glucose response to meals, exercise, stress, or even sauna sessions.

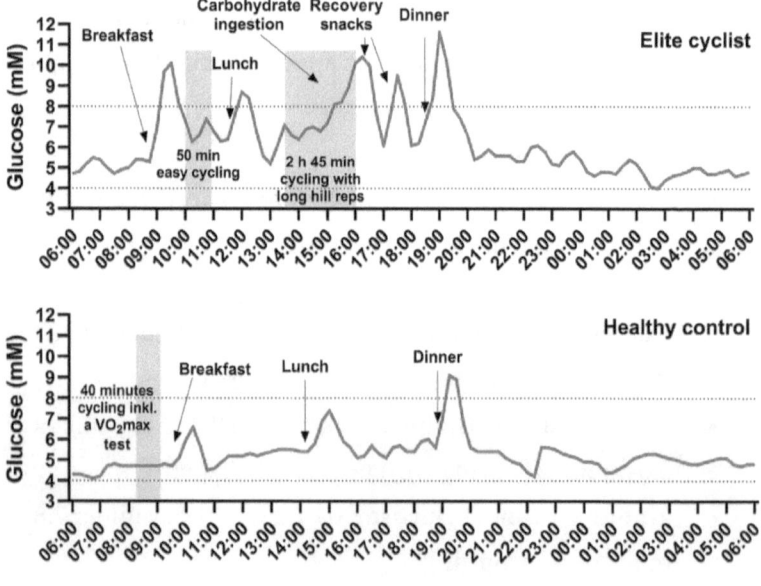

Continuous Glucose Monitoring (CGM): The top CGM record shows significant sugar spikes (over 7.8) in an elite cyclist, likely due to stress and high-carb meals and snacks. The bottom record shows steady blood sugar in a healthy control with one spike at dinner time.

Some people are shocked to see their glucose spike during intense workouts or saunas. This isn't a food issue - it's adrenaline at work, releasing stored glucose from the liver. Understanding this empowers you to:

- Adjust exercise intensity
- Manage stress
- Prioritise sleep
- Combine carbs with protein or fat for smoother glucose curves

In short

The question **"Do you have a blood glucose problem?"** isn't reserved for those already diagnosed. It's relevant for anyone who feels tired, foggy, or "off."

Blood sugar imbalances are not a switch that flips from normal to diabetic - they're a slow progression. Recognising the signs early gives you the chance to course-correct, rebalancing your body before disease sets in.

Sugar may be sweet, but its effects are anything but. Listen to the clues your body is giving you - they might save your life.

Know Your Fuel Type: Sugar Burner, Fat Burner, or Hybrid?

Imagine your body as an engine. Some engines run only on petrol, others on electricity - but the most advanced ones run on both. Your body is no different. You can run on sugar, fat, or ideally, both - like a hybrid vehicle that shifts seamlessly between fuel types depending on availability and need.

Most people in modern society are primarily sugar burners. Their bodies rely almost exclusively on carbohydrates for energy. This might sound efficient, but it has a hidden cost. When sugar (glucose) is plentiful, all seems fine. But when sugar intake drops -

whether from skipping a meal or reducing carbs - the sugar burner's engine starts sputtering. To compensate, the body breaks down muscle tissue to create glucose in the liver through a process called **gluconeogenesis**, converting amino acids into an emergency fuel source. This is a last resort, not a sustainable way to live.

But there's a better way - **metabolic flexibility**. Metabolically flexible individuals are like hybrid engines. They burn sugar when it's available but effortlessly shift to burning fat when sugar levels are low. They don't experience energy slumps when skipping meals or switching to a low-carb diet. They don't need constant refuelling with snacks. Their insulin levels remain balanced, and their bodies efficiently access stored fat for energy.

Unfortunately, metabolic flexibility is rare among people who eat a standard Western diet - the key roadblock is **chronically high insulin** levels. When insulin levels are elevated, fat burning is inhibited, and sugar remains the dominant - if not the only - fuel. Reclaiming your metabolic flexibility means retraining your body to access both energy systems.

Here's how to do it:

Three Pillars to Restore Metabolic Flexibility

- **Upgrade Your Food Quality**
  Return to real food. The industrial diet - characterised by ultra-processed snacks, sugary drinks, and refined grains - disrupts your metabolism and keeps insulin levels chronically elevated. Instead, eat whole, nutrient-dense foods that come from nature, not factories: fresh vegetables and fruits, legumes, nuts and seeds, eggs, poultry, meat, and fish. This naturally stabilises blood sugar and reduces the burden on insulin.

- **Control the Eating Window**
  Every time you eat, your body signals the release of insulin. That's fine in moderation - but if you're grazing all day (three meals, three snacks, and maybe dessert), your insulin never gets a break. Enter **intermittent fasting**. A popular method is the 16:8 pattern, where you eat during an 8-hour window and fast for 16 hours. This trains your body to rely more on fat during the fasting period, rebuilding your ability to switch fuels.

- **Move More, Move Often**
  Physical activity is one of the most powerful tools for improving insulin sensitivity. It doesn't have to be intense - walking, strength training, or any movement helps your muscles use glucose efficiently and enhances fat metabolism. The more you move, the better your body becomes at managing energy.

Understanding the Glycaemic Index and Glycaemic Load

You've already been introduced to the **glycaemic index (GI)** and **glycaemic load (GL)** earlier in this book. Let's now unpack these concepts with a bit more clarity and context.

The **glycaemic index** is a ranking of how quickly a carbohydrate-containing food raises blood sugar levels. It's a scale from 0 to 100:

- **Low GI (1–55):** Slow, steady release of glucose (e.g., lentils, most fruits, oats)
- **Medium GI (56–69):** Moderate rise in blood glucose (e.g., ripe bananas, couscous)
- **High GI (70+):** Rapid spike in blood glucose (e.g., white bread, cornflakes, sugary sodas)

Pure glucose sits at the top with a GI of 100.

However, **glycaemic load** adds nuance. It considers not just how fast glucose enters your blood, but how much sugar is delivered in a typical serving. It's calculated like this:

GL = (GI × grams of carbohydrate per serving) ÷ 100

A food can have a high GI but a low GL if it contains only a small amount of carbohydrate per serving. Take **watermelon,** for example: its GI is high (around 72), but its GL is low because a typical portion has little carbohydrate. Therefore, it won't significantly spike your blood sugar in practice. That's why both GI and GL matter.

Even fruits can vary significantly in terms of ripeness. For example:

- **Green bananas** (low GI ~30): slower glucose release due to resistant starch.
- **Ripe bananas** (higher GI ~60): starch converts into sugar, raising blood glucose faster.

And then there are surprising stars: **dates**, often feared for their sweetness, have a relatively low GI of 42, thanks to their natural fibre and slower sugar release.

In general, **whole foods win**. They offer a gentler impact on blood sugar than processed equivalents. Nature packages its sugars with fibre, water, and nutrients that slow digestion and soften the glucose impact.

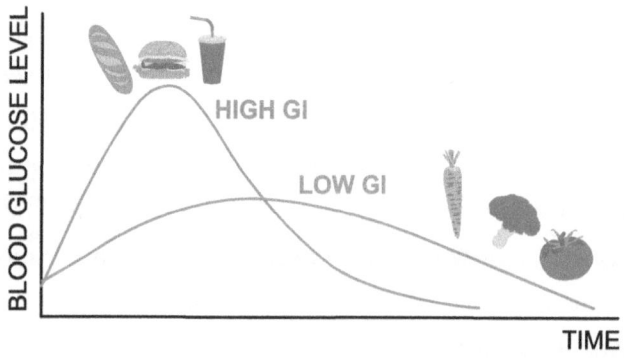

Bottom Line

Fuelling your body wisely means knowing what kind of engine you're running and how to optimise it. Sugar burners rely on constant carb refills. Metabolically flexible individuals can go the distance on fat, sugar, or both - without crashing. Achieving metabolic flexibility isn't about eliminating all carbs or fasting indefinitely. It's about eating smarter, moving regularly, and allowing insulin to reset so your body can function the way it was designed to - like a finely tuned hybrid.

Sugar Addiction and Cravings – Hijacked by Hunger

Imagine a hostage situation. You're not tied to a chair or locked in a room - but your biology is being manipulated in a quiet, calculated way. Every time you reach for that mid-morning biscuit, that soft, sticky chocolate bar in the afternoon, or that comforting late-night bowl of cereal, your brain is reacting not just to habit or convenience but to a deeply rooted survival signal. This chapter isn't just about cravings - it's about reclaiming control from a captor that's hiding in plain sight: sugar.

When Biology Becomes Betrayal

Cravings are not random. They are urgent, precise, and biologically choreographed signals often disguised as emotional whims or weakness of will. These sharp desires - especially for sugar - are desperate calls from the brain to stabilise its fuel supply.

For a brain that relies heavily on glucose and can't yet efficiently burn fat, a dip in blood sugar is interpreted as a life-or-death scenario. Your body doesn't ask politely. It demands – urgently - for sweet reinforcements. That's why you find yourself rummaging through the kitchen at 3 p.m., even though you had lunch just two hours ago.

This isn't your fault. You've been biochemically conditioned. That cinnamon roll is not just a treat - it's a biochemical rescue mission. But the rescue becomes the problem.

The Rollercoaster of Addiction

Start your day with cereal and toast, and you'll feel the difference. The breakfast that was meant to energise you becomes the ticket to a blood sugar spike - and then the crash. Your body overcompensates, releasing too much insulin, and the subsequent drop is steep and brutal. Cue the cravings. This pattern - rise, crash, rescue - is the classic sugar rollercoaster.

Repeated often enough, it wires your brain for dependency. And here's the disturbing part: sugar doesn't just *behave* like a drug - it *uses the same neural pathways* as highly addictive substances like cocaine. And just like cocaine, the more sugar you consume, the more you need to get the same dopamine hit. Your brain rewires itself for the next fix.

In studies with rats, sugar has outcompeted cocaine as the preferred reward. And unlike cocaine, sugar is everywhere: it hides in sauces, salad dressings, yoghurt, juices, and "healthy" bars. It's legal. It's normalised. And it's socially encouraged.

When Cravings Are a Cry for Help

You don't crave just because you're weak. You crave because your biology is dysregulated.

Some people burn sugar all day long and have completely

lost metabolic flexibility. When their glucose dips - often from a previous sugar spike - they panic, internally. Craving becomes a life jacket in turbulent biochemical waters. That's why cravings often intensify under stress, fatigue, or emotional upheaval. In those moments, the body wants one thing: quick glucose.

And cravings don't just affect people with diabetes or metabolic issues. Even "healthy" people experience sugar crashes. The difference is often just the threshold at which the alarm goes off.

Men, Women, and Cravings: The Hormonal Landscape
Craving patterns vary. Men are more likely to crave savoury, salty snacks - chips, crackers, crisps. Women often crave sweet, fatty foods - especially during pregnancy or hormonal fluctuations. This is not just psychology; it's endocrinology. Hormonal changes affect neurotransmitters, which in turn influence cravings. Understanding these patterns can help normalise them - and make them easier to manage without shame or guilt.

Breaking Free: The Path to Liberation
There are two main escape strategies: the **gradual taper** and the **cold-turkey revolution**.

- **Gradualists** choose a gentler path. They swap sweets for fruits, fruits for nuts, and eventually retrain their taste buds to appreciate the forgotten flavours of real food - bitter greens, sour lemon, umami-rich seeds and beans. Their victories are quiet, sustainable, and permanent.
- **Radicals** throw the kitchen into disarray. Sugar: Out. Pasta: Gone. The chocolate stash: Donated or dumped. They brace for the withdrawal storm: irritability, headaches, and a foggy mind. But they know it's

temporary. Like a fever breaking, they push through, emerging clearer, stronger, and metabolically reborn.

There's no one-size-fits-all. What matters is your *resolve*, your *plan*, and your *support system*.

Build a Craving-Proof Life

You don't defeat sugar cravings with willpower alone. You outsmart them. You build a life where sugar has no space to hide. Here's how:

- **Start strong**: A breakfast with eggs, avocado, seeds, or full-fat yoghurt stabilises blood glucose and reduces mid-morning crashes.
- **Stay hydrated**: Dehydration mimics hunger. A glass of water may silence what feels like a craving.
- **Replenish minerals**: Magnesium, zinc, chromium, B vitamins - if deficient - can mimic hunger or sugar needs.
- **Don't skip fats**: Healthy fats (from oily fish, nuts, seeds, and olive oil) are essential to satiety.
- **Identify stress triggers**: Stress creates the illusion of hunger. Address the root cause, not just the response.
- **Use comfort alternatives**: Herbal teas, sugar-free chewing gum, a crunchy snack like cucumber and hummus - these can satisfy the oral fixation without feeding the addiction.

Mind Over Mechanism

Cravings are not just biological - they're emotional. A craving is often your brain's way of asking, *"What's missing?"* Sometimes it's joy. Sometimes, rest. Sometimes, safety. When you listen to the craving instead of fighting it blindly, you can uncover its real message.

Use that knowledge. Replace doom-scrolling with a nature walk. Replace worry with deep breathing. Practice gratitude instead of guilt. Your body is talking. Sugar is just the translator.

Key Takeaways: Taming the Beast

- Cravings are survival messages, not character flaws.
- Sugar addiction is neurological - more potent than many drugs.
- You can retrain your biology with a balanced diet of protein, fats, minerals, and proper planning.
- Hydration and emotional regulation are crucial.
- Gradual or radical, choose a path and commit to it.

You're not weak. You're wired. But wiring can be changed. Reclaim the steering wheel from sugar - and drive toward the life you were meant to live.

Final Thoughts

The sweet allure of sugar masks a bitter truth: it can wreak havoc on your health. Elevated blood glucose levels - primarily driven by the dominance of ultra-processed foods in our modern diet - damage nearly every system in the body. Our reliance on factory-made food has come at a steep cost.

To reclaim our health, we must return to our roots. Whole, farm-fresh foods - untouched by industrial processing - offer the ideal fuel for the human body. By embracing nature's original design, we can restore vitality, optimise well-being, and prevent and reverse many forms of metabolic disease.

Equally important is avoiding insulin resistance, a silent disruptor that keeps insulin levels chronically high, fooling our bodies into thinking we're in a constant state of feasting, much like our hunter-gatherer ancestors during times of abundance. This triggers the liver to produce cholesterol to support new cell growth, leading to elevated cholesterol, triglycerides, and a decrease in HDL - the so-called "good" cholesterol.

These are not just numbers on a blood test - they are warning signs of deeper metabolic dysfunction. In the next chapter, we'll explore these markers in more detail and uncover how to correct them before they spiral out of control.

CHAPTER 7

Cholesterol – Friend, Foe, or Misunderstood?

Does high cholesterol cause heart attacks? For decades, the answer seemed obvious. After all, cholesterol was found in the arterial plaques of heart disease victims, and those waxy buildups became synonymous with cardiovascular doom. But the truth - like cholesterol itself - is far more nuanced than the headlines ever suggested.

In this chapter, we'll unravel cholesterol's tangled reputation, explore the critical differences between various types of cholesterol and blood lipids, and explain how a deeper understanding of their interplay with your metabolism can help you reduce your cardiovascular risk - possibly without fearing every egg yolk or skipping your favourite cheese.

The Cholesterol Myth and Metabolic Reality
The year was 1955. When President Dwight D. Eisenhower suffered a heart attack, panic swept across the United States - not just over his health, but about the mystery of what caused such a seemingly sudden and devastating event. Doctors, eager to explain, pointed the finger at cholesterol, especially since it was present in the

arterial blockages of patients who had died from cardiovascular disease. From that moment, cholesterol became public enemy number one.

The American Heart Association doubled down. Fat - especially saturated fat - was vilified. Butter, red meat, and eggs were replaced by margarine, skim milk, and highly processed "heart-healthy" grains. For the next sixty years, this low-fat dogma shaped food policy, public health messaging, and family dinner plates across the Western world.

But science, thankfully, evolves.

We now understand that cholesterol is not inherently dangerous. In fact, it's indispensable. Cholesterol forms roughly one-third of every cell membrane in your body. It enables the production of bile (critical for fat digestion), vitamin D, and key hormones including cortisol, oestrogen, progesterone, and testosterone. In short, without cholesterol, life itself would unravel.

So, if cholesterol isn't the villain, what is it?

The Lipid Landscape: HDL, LDL, and Triglycerides

To understand cardiovascular risk, we need to stop asking *"Is cholesterol bad?"* and start asking *"Which kinds of lipids signal danger, and in what context?"*

There are several key players in your lipid panel:

- **HDL (High-Density Lipoprotein)** - Often called "good cholesterol," HDL is protective. It scavenges damaged cholesterol from your bloodstream and carries it back to the liver for recycling or disposal. Higher HDL levels generally correlate with a lower risk of heart disease.
- **LDL (Low-Density Lipoprotein)** - Branded the "bad cholesterol," but not all LDL is created equal. Small, dense

LDL particles are more likely to penetrate arterial walls and contribute to plaque formation, especially in the presence of inflammation. Larger, buoyant LDL particles are considered less harmful.
- **Triglycerides** - the common type of fat circulating in the bloodstream, triglycerides spike after carbohydrate-rich meals. Chronically high triglycerides are a hallmark of insulin resistance and are strongly linked to metabolic syndrome and cardiovascular risk.

Here's the twist: *it's not necessarily high total cholesterol that's dangerous, but a combination of high triglycerides, low HDL, and small, dense LDL particles that form the metabolic storm brewing beneath the surface.*

This trio is particularly dangerous in people with metabolic syndrome - a condition often driven by poor diet, sedentary behaviour, chronic stress, and sleep disruption. If you've been following this book, you'll recognise this familiar theme: what damages your metabolism also endangers your heart.

Why Lifestyle, Not Just Labs, Matters

In a healthy person, the liver tightly regulates cholesterol production. About 80% of your body's cholesterol is made by the liver, while only 20% comes from food. When dietary cholesterol increases, liver production generally decreases to keep the balance - a marvel of biological self-regulation. This is why dietary cholesterol, on its own, has a modest effect on blood cholesterol in most people.

However, that balance breaks down when your metabolism is compromised.

High insulin levels (from chronically elevated blood sugar), for instance, upregulate the liver's triglyceride production and increase the output of small LDL particles. This is the metabolic milieu in which cholesterol becomes dangerous: not because of its presence, but because of how it's being processed, packaged, and transported.

In practical terms, a bagel and juice breakfast, followed by a sedentary day and poor sleep, can be far more damaging to your lipid profile than a steak and eggs dinner.

When Cholesterol Isn't the Whole Story
The Curious Case of Andy

I'd like to begin this chapter not with a theory or a principle, but with a patient. One whose case both confounded expectations and brought into sharp focus the limitations of how we think about cardiovascular risk. His name was Andy.

Andy, a 53-year-old gentleman, walked into the Vitality Clinic with an anxious heart and a long list of numbers. The one number that haunted him was his cholesterol level - high, frighteningly high. His fear was straightforward: *"Am I going to have a heart attack?"*

At first glance, Andy's case seemed like a familiar one. He had high blood pressure, diagnosed over a decade ago, and it had been well controlled on a single medication. But like many seemingly straightforward stories, this one soon became tangled. Andy also had gout - a sign of chronic metabolic disturbance. His blood pressure quietly worsened over the years, eventually leading to chronic kidney disease (CKD). Curiously, this was left untreated. Whether it was due to oversight or resignation, the silence surrounding his kidneys would echo loudly in the years to come.

Two years before we met, a routine blood test flagged high cholesterol and elevated triglycerides. His doctor prescribed a statin, the gold-standard treatment. But Andy couldn't tolerate it.

He developed severe muscle pain and weakness, especially in his legs. Within weeks, walking became difficult, and the medication had to be stopped. What should have been a simple intervention turned into another dead end.

Then things took a darker turn. Andy was assaulted, sustaining a head injury. In the aftermath, his blood pressure became chaotic, spiking to dangerous levels despite multiple medications. He began experiencing visual hallucinations, surreal intrusions that emerged every time his pressure climbed too high. Eventually, his kidneys gave up the fight. Andy entered end-stage renal failure and began nightly peritoneal dialysis at home. He was tethered to a machine, but his mind remained tethered to his cholesterol levels.

Looking at Andy, it was hard to ignore the constellation of visible and invisible signs pointing to a deeper problem. He was overweight, with a BMI of 27.5 kg/m^2 and a waist-to-hip ratio of 0.97 - a classic pattern of abdominal obesity. His blood pressure, despite maximal therapy, remained stubbornly high at 170/100 mmHg. His liver was enlarged, another telltale sign: fatty liver disease. These were not isolated issues. They were chapters of the same book - the metabolic syndrome.

By this point, the diagnosis was clear. Andy's body was a battlefield of dysregulated systems: abdominal obesity, insulin resistance, hypertension, dyslipidaemia, and renal compromise. Yet Andy himself remained focused on one enemy: cholesterol.

Let's look at the numbers that terrified him. His total cholesterol was a startling 9.0 mmol/L. His LDL - the so-called "bad cholesterol" - was 6.15 mmol/L. These figures would raise concern in any cardiologist's office. But here's where the story takes an interesting turn. Andy's HDL - the "good" cholesterol - was 1.90 mmol/L. That's normal, even favourable. In theory, this offered him some protection.

So, what went wrong?

Here lies the central puzzle of this chapter. Despite his high LDL, Andy's risk of heart disease wasn't solely - or even primarily dictated by that number. In fact, by the time we calculate risk in someone like Andy, we must go beyond the cholesterol panel. He was a classic example of someone whose *overall metabolic terrain* - not just one lab result - dictated his cardiovascular risk.

This forces us to ask a deeper question: **What other factors were silently shaping Andy's fate?**

Let's consider the following possibilities:

- **Small, dense LDL particles**: Even though Andy's LDL level was high, what truly matters is the *quality* and *pattern* of those LDL particles. Small, dense LDL is far more atherogenic - more likely to penetrate the endothelium and cause inflammation - than large, buoyant particles. Andy's metabolic syndrome increased the likelihood of the former.
- **Insulin resistance**: Often the hidden conductor of the metabolic orchestra, insulin resistance fuels high triglycerides, low HDL, and the transformation of LDL particles into their more dangerous form. Although Andy's fasting glucose was not recorded here, we can infer from his abdominal obesity, fatty liver, and chronic kidney disease (CKD) that insulin resistance was a significant factor.
- **Inflammation**: Andy's chronic kidney disease and fatty liver suggest a state of systemic inflammation - a key promoter of atherosclerosis, independent of LDL.
- **Oxidative stress and endothelial dysfunction**: These often accompany hypertension, diabetes, and CKD, and accelerate vascular damage. In Andy's case, visual hallucinations at peak blood pressure hinted at underlying

neurovascular strain.
- **ApoB and Lp(a)**: These advanced lipid markers were never measured in Andy, but they could have provided valuable insights. ApoB tracks the number of atherogenic particles, and lipoprotein(a) is an independent genetic risk factor for cardiovascular disease. Patients like Andy may have a normal HDL and still be at high risk if these markers are elevated.

Andy's story teaches us something essential: high cholesterol doesn't act in a vacuum. It interacts with dozens of metabolic variables, lifestyle factors, and genetic predispositions. In his case, high LDL was only one part of a much larger and more dangerous picture.

By the time Andy came to us, he wasn't just dealing with a lipid problem. He was living the endgame of uncontrolled metabolic dysfunction. And yet, had we focused only on the cholesterol, we might have missed the broader narrative - the one that could have rewritten his story much earlier.

The Real Culprits Behind High Cholesterol

In a paradox that continues to baffle both patients and practitioners, cardiovascular disease remains the leading cause of death in the modern world - despite decades of aggressive low-fat dietary guidelines and the widespread use of cholesterol-lowering statins. The numbers haven't budged; if anything, they've risen. There's more to this story than just "bad fat."

We now know that high cholesterol is often not the simple byproduct of eating cholesterol-rich foods. Instead, it's entangled in a web of metabolic disturbances, hormonal imbalances, genetic mutations, and lifestyle choices. The truth is both more complex and more compelling than conventional wisdom would have us believe.

Sugar: The Sweet Villain in Disguise

Far more than dietary fat, it is the excess intake of sugar and refined carbohydrates that plays the lead role in disrupting lipid metabolism. The Western diet - high in added sugars, low in fibre, and dominated by ultra-processed foods - acts like a slow poison, damaging the metabolic machinery from within.

A key player in this metabolic disruption is high-fructose corn syrup (HFCS). Once a cheap, industrial substitute for sugar, HFCS now sweetens everything from soft drinks to salad dressings. Unlike the natural fructose found in fruits, which comes packaged with fibre, antioxidants, and micronutrients, HFCS bombards the liver in an unregulated rush. The liver, overwhelmed, converts the surplus into triglycerides and stores them as fat. Over time, this leads to non-alcoholic fatty liver disease, an ominous precursor to insulin resistance, type 2 diabetes, and - yes - high cholesterol.

Worse yet, this cascade alters our lipid profile for the worse: LDL (low-density lipoprotein) cholesterol climbs, especially the small, dense, inflammatory kind, while HDL (high-density lipoprotein) - the so-called "good cholesterol" - diminishes. The body, in effect, becomes a cholesterol mismanagement machine.

The Liver's Secret Life

Beyond dietary input, the liver plays a complex role in regulating cholesterol. It's the body's metabolic control tower - and when it malfunctions, cholesterol often spirals out of control.

One subtle disruptor is hypothyroidism - an underactive thyroid. This hormonal slowdown decreases the liver's ability to clear LDL cholesterol efficiently. Patients with untreated hypothyroidism may feel constantly cold, foggy, tired, and constipated - all while gaining weight despite unchanged diets. Historically, thyroid hormone (thyroxine) was used to lower cholesterol levels, even in individuals without thyroid disease. It worked - but with serious side effects. It's no longer used for this purpose, but its history reveals how deeply metabolism and cholesterol are intertwined.

Other liver-related issues, like primary biliary cirrhosis (a rare autoimmune condition), can also impede cholesterol clearance and lead to abnormal lipid deposits — around the eyes (xanthelasma), within the cornea (arcus senilis), or even on tendons (tendon xanthoma). These are more than cosmetic nuisances; they are often early warning signs of systemic cardiovascular risk.

Cholesterol, Immunity, and Inflammation

Emerging evidence suggests that elevated total cholesterol (above 5 mmol/L) and LDL cholesterol (above 3 mmol/L) may compromise immunity and exacerbate systemic inflammation. This chronic low-grade inflammation is the silent accomplice of many cardiometabolic diseases - quietly damaging arterial linings, thickening the blood, and promoting plaque buildup.

This is particularly troubling in the context of metabolic syndrome, where high cholesterol is just one component of a larger constellation that includes insulin resistance, abdominal obesity, and hypertension. It's not just one thing - it's everything at once.

When the Genes Get Involved

Not all cases of high cholesterol can be blamed on lifestyle. Sometimes, it's in your DNA.

If your father had a heart attack at 52 or your mother at 61, your risk is significantly higher.[1] But it's worth pausing to consider: did you inherit a faulty gene, or just the family's dietary and lifestyle habits?

One inherited culprit is familial hypercholesterolaemia (FH), a genetic disorder that severely impairs your ability to clear LDL cholesterol. If one parent carries the mutation, your risk of developing the condition is 50%. If both do (rare, but not impossible), your fate is sealed at birth. FH can result in cholesterol levels more than twice the normal range - and in heart attacks before the age of 30. Statins are particularly effective in familial hypercholesterolemia (FH), and early diagnosis can be lifesaving.

Then there's **Lipoprotein(a)** [Lp(a)], a little-known but powerful risk factor. Structurally similar to LDL, Lp(a) is genetically determined and largely unaffected by lifestyle. Elevated Lp(a) thickens the blood and promotes plaque formation. If heart disease strikes early in your family, this is one of the first things your doctor should test for.

Another molecule to watch is **homocysteine**, an amino acid that accumulates in some individuals with mutations in the **MTHFR** gene. High homocysteine levels irritate blood vessels and increase the risk of clot formation. Fortunately, with the right nutritional interventions (like B vitamins), homocysteine can often be brought under control.

Finally, there's **APOE**, a gene with profound implications not only for heart disease but also for Alzheimer's. People with the APOE4 allele are at a significantly higher risk of both. This gene alters how your body processes lipids, often leading to elevated cholesterol levels and disrupted vascular health.

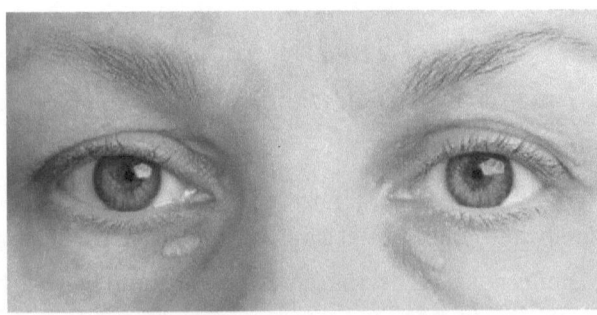

Xanthelasma is a soft, yellow bump caused by the deposition of cholesterol around the eyelids. They can be flat and are often a sign of raised cholesterol, diabetes or thyroid disease.

Pulling Back the Curtain

So, what does this all mean for the average person concerned about their cholesterol levels? It implies that blindly following "low-fat" advice is unlikely to help. It means that if you're serious about preventing heart disease, you must look at cholesterol through a metabolic, genetic, and lifestyle lens.

- Are you insulin resistant?
- Are you eating too many processed carbs or consuming HFCS?
- Is your thyroid sluggish?
- Do you have a family history of early heart disease?
- Could you be carrying a gene that puts you at risk?

Answering these questions is far more critical than focusing solely on the cholesterol number printed on your blood test. After all, cholesterol itself is not the enemy. It's an essential molecule used in every cell membrane and in the production of hormones and vitamin D. What matters is *how* your body processes and manages it - and what that tells us about your overall metabolic health.

Heart Disease and Heart Attacks – More Than Just Cholesterol

Heart disease is often painted with a broad brush, with cholesterol cast as the primary villain. However, the truth is more complex and, in many ways, more intriguing. Heart disease doesn't arrive like a bolt of lightning; instead, it builds slowly and stealthily over time, with a series of biochemical missteps, lifestyle factors, and genetic predispositions laying the groundwork. By the time a heart attack strikes, it is merely the final act in a drama that may have started decades earlier.

The Hidden Beginnings

As we saw in Chapter 3, chronic low-grade inflammation plays a critical role in setting the stage. This persistent, subtle fire within the arterial wall isn't loud or immediately symptomatic, but it is relentless. One of its many consequences is the development of insulin resistance - a metabolic disruption that affects how glucose and lipids are handled in the body.

With elevated blood glucose, LDL (low-density lipoprotein) cholesterol particles undergo glycation and oxidation - transformations that turn these otherwise neutral carriers of cholesterol into inflammatory triggers. These damaged LDL particles are more likely to penetrate the inflamed endothelium (the inner lining of arteries), become embedded, and trigger a cascade of immune responses. Over time, this leads to the formation of atherosclerotic plaques, which narrow the arteries and silently set the stage for coronary artery disease.

A Crisis Years in the Making

A heart attack doesn't typically result from a single event but from a prolonged progression. The narrowed arteries compromise oxygen delivery during physical exertion, often manifesting as effort-induced chest pain - known as angina. But the true danger lies in what happens when a plaque ruptures. This rupture exposes the inner contents of the plaque to the bloodstream, triggering the formation of a clot. If the clot blocks an already narrowed artery completely, the oxygen supply to part of the heart is cut off, resulting in a heart attack (myocardial infarction).

It's crucial to understand that this is not merely a "plumbing problem." It's an inflammatory, metabolic, and vascular condition with deep systemic roots.

The Unexpected Culprit: Low HDL

We've long been told that "high cholesterol" causes heart attacks, and while elevated LDL may contribute, the story is not so straightforward. A massive study of over 136,000 patients admitted for heart attacks revealed a surprising twist: **three-quarters of the patients had normal LDL cholesterol**, and half had LDL levels considered optimal.[2] Something was missing from the traditional narrative.

Digging deeper, researchers discovered a startling pattern - **90% of these patients had low levels of HDL (high-density lipoprotein) cholesterol**, the so-called "good cholesterol." This finding suggests that low HDL may be an even more significant predictor of cardiovascular risk than high LDL.

Why? Because HDL does more than just transport cholesterol - it's part of the body's clean-up crew. HDL particles collect oxidised LDL and carry it back to the liver for disposal. In this sense, HDL is not just "good," it's protective. When HDL levels are low, this cleanup mechanism is impaired, allowing oxidised LDL to linger and continue its damaging work. The total cholesterol and HDL ratio is even more accurate in assessing the risk of a heart attack.[3]

When "More" Isn't Better

If some HDL is good, more must be better. But even here, biology resists oversimplification. Very high levels of HDL - above 1.4 mmol/L, especially over 2.3 mmol/L - may correlate with an **increased** cardiovascular risk. This paradoxical effect may result from dysfunctional HDL particles, often seen in genetic disorders, chronic alcoholism, or as a side effect of certain medications like steroids, anticonvulsants, or hormonal treatments.

So, when it comes to HDL, **quality and function may matter as much as quantity**.

A Case in Point

Take Andy, a patient concerned about his cardiovascular risk. His HDL levels were within the normal range, which provided some initial reassurance. But numbers alone don't tell the whole story. Further investigation revealed that Andy's LDL particles were predominantly small and dense - more likely to oxidise and promote clot formation. We'll explore the importance of LDL particle size and quality later in this chapter, but suffice it to say: Andy's risk was not what it first appeared.

Rethinking the Role of Diet

For years, the public was told to avoid fat like the plague. Butter became taboo, egg yolks were vilified, and low-fat margarine was the supposed salvation. However, science has progressed, and the truth is far more complex.

A landmark meta-analysis involving over 350,000 participants found **no significant association between total or saturated fat intake and the risk of heart disease**. In contrast, **trans fats** - found in many processed foods - remained harmful.

What about the long-endorsed low-fat, high-carb diet? Multiple studies have shown that this approach may **worsen** key heart disease risk factors.[4] High carbohydrate intake can lead to elevated triglycerides, reduced HDL levels, and the proliferation of small, dense LDL particles - all of which spell trouble.

In one large-scale study of 50,000 post-menopausal women, researchers found **no difference** in the rate of heart attacks or strokes between those on a low-fat diet and those eating normally.[5] This prompted the U.S. Dietary Guidelines Advisory Committee to dramatically shift its stance, lifting the long-standing restriction on dietary cholesterol and classifying it as a "nutrient of no concern."

The Bigger Picture

Heart disease isn't caused by a single nutrient or cholesterol level. It's the result of a complex interplay between inflammation, insulin resistance, lipid quality (not just quantity), and lifestyle. The earlier we shift our focus from simplistic cholesterol metrics to a broader metabolic lens, the more effective we'll be at prevention and treatment.

In the following sections, we'll delve into the roles of LDL particle size, lipoprotein(a), and the emerging biomarkers that offer a more precise picture of cardiovascular risk - allowing us to move beyond guesswork and into the realm of tailored, evidence-based care.

When Genes Trump Fitness - Tom's Story

Despite our best efforts to eat well, stay active, and manage stress, sometimes the deck is stacked against us. The story of Tom, a lean, athletic 41-year-old professional, reminds us that cardiovascular disease isn't always the predictable outcome of poor choices. Sometimes, it's the silent hand of genetics that plays the deciding card.

Tom was the picture of health - or so it seemed. With a VO_2 max of 60 mL/kg/min and a body fat percentage of just 9%, his fitness level was what most people strive to achieve. He looked younger than his age, never smoked, and was mindful of his diet. To any casual observer, Tom was "fit as a fiddle." But under the surface, something far more sinister was brewing.

His journey began, oddly enough, in the ear, nose, and throat (ENT) department. Tom had started experiencing bouts of vertigo - an unsettling sensation that the room was spinning even while he remained perfectly still. The ENT consultant suspected benign positional vertigo and prescribed vestibular exercises, reassuring him it was nothing to worry about. Tom, ever diligent, incorporated the exercises into his morning routine. However, the dizziness persisted, gradually evolving into something more ominous over time.

Within six months, new symptoms crept in - palpitations, episodes of light-headedness, and headaches that felt too intense to be shrugged off. Tom was no hypochondriac, but he had a deep awareness of his family history. Several close relatives had succumbed to heart disease, and his father had suffered a heart attack before the age of 50. Spurred by this concern, Tom began tracking his blood pressure at home - and the readings were consistently high. A blood test confirmed another red flag: his LDL cholesterol was elevated, spiking after a particularly stressful business ordeal.

His general practitioner wasted no time. Tom was started on antihypertensive medication and a statin. The response was swift and encouraging - his LDL cholesterol plummeted from a risky 160 mg/dL (4.1 mmol/L) to a much safer 65 mg/dL (1.6 mmol/L). Numbers like that would comfort any cardiologist, but in Tom's case, they didn't tell the whole story.

Outwardly, Tom continued to thrive - training regularly, maintaining a healthy weight, and outperforming his peers in fitness metrics. Yet his clinical profile now included two significant risk factors: hypertension and hyperlipidaemia. Given his family history, we decided to take a closer look. The results were startling.

A coronary calcium scan - a test that detects hardened plaque in the arteries - revealed a score of 398. For his age, this was alarmingly high, strongly indicative of significant atherosclerotic burden. One of his coronary arteries showed a 35% blockage. A carotid ultrasound, often used to assess stroke risk, revealed 45% stenosis of the main artery feeding his brain on one side. These weren't trivial findings. This was silent heart disease, quietly evolving beneath his well-toned exterior.

Naturally, Tom wanted answers. How could someone so fit, so careful, and so young already be dealing with advanced vascular disease? The answer lay in his genes.

We conducted a comprehensive genetic work-up - something we don't do lightly, but in cases like Tom's, it can be illuminating. What we found was a constellation of gene variants that made his body more prone to inflammation, less efficient at clearing cholesterol, and more vulnerable to oxidative stress - all potent drivers of cardiovascular disease. These weren't lifestyle-induced weaknesses; they were baked into his biology.

So, we adjusted our strategy. Lifestyle optimisation remained foundational - no pill or intervention can outdo the power of a healthy lifestyle - but now we focused on targeted support for his genetic vulnerabilities. Nutrigenomic interventions, tailored supplementation, and stress modulation were added to his treatment plan. More importantly, we developed a roadmap aimed not just at management, but at **reversal** - halting the progression of disease and safeguarding him from acute events like heart attacks or strokes.

Tom's case reminds us of an uncomfortable truth: fitness is not immunity. While regular exercise and a balanced diet are non-negotiable pillars of cardiovascular health, they don't always protect us from what's encoded in our DNA. For those with a strong genetic predisposition, especially when compounded by stress or inflammation, early intervention is crucial - even when outward health seems impeccable.[5]

Frank's Sign, diagonal ear lobe crease

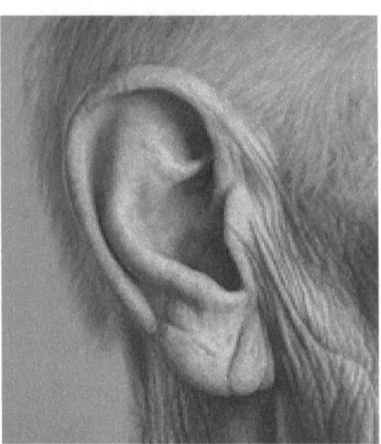

Frank's sign, a diagonal crease across the earlobe, is associated with an increased risk of heart disease, particularly if it's deep and on both sides.

"I've Got a Sweet Tooth"

Helen often joked about her lifelong love affair with sugar. "I've got a sweet tooth," she'd say, with a smile that barely concealed the decades of frustration behind it. But what began as an innocent indulgence in childhood sweets gradually morphed into a cascade of health issues that culminated in a life-altering cardiac event.

At 57, Helen presented to our clinic with persistent migraines - sharp, throbbing episodes that had become more frequent and debilitating. But the migraines were only the tip of the iceberg. Her medical history read like a textbook case of metabolic unravelling: obesity, high blood pressure, prediabetes, and a strikingly high cholesterol level of 7.2 mmol/L. Beneath these numbers lay a complex interplay of factors - many familiar from earlier chapters, but here they converged with alarming clarity.

Despite many attempts over the years - low-fat fads, detoxes, keto cycles, and more - Helen's efforts to lose weight never stuck. Sugar cravings haunted her like clockwork, especially after meals, late at night, and during periods of stress. It wasn't simply poor willpower. Her body had become metabolically wired for sugar dependency, and her physiology was paying the price.

But Helen's story also had some underappreciated threads, such as her oral health, for example. Decades of gum disease had left her with persistent bleeding gums, tooth sensitivity, and a low-grade inflammation that simmered quietly in the background. She had 17 silver amalgam fillings - those once-standard dental restorations now known to contain mercury, a heavy metal with toxic implications. Her gum disease had been treated intermittently, mostly with repeated courses of antibiotics, which not only disrupted her gut microbiota but may also have impaired cholesterol metabolism. Each round of antibiotics brought short-term relief, but over time, they may have contributed to a troubling shift in her gut flora - decreasing protective HDL cholesterol and allowing pro-inflammatory pathways to flourish.

Adding another layer, Helen tested positive for *Helicobacter pylori*, a common stomach bacterium linked to ulcers but also associated with systemic inflammation. Chronic infections like this don't just irritate the digestive tract - they can trigger the immune system in ways that contribute to atherosclerosis and elevate cholesterol.

Then came the heart symptoms. Helen began experiencing chest tightness on mild exertion - classic angina. Tests confirmed narrowing of her coronary arteries, and she underwent a stenting procedure to restore blood flow. The procedure brought relief, but it was a wake-up call.

In Helen's case, heart disease wasn't the result of a single bad habit or an unlucky gene. It was the convergence of chronic sugar exposure, persistent low-grade infections, metabolic derailment, antibiotic overuse, and toxic heavy metals. It was a perfect storm -

a story hiding in plain sight, obscured by the idea that heart disease is only about fat and cholesterol.

We designed a comprehensive recovery plan. It focused on reducing her sugar intake while nourishing her body with whole foods rich in antioxidants and nutrients. Addressing her mercury burden became a key priority, as did rebalancing her gut microbiota and tackling the gum disease that had quietly persisted for decades.

Helen's journey reminds us that high cholesterol is not always just a dietary issue - it's often a signpost pointing toward deeper imbalances in the body. In her case, those imbalances had been present since childhood, woven together through years of metabolic stress and an inflammatory load.

We'll return to Helen's progress in Chapter 10. Still, her case stands as a vivid illustration of how seemingly unrelated issues - dental health, gut bugs, sugar habits, and toxic metals - can unite to sabotage the heart. And perhaps most importantly, how addressing them together offers a path back to healing.

The Real Culprit Behind Heart Disease:
The Passenger Myth and the Vehicle Truth

Imagine you're watching traffic from a helicopter above a busy highway. Each car is a vessel in motion, transporting people to various destinations. Now, let's say you want to predict the likelihood of accidents on this highway. Would you count the number of passengers or the number of cars? Most of us would agree it's the number of vehicles that determines congestion and crash potential, not just how many people they carry.

Surprisingly, in medicine, we often do the opposite.

We routinely measure **LDL cholesterol** - the "passengers" - but often overlook **LDL particles** - the "cars." And just as crowded highways with more cars lead to more accidents, more LDL particles crowd our arteries, increasing the risk of plaque build-up and, eventually, vascular catastrophes like heart attacks and strokes. It's time we shift our focus to the actual number of LDL cars on the road, not just how full each one is.

The Dangerous Distinction:
Fluffy Beach balls vs. Sticky Golf Balls

Not all LDL particles are created equal. Some are large and buoyant - imagine beachballs bobbing in water. These are relatively harmless. Others are small, dense, and sticky - like golf balls rolling around with a tendency to clump. It's these compact particles that can wedge into the delicate lining of blood vessels, sparking inflammation and clot formation. This subtle transformation marks the beginning of atherosclerosis - the invisible fire that slowly narrows arteries.

So, what determines whether your body makes beachballs or golf balls?

The Origins of Particle Chaos: Metabolic Syndrome and More

Enter **metabolic syndrome**, the perfect storm to produce harmful LDL particles. Picture a ticking time bomb made of five interlocking factors:

- Central obesity (belly fat)
- High blood pressure
- Elevated triglycerides
- Low HDL (good) cholesterol
- Insulin resistance or elevated blood sugar

Together, these forces tilt your metabolic machinery toward danger, flooding your bloodstream with small, dense LDL particles.

But that's not all. An underactive thyroid, persistent infections, and even an imbalanced gut microbiome (dysbiosis) can tip the scales, subtly increasing particle count and risk. Yes, the bacteria in your intestines can influence your heart health - proving once again that the body is an interconnected ecosystem, not a set of silos.

Trans Fat: The Industrial Saboteur
No modern villain wreaks as much cardiovascular havoc as **trans-fat**. Created by chemically altering vegetable oil to make it solid, trans fat hides in margarine, fast food, doughnuts, and packaged snacks. It increases LDL, lowers HDL, raises triglycerides, and inflames blood vessels - all at once.

Trans fats are banned or restricted in many countries, but loopholes and lingering products still expose millions to their damage. They don't just cause cholesterol problems - they actively **ignite** atherosclerosis by generating oxidative stress and impairing your body's natural defences.

Screening and Surveillance: Know Your Numbers
Current guidelines recommend:

- **Every 2 years**: cholesterol screening for men aged 45-65 and women aged 55-65.
- **Annually**, for individuals over 65 or those with a high risk.

However, consider going beyond routine LDL cholesterol levels. Ask your doctor about **LDL particle number (LDL-P)** or **ApoB**, a protein present on every atherogenic particle. These advanced markers may better predict your cardiovascular risk than standard lipid panels.

Dietary Offenders: What's Clogging the Engine?

Let's cut through the confusion. Cholesterol in food doesn't always translate to cholesterol in blood, but some foods still push your metabolic system into overdrive:

- **Red meat** (more than 100g daily): may increase uric acid levels and contribute to joint issues or the formation of kidney stones.
- **Processed meats** (sausages, burgers): saturated fat bombs that increase LDL cholesterol.
- **Fried foods**: toxic oils and glycation products harm blood vessels and increase calorie density.
- **Sugary and refined carbs** (pastries, pasta, pizza): drive liver fat production and LDL particle formation through **lipogenesis**.
- **HFCS** (high-fructose corn syrup): a master manipulator of triglycerides and liver health.

Dietary Defenders: What Clears the Road?

Here's your **cholesterol-lowering toolkit**—simple, natural, powerful:

1. **Fibre**:
   - Found in oats, beans, seeds, and vegetables. Slows sugar and fat absorption, reduces LDL.
2. **Healthy fats**:
   - **Olive oil**: rich in omega-9s.
   - **Avocados**: lower LDL, triglycerides; raise HDL.
   - **Nuts & seeds**: full of polyunsaturated fats and plant sterols.

3. **Omega-3 fatty acids:**
   - Eat fish like sardines, mackerel, and salmon.
   - Supplement up to 2g/day if needed.
4. **Dark, leafy greens**: Spinach and kale provide **lutein** and antioxidants that mop up oxidised LDL.
5. **Tomatoes**: rich in **lycopene** - aim for 30mg/day.
6. **Garlic**: contains **allicin**, a natural cholesterol-fighter.
7. **Blueberries** are rich in antioxidants that help protect LDL from oxidation.
8. **Tea & wine (in moderation):**
   - **Green tea**: EGCG lowers blood pressure.
   - **Red wine**: Polyphenols reduce LDL oxidation.

Exercise: The Unsung Hero

It's not just what you eat - it's also what you **burn**. Regular physical activity:

- Increases HDL cholesterol (the scavenger).
- Lowers triglycerides and body fat.
- Improves insulin sensitivity—fighting metabolic syndrome at its root.

Medications: A Double-Edged Sword

Statins remain the cornerstone of cholesterol-lowering drugs, effective in reducing LDL cholesterol and cardiovascular events. But they aren't perfect:

- They do **not** lower **Lipoprotein(a)**, a stubborn, genetically influenced particle.
- Potential side effects: muscle pain, liver enzyme changes, increased risk of diabetes, and possible cognitive effects.

That said, for high-risk individuals, statins may be lifesaving - just be sure to pair them with lifestyle changes rather than rely on them as a magic pill.

Final Thoughts: Where Prevention Begins
Prevention isn't about cutting cholesterol - it's about understanding **how and why** it becomes a threat. LDL particles, metabolic imbalances, dietary missteps, and inflammation all converge to create the perfect storm. Shift your attention from passenger counts to traffic flow. Prevent the jam before the crash.

Instead of chasing numbers, pursue **balance**. A whole-food, fibre-rich diet. Movement every day. Conscious choices about what you fuel your body with. Your arteries will thank you.

These aren't just cholesterol-lowering strategies - they're metabolic healing tools.

From Awareness to Action:
With this chapter complete, you've now mastered the core of Section 1 - an in-depth look at the five key metabolic risk factors: central obesity, high blood pressure, elevated blood sugar, high triglycerides, and low HDL cholesterol. These silent drivers of metabolic syndrome often go unnoticed until they lead to serious health issues. Before moving on to Section 2, take a moment to reflect: which of these factors affects you most, and what first step could you take today toward better health?

In the next section, we'll explore common yet often overlooked conditions closely tied to metabolic syndrome - fatty liver, sleep apnoea, periodontal disease, benign prostatic hyperplasia (BPH), polycystic ovary syndrome (PCOS), osteoarthritis, and varicose veins. Understanding their connection to metabolic health may change the way you see these familiar conditions - and how you choose to respond.

SECTION 2

METABOLIC SYNDROME-RELATED CONDITIONS

CHAPTER 8

Fatty Liver Disease – The Silent Invasion

In the great unfolding of metabolic syndrome, fatty liver disease stands as a quiet but ominous sentinel. While it rarely shouts in its early stages, it whispers relentlessly, embedding itself in the lives of millions. By the time it speaks clearly - often through organ damage - it is already deeply entrenched. It is the liver's subdued cry for help in a world that has fed it too much of the wrong thing.

At its core, fatty liver disease is the unnatural accumulation of fat in the liver - a paradox, considering this organ is evolutionarily designed to process fat, not store it. When this fat exceeds 5% of the liver's weight, it begins to tip the balance from benign to dangerous. Today, up to **30% of adults** in developed nations carry this burden. Even more concerning: **1 in 10 children** in the UK already have fatty livers, a silent testimony to our changing food environment and sedentary culture.

A Clinical Skill Rooted in the Tropics

I learned to read the liver long before I saw my first case of NAFLD. Four decades ago, while working in the heart of tropical Africa, I developed a deep familiarity with hepatomegaly - enlargement of the liver. There, the causes were distinctly infectious: malaria, typhoid, schistosomiasis. In those settings, the liver was under siege from pathogens. My hands learned to feel those changes, to sense the shifting texture and edge of an organ under distress.

Today, in the UK, I still palpate livers. But what I find is not the rugged, inflamed tissue of infection, but the smooth and swollen liver of indulgence - bloated not with parasites or fever, but with triglycerides and regret. The enemy has changed. It is no longer a parasite from a riverbank, but a sugar-sweetened beverage, a packet of crisps, an extra slice of pizza.

Stress - so often the root of modern illness - plays its part too. Pressured lives, remote work, emotional eating, and increasingly sedentary days form the perfect storm. As lifestyle stress rises, so do our habits of comfort: overeating, inactivity, and alcohol. The result is a liver overwhelmed and inflamed, slowly moving toward its demise.

From Alcohol to Sugar: A Shift in Culprits

Historically, fatty liver was almost exclusively the domain of alcoholics. **Alcoholic Fatty Liver Disease (AFLD)** was common in those who drank excessively. But in recent decades, a new form has quietly overtaken it: **Non-Alcoholic Fatty Liver Disease (NAFLD)**. It mimics the same progression, the same endgame - cirrhosis and liver failure - but arises from a different kind of abuse: **chronic overconsumption of refined carbohydrates and sugar**.

NAFLD is now a nutritional disease, born in the kitchen rather than the pub. Its drivers include white bread, breakfast cereals, sweetened drinks, and, particularly, **high-fructose corn syrup (HFCS)** - the ubiquitous sweetener we explored in Chapter 3. HFCS hijacks liver metabolism, fuelling **de novo lipogenesis** - the creation of fat from sugar - and lays the foundation for insulin resistance.

Alcohol and sugar, once distant cousins in liver pathology, now converge. Both lead to fat buildup. Both trigger inflammation. Both, if ignored, march toward cirrhosis. AFLD and NAFLD are, in many ways, two sides of the same metabolic coin.

The Four Stages: From Fatty to Failing
Fatty liver disease follows a predictable path, though not all will journey to the end:

- **Steatosis** (Simple Fatty Liver): This is the earliest and most silent stage. Fat infiltrates liver cells without inflammation or fibrosis. Often found incidentally on imaging or through abnormal liver enzyme tests.
- **NASH** (Non-Alcoholic Steatohepatitis): The liver becomes inflamed. It is no longer just storing fat - it is reacting to it. Roughly **5% of the UK population** has progressed to this stage, where damage becomes more serious and persistent.
- **Fibrosis**: In response to ongoing inflammation, scar tissue forms. At this point, liver function may still appear normal, but the liver's structure is changing.
- **Cirrhosis**: The final and irreversible phase. The liver becomes nodular, shrunken, and severely scarred. It begins to fail in its duties - filtering blood, producing proteins, and managing energy. Some patients may also develop **hepatocellular carcinoma**, a form of liver cancer.

Nature or Nurture? The Genetic Overlay
While lifestyle is the primary driver, **genes set the tone**. Some individuals are genetically predisposed to develop fatty liver more easily, even on a relatively moderate diet.

One key genetic player is the **PEMT gene**, responsible for the enzyme phosphatidylethanolamine N-methyltransferase. This enzyme is vital in synthesizing **phosphatidylcholine**, a molecule essential for fat export from the liver and membrane integrity. Mice lacking this gene develop fatty livers swiftly, and human variants of the gene appear to slow fat metabolism, leading to accumulation within liver cells.

In other words, some people are born with a liver that struggles to offload fat. When paired with a modern diet, it becomes a dangerous combination.

A Tale of Two Livers: Tropical vs. Western
In tropical medicine, liver disease often presents in a distinct form. **Schistosomiasis**, caused by waterborne parasitic worms, can lead to **rapid portal fibrosis**, which blocks liver blood vessels and produces severe complications. I've seen patients - young, vibrant people - collapse in a cascade of blood from ruptured **gastro-oesophageal varices**. The image of a person vomiting litres of fresh blood, the team rushing, transfusing, resuscitating, and still failing to save them - it stays with you.

In contrast, Western fatty liver disease is insidious. It doesn't arrive with a splash, but with a whisper. Most patients have no symptoms for years. Yet over decades, NAFLD carves a slow path to liver failure and cancer. It rarely causes acute bleeding like tropical schistosomiasis, but it steals lives nonetheless - quietly, predictably, and with increasing frequency. NAFLD is now the **leading cause of liver transplantation** in countries like the UK and the US.

The Silent Sirens of a Fatty Liver
The liver, our body's biochemical powerhouse, rarely complains until it's on the verge of failure. By then, the signs it sends - subtle,

scattered, often misread - are often drowned out by more pressing distractions of modern life. But for those tuned in, the early whispers of fatty liver disease can be recognised, and its course, potentially reversed.

Early Clues from a Sugar-Sick Liver

The earliest symptoms of fatty liver disease are not always specific to the liver. Instead, they emerge from the chaos of metabolic disruption. Patients often speak of relentless fatigue, a dragging sense of low energy, mid-afternoon slumps, and the frustrating inability to sleep through the night. These are not random complaints - they're red flags of a system struggling to manage energy efficiently.

At a more advanced stage, the signs become more telling. Men may notice gynecomastia- enlarged breast tissue - triggered by altered oestrogen/testosterone ratio. Some individuals feel bloated or experience discomfort in the area under the right rib cage, where the liver is located, and it silently swells. As detoxification falters, jaundice creeps in, skin turns yellow, the whites of the eyes lose their clarity, and confusion begins to cloud cognition - a condition ominously known as hepatic encephalopathy.

Look closely and you may find the telltale "liver palms," red and warm to the touch, or see veins spreading like tributaries across the chest and abdomen. Ankle swelling, an enlarged spleen, and bleeding tendencies are all late-stage warnings of a liver teetering on collapse.

A Failing Factory

The tragedy of fatty liver is that it repurposes a high-performing organ into an inefficient storage depot. Instead of executing over 500 metabolic tasks, a liver saturated with fat becomes sluggish, overwhelmed, and inflamed. The same happens to the pancreas - another metabolically vital organ. These organs don't just lose functionality; they sabotage your body's ability to generate and regulate energy.

Imagine trying to run a city where the power plant is overloaded, the water treatment facility is leaking, and the emergency response team is underfunded. This is the internal reality of advanced fatty liver disease.

The Hidden Battle in Peter's Body

Peter's story illustrates this insidious transformation. At 33, he should have been thriving - his youth, his gym commitment, even his personal trainer seemed to suggest vitality. But appearances deceive. Behind the protein shakes and kettlebells, Peter's body was deteriorating.

He complained of fatigue, brain fog, and declining exercise capacity. Yet he was slim-limbed, muscular even, and active. The problem lay deeper. Despite physical activity, his high-carb diet - rich in cereals, bread, pasta, pizza, sugary snacks, and sports drinks - kept his insulin levels elevated. His blood pressure hovered at prehypertensive levels, and his blood work was a catalogue of metabolic distress: high insulin, low HDL cholesterol, dangerously high triglycerides, elevated liver enzymes, and fatty liver on ultrasound.

Peter's muscles were starving for glucose, but insulin resistance blocked the gates. His liver, already inflamed and enlarged, could no longer manage toxins or regulate metabolism. Even his pancreas - an organ rarely noticed until it fails - was quietly succumbing to fatty infiltration.

Fat in the Pancreas: A Silent Saboteur

The pancreas, nestled behind the stomach, plays dual roles:

producing insulin for glucose control and enzymes for digestion. When fat infiltrates it, both these functions falter. A fatty pancreas is often discovered incidentally on ultrasound but carries serious implications: a higher risk of pancreatitis, loss of insulin-producing cells, poor digestion, and even pancreatic cancer.

In essence, a fatty pancreas is a ticking time bomb - each gram of fat is a fuse shortening your metabolic resilience.

Diagnosing the Invisible

Routine blood tests can reveal the truth before symptoms arise. Elevated liver enzymes - ALT, AST, and GGT - suggest hepatic inflammation. Elevated triglycerides, HbA1C, fasting glucose, and hs-CRP add further evidence of metabolic dysfunction. An ultrasound may detect fat, but it cannot assess the severity of the disease. Liver biopsy remains the definitive test, but its risks - especially bleeding due to impaired clotting factor production - make it a last resort.

When the Liver Fails

As fatty liver disease advances, it's not just detoxification that halts. Complications like hepatic encephalopathy and internal bleeding from ruptured varices become life-threatening. Liver cancer may develop silently, and the only hope for some becomes a transplant. The cost - physically, emotionally, and financially - is profound.

Who's at Risk?

If you have central obesity, prediabetes or type 2 diabetes, high blood pressure, elevated triglycerides, or low HDL cholesterol, you are already standing in the shadow of fatty liver disease. It strikes people over 50 more frequently, but as Peter's case shows, youth is no safeguard. A fatty liver almost certainly means fat accumulation in other organs, especially muscle and pancreas, where it disrupts insulin signalling and energy production.

Can It Be Reversed?

Yes - but only if we change the inputs.

Avoiding alcohol helps, but the real culprit in non-alcoholic fatty liver disease (NAFLD) is not dietary fat - it's sugar, especially in its high-fructose corn syrup (HFCS) form. HFCS-laced beverages and refined carbohydrates are potent drivers of liver fat accumulation.

Artificial sweeteners, often marketed as healthy alternatives, can worsen the issue by disrupting the gut microbiome and promoting insulin resistance. So swapping sugar for aspartame is not a solution - it's a detour that still leads to disease.

Instead, reversal begins with removing the source: processed carbs, sugary drinks, and insulin-spiking snacks. Restoring insulin sensitivity through a whole-foods diet, regular physical activity, and improved sleep habits can help turn the tide.

Eat Whole Food, Move More - Your Treatment Strategies

Imagine your liver not as a passive organ tucked away in the upper right of your abdomen but as a vigilant conductor orchestrating your body's metabolic symphony. Now imagine what happens when fat infiltrates this conductor's podium - disrupting the rhythm, causing chaos in the orchestra. This, in essence, is what happens in fatty liver disease. But here's the good news: the conductor can be restored to harmony, and the orchestra can play beautifully again. The tools are Food and movement.

A Revolution from Within

In the early 2010s, Professor Roy Taylor of Newcastle University conducted a study that sent ripples through the medical community. Using advanced MRI scans, he visualised the reversal of type 2 diabetes - yes, reversal - in people who followed a strict low-calorie diet. The imagery was striking; fat once clogging the liver and pancreas, visibly diminished. With this internal detox came a miraculous return to normal blood glucose levels in most participants. What this proved was profound: by reducing ectopic fat, particularly in the liver and pancreas, one could reset the very machinery of insulin regulation.

And how was this achieved? Not with a new pill. Not with surgery. But through food. Through movement. Through will.

Food as Code: Rethinking What Nourishes Us

Too often, dietary advice is reduced to calories and restrictions when the true power lies in the **composition** of food. Think of whole food not just as sustenance, but as biological software - data that programs your metabolism. Highly processed foods overload and misinform the system; whole foods recalibrate it.

Your strategy: Choose a diet rich in fibre, antioxidants, and nutrients - a pattern of eating that is high in fruits, vegetables, legumes, nuts, seeds, and healthy fats. While many names exist - Mediterranean, paleo, low-carb - the core is the same: real food, unprocessed, plant-forward, and rich in monounsaturated fats. Avocados, olive oil, walnuts, almonds - these aren't just tasty additions. They're biochemical allies that promote insulin sensitivity and fat oxidation.

Green tea is more than a trendy drink. It contains **epigallocatechin gallate (EGCG)**, a compound that has been shown to reduce liver inflammation and lipid accumulation. Incorporating two to three cups a day may quietly tip your liver's balance from inflamed to healing.

Exercise: The Unsung Liver Tonic

The liver is a resilient organ, but it responds remarkably to movement. You don't need to run marathons or train like an athlete - just move consistently. Both aerobic and resistance exercises reduce hepatic fat, and the effect appears to be dose-independent; even moderate activity works.

What matters is not how hard you go, but how often. Like brushing your teeth, daily movement is hygiene for your metabolic health. Exercise improves insulin sensitivity, burns visceral fat early in the weight-loss process, and even alters gene expression in ways that favour liver repair.

Helpful Supplements: Tools from Nature's Cabinet

Supplements are not shortcuts - but they can amplify your efforts. The following have shown promise:

- **Berberine**: Derived from plants, berberine acts like a natural metformin. In clinical studies, 500 mg taken three times daily alongside physical activity reduced liver fat by over 50% in just 16 weeks. It also helps with blood sugar, insulin, and lipid control.
- **Fish Oil (EPA & DHA)**: Found in fatty fish like sardines and salmon, these omega-3 fatty acids are potent anti-inflammatory agents. A dose of 2 to 4 grams daily has been shown to reduce liver fat by up to 33%.
- **Probiotics**: In cases of fatty liver linked to gut dysbiosis, probiotics can re-establish microbial balance and reduce inflammation.
- **Soluble Fibre**: High in oats, psyllium husk, flaxseed, and legumes. Consuming 10 to 15 grams of fibre daily enhances insulin sensitivity and reduces liver enzymes - a sign of less hepatic stress.

Why This Matters: The Metabolic Nexus

When fat crowds the liver, it slows down your entire metabolic engine. You gain weight more easily - your energy production lags. And worst of all, you develop **central obesity**, the type most associated with insulin resistance and cardiovascular risk.

This becomes especially relevant when considering related conditions, such as **obstructive sleep apnoea (OSA)**. Fat in the upper airway and abdomen increases the risk of nighttime hypoxia episodes, where oxygen levels dip repeatedly. These not only exhaust the body but also fuel liver inflammation and fibrosis. This vicious cycle of fat, inflammation, and hormonal disruption sets the stage for liver scarring and advanced disease.

Understanding this connection is crucial. It allows you to see OSA not just as a breathing disorder but as a **metabolic amplifier**, with fatty liver as both a cause and consequence. The next chapter will delve into OSA in greater depth.

Key Takeaways

- **Whole food diets** rich in fibre and monounsaturated fats reduce liver fat and improve insulin sensitivity.
- **Consistent physical activity**, regardless of intensity, reduces liver fat content and supports weight loss.
- Supplements such as **berberine, omega-3 fish oils, probiotics, and soluble fibre** can reinforce your lifestyle efforts.
- Addressing fatty liver early can not only reverse insulin resistance but also prevent downstream complications like type 2 diabetes and OSA.

In essence, the liver responds well to love. Feed it wisely, move your body, manage stress, and the silent invader retreats.

CHAPTER 9

A Breath of Insight – Sleep Apnoea and the Metabolic Maze

The first time I truly encountered obstructive sleep apnoea (OSA), I wasn't looking for it.

It was over 25 years ago, during my time at King's College Hospital in London. I was still relatively early in my clinical journey, navigating the tides of complex presentations and piecing together the mosaic of metabolic syndrome in real patients. A case from that period, seemingly routine at first, remains etched in my mind - not for its drama, but for its subtle unravelling of a hidden condition.

She was 35, morbidly obese, and had recently moved from Portugal to London - her chief complaint: a persistent, unrelenting headache. There had been no trauma, no fever, no signs of infection - but the headache was severe, and her lethargy was unmistakable. More striking, though, was how easily she drifted off during our conversation. A nap seemed to hover just under her eyelids, tugging her into sleep. Her blood pressure was slightly elevated, and in a precautionary sweep for a possible stroke, I ordered a head CT. It came back clear. Still concerned, I admitted her for observation.

She was mistakenly placed in the high-dependency unit - a

clinical misstep that turned out to be serendipitous.

The next morning, I was greeted by a flurry of notes from the night nurse. The patient has had multiple oxygen desaturations during the night - episodes where her oxygen levels dropped dramatically. These dips were not subtle. They were stark, alarming, and cyclic. Her blood pressure, too, had fluctuated wildly, at times reaching dangerous highs. The nurse mentioned something else almost in passing: the patient had snored so loudly that other patients had complained.

A senior respiratory consultant happened to be in the unit. I approached him with curiosity, and as soon as I mentioned the oxygen drops and the nocturnal symphony of snores, his interest was piqued. "Could be sleep apnoea," he said, almost reflexively, as if this clinical puzzle had only one solution. At the time, it wasn't a term I'd used often. But that was about to change.

I returned to the patient's bedside and gently reopened the conversation. She admitted something personal - she had recently separated from her boyfriend in Portugal. It wasn't just the usual drift of relationships, she said. "He couldn't take the snoring anymore." Her voice cracked with a mix of frustration and embarrassment. "It was ruining our sleep - and our lives."

This turned the case on its head. We arranged a sleep study, and it confirmed what we had suspected: she had moderate-to-severe obstructive sleep apnoea. CPAP (continuous positive airway pressure) was recommended, and although she tried it, she was hesitant to commit. She longed for a natural solution.

With my growing interest in holistic approaches and metabolic health, I proposed something that seemed deceptively simple but was profoundly challenging: weight loss. I believed - strongly - that her sleep apnoea was not just a standalone respiratory condition but a downstream manifestation of metabolic syndrome. Excess visceral fat, insulin resistance, systemic inflammation - these were not just abstract concepts. They were suffocating her every night.

The Hidden Link: Sleep Apnoea and Metabolic Syndrome

In hindsight, her case was a classic - but at the time, it was a revelation.

Obstructive sleep apnoea and metabolic syndrome are partners in a quiet but destructive dance. The relationship is bidirectional. OSA can aggravate insulin resistance, elevate blood pressure, and worsen dyslipidaemia. Conversely, the components of metabolic syndrome - especially central obesity - physically predispose individuals to OSA by altering airway anatomy and impairing neuromuscular control during sleep.

More intriguingly, sleep apnoea acts like a metabolic amplifier. Intermittent hypoxia from apnoeic episodes increases sympathetic tone, stimulates the release of inflammatory cytokines, and contributes to oxidative stress. This cascade not only perpetuates insulin resistance but also contributes to endothelial dysfunction and atherogenesis - further entrenching cardiovascular risk.

In patients like my Portuguese patient, the cycle becomes self-sustaining. Poor sleep worsens appetite regulation (think ghrelin and leptin), leading to increased caloric intake and further weight gain. The metabolic milieu becomes more hostile. Fatigue leads to sedentary habits. Blood pressure creeps up, and glucose control slips. And the syndrome deepens.

What is Obstructive Sleep Apnoea?

Obstructive sleep apnoea (OSA) has ancient roots - references to sleep-related breathing disorders date back to 4000 BC. Charles Dickens gave it a name, in a way, through his character Joe in *The Pickwick Papers*, a perpetually drowsy boy whose noisy slumber later inspired the term "Pickwickian syndrome." It wasn't until the 1960s that the term "sleep apnoea" was formally introduced, describing the partial or complete blockage of the upper airway during sleep, particularly in people with obesity.

At its core, OSA is a nightly tug-of-war between airflow and obstruction. The airway narrows or collapses repeatedly during sleep, cutting off oxygen (a condition known as intermittent hypoxia), which prompts brief awakenings - often unnoticed - and results in loud snoring, poor sleep quality, and chronic fatigue. Over time, these disruptions take a toll on the body and mind.

In the UK, one in six people are affected - a figure that has climbed with the rise in obesity. As discussed earlier in the book, the relationship between OSA and metabolic syndrome is reciprocal: one condition feeds into the other. OSA increases the risk of developing obesity, diabetes, and cardiovascular disease, and in turn, these metabolic conditions can worsen OSA.

The effects aren't limited to the night. Poor-quality sleep can make daytime feel like wading through mud - lethargy, irritability, poor concentration, and even moments of "microsleep" where the brain dozes off for a few seconds, which can be especially dangerous while driving. Immunity weakens too, making infections more frequent. In the long run, untreated OSA shortens lifespan. A significant study from Wisconsin found that those with untreated OSA had a nearly fourfold increase in all-cause mortality and a fivefold increase in death from cardiovascular causes.

Not All Snoring is Equal

Snoring is a hallmark of OSA, but not all snorers have sleep apnoea. About 60% of adults snore habitually, yet only a fraction - 13% of men and 6% of women in the UK - are diagnosed with OSA. The difference lies in what happens between the snores.

Benign or "simple" snoring occurs when airflow vibrates relaxed throat tissues but doesn't stop breathing. On the other hand, "pathological" snoring - marked by gasping, choking, or pauses in breathing - signals the presence of OSA and needs attention.

Snoring tends to worsen with age and weight gain. Men snore more than women, although postmenopausal women catch up. Alcohol, sedatives, and smoking all increase the risk by relaxing throat muscles or irritating the airway, making collapse more likely. Even family anatomy can play a role: narrow airways, large tonsils, or nasal blockage can all lead to snoring. Sleeping on your back is also a common culprit, as gravity pulls the tongue backwards into the airway. Simply turning onto your side can make a noticeable difference.

When to Be Concerned

Snoring that's getting louder, interrupted by silences or choking sounds. It's time to ask a bed partner for details. According to the British Snoring and Sleep Apnoea Association, OSA is suspected when breathing stops for more than 10 seconds at least five times per hour of sleep. These pauses often end with a loud snort or gasp as the brain briefly wakes the person to resume breathing.

Those with OSA often wake dozens - even hundreds - of times per night, though they rarely remember it. What they do notice is the aftermath: daytime sleepiness, headaches, poor mood, low libido, and flagging concentration. Falling asleep in meetings, during conversations, or while driving may become a common occurrence.

Why Neck Size Matters

In children, OSA is often caused by large tonsils and adenoids. Left untreated, it can affect growth, learning, and behaviour, especially in children with obesity. In adults, neck circumference provides a valuable clue. As mentioned in Chapter 1, it's a simple but powerful measurement. A neck wider than 38 cm (15 inches) in men or 32 cm (12.6 inches) in women suggests a higher risk of OSA,

not just due to overall weight, but because excess fat around the neck narrows the airway.

Diagnosing Sleep Apnoea

The gold standard for diagnosing OSA is a **sleep study**, or polysomnography. This comprehensive test tracks brain waves, eye movement, breathing patterns, heart rate, blood pressure, and oxygen levels overnight. While traditionally done in a sleep clinic, home-based versions using portable monitors are increasingly common and reliable.

During the test, the number of apnoea events per hour determines the severity:

- **Mild:** 5–15 episodes
- **Moderate:** 16–30 episodes
- **Severe:** More than 30

In severe cases, oxygen levels can drop to 75% or lower, placing enormous strain on the heart and brain.

Case Study: When Lifestyle Alone Isn't Enough

Barbra, 55, arrived at the clinic perplexed. Despite her determined efforts to overhaul her lifestyle, her blood glucose levels remained stubbornly elevated. She had adopted a low-carbohydrate, low-sugar diet rich in fibre from vegetables, legumes, and heart-healthy fats found in avocados, nuts, and seeds. Her commitment extended beyond the plate - she regularly practised yoga and Pilates and kept active with walking and swimming.

Her dedication paid off in many respects. Barbra's weight dropped significantly, and her body mass index stabilised at a healthy 24.5 kg/m². But despite this, metabolic red flags persisted. Her waist circumference remained elevated at 96.5 cm, and her waist-to-hip ratio stood at 0.95 - well above the recommended threshold for women. Her neck circumference, another subtle yet telling marker of metabolic strain, measured 36.8 cm. Blood pressure hovered at the upper limit of normal, at 135/85 mmHg. Most telling of all, her fasting glucose lingered at 6.5 mmol/L - a persistent prediabetic level.

Intrigued by this disconnect between lifestyle improvements and metabolic outcomes, we turned to continuous glucose monitoring (CGM). The results were revealing. Barbra's glucose levels were relatively stable during the day, but at night, they fluctuated unpredictably. This nocturnal pattern, combined with reports of loud snoring, pointed to a frequently overlooked culprit: obstructive sleep apnoea (OSA).

A formal sleep study confirmed the suspicion. Barbra experienced apnoea events - brief pauses in breathing - 30 times per hour during sleep. This fragmented her rest, explaining her persistent fatigue despite sleeping 7 to 8 hours each night. With the initiation of nasal CPAP therapy, the transformation was striking. Barbra began sleeping deeply and waking refreshed. Her blood pressure normalised, and most importantly, her glucose levels stabilised both day and night.

Barbra's story serves as a reminder that metabolic health is multifaceted. Weight loss, dietary discipline, and exercise are powerful tools - but sometimes, underlying issues like sleep-disordered breathing must be addressed before the full benefits of lifestyle change can be realised.

The Metabolic Consequences of Obstructive Sleep Apnoea

Obstructive sleep apnoea (OSA) is far more than a sleep disorder - it is a systemic condition with wide-reaching metabolic implications. Among its most concerning consequences is its role in the development and progression of metabolic syndrome, a cluster of conditions including high blood pressure, elevated blood glucose, abnormal lipid levels, and central obesity. At the core of this link lies a cascade of physiological disruptions triggered by repeated episodes of breathing cessation and oxygen deprivation during sleep.

Hypoxia, the Stress Response, and Glucose Dysregulation

In individuals with OSA, the airway intermittently collapses during sleep, leading to recurrent apnoea (pauses in breathing) and consequent nocturnal hypoxemia (low blood oxygen levels). These events activate the sympathetic nervous system - the body's acute stress response mechanism. Each apnoeic episode mimics a physiological emergency, causing the body to release stress hormones, particularly adrenaline.

This surge in adrenaline has a direct metabolic impact. It prompts the liver to break down glycogen (its stored form of glucose) and engage in gluconeogenesis, the synthesis of glucose from non-carbohydrate sources. The result is a rise in circulating blood glucose levels, even during rest. Unlike the controlled glucose fluctuations seen in healthy individuals, these nocturnal spikes are abnormal and sustained, contributing over time to insulin resistance - a hallmark of metabolic syndrome.

If left untreated, this chronic dysregulation of blood glucose can evolve into type 2 diabetes. Fortunately, effective treatment strategies such as continuous positive airway pressure (CPAP) therapy and weight loss have been shown to restore more stable glucose metabolism, reduce insulin resistance, and significantly lower the risk of diabetic complications.

Leptin Resistance: The Hormonal Bridge

Another key player linking OSA to metabolic syndrome is leptin, a hormone secreted by adipose (fat) tissue that regulates appetite and energy balance. Under normal conditions, leptin signals satiety, helping to suppress appetite and reduce food intake. However, in individuals with obesity and OSA, leptin levels are paradoxically elevated - a condition known as leptin resistance.

This resistance renders the body unresponsive to leptin's regulatory effects, perpetuating overeating and further weight gain. Moreover, elevated leptin levels are associated with increased insulin resistance, compounding the metabolic dysfunction initiated by glucose instability. Research has consistently demonstrated that patients with OSA exhibit higher circulating leptin levels, even when adjusted for body mass index, suggesting that OSA contributes independently to leptin dysregulation.

Cardiovascular Strain and Hypertension

Beyond its metabolic effects, OSA imposes significant stress on the cardiovascular system. Each apnoeic event triggers a sympathetic surge, not only elevating glucose levels but also increasing heart rate and blood pressure. Over time, the body adapts to these nocturnal stress signals by maintaining higher daytime blood pressure, which can lead to sustained hypertension.

Persistent high blood pressure, in turn, is a major contributor to the cardiovascular component of metabolic syndrome. OSA is now recognised as an independent risk factor for a range of serious cardiac conditions, including myocardial infarction (heart attack), stroke, heart failure, and cardiac arrhythmias. In severe cases, the disrupted breathing patterns of OSA may even lead to bradycardia (abnormally slow heart rate), cardiac arrest, or ventricular asystole (complete cessation of heart activity).

Treatment of Obstructive Sleep Apnoea (OSA)

Beyond Machines: The Holistic Lens

Today, OSA is more widely diagnosed and managed - often with remarkable results using CPAP. But I remain an advocate for upstream interventions. Addressing root causes, especially weight loss through nutritional changes, physical activity, and insulin sensitivity restoration. Several non-invasive strategies can markedly reduce symptoms in mild to moderate cases and enhance the efficacy of more advanced therapies in severe cases.

It's a point worth emphasising while machines manage the mechanics of breathing, lifestyle changes alter the biology of disease.

Foundational Lifestyle Adjustments

Simple behavioural changes can significantly impact the severity of OSA. These include:

- **Smoking cessation** reduces airway inflammation.
- **Avoiding alcohol**, especially in the evening, to prevent airway muscle relaxation.
- **Nasal decongestion**, using nasal strips or sprays to promote airflow.
- **Sleep positioning**, particularly side-sleeping, helps prevent the tongue from collapsing backwards into the airway.

Patients should also avoid medications that relax the upper airway musculature - such as sedatives, muscle relaxants, antihistamines, and sleeping pills - which can worsen airway collapse during sleep.

Oral Devices and Surgical Options

In cases where anatomical factors contribute to airway obstruction, simple intraoral appliances can help. These devices reposition the jaw and tongue forward to maintain airway patency during sleep. For individuals with enlarged tonsils, nasal polyps, or a deviated septum, surgical intervention may be necessary to open nasal or pharyngeal passages and facilitate airflow.

Continuous Positive Airway Pressure (CPAP)

CPAP therapy remains the cornerstone of treatment for moderate to severe OSA. By delivering a continuous stream of pressurised air via a nasal or full-face mask, CPAP prevents airway collapse during sleep, dramatically reducing apnoeic events. Its benefits are systemic and include:

- **Improved blood pressure control**,
- **Enhanced insulin sensitivity**, and
- **Reduced risk of cardiovascular and metabolic disease**.

Importantly, CPAP has demonstrated efficacy in normalising cardiac rhythms. In one clinical study, CPAP therapy corrected asymptomatic bradyarrhythmias in 7 out of 8 patients with OSA, obviating the need for permanent pacemaker insertion.

Despite its effectiveness, **compliance remains a significant challenge**. Only about half of CPAP users adhere to the recommended use, at least four hours per night on five or more nights per week. Addressing discomfort, claustrophobia, and dry mouth can improve long-term adherence.

Obesity: The Modifiable Risk Factor

Excess body weight is the strongest modifiable risk factor for OSA.

A 10% reduction in body weight can lead to substantial improvements in airway patency and a decrease in symptom severity. Thus, **comprehensive weight management** is a foundational component of OSA treatment.

Lifestyle modifications, including a whole-food, plant-forward diet and regular physical activity, not only reduce OSA severity but also improve overall cardiometabolic health. When combined with CPAP, these changes yield synergistic benefits.

Diet and Exercise Interventions

Adopting a dietary pattern like the **Mediterranean diet** - rich in fruits, vegetables, legumes, fish, and poultry, and low in red meat and saturated fats - has been shown to have independent benefits in reducing OSA symptoms, regardless of weight loss or CPAP use. Specific foods, such as cherries, broccoli, and cucumbers, may also contribute to anti-inflammatory and antioxidative effects, whereas excessive intake of red meat and dairy may exacerbate airway inflammation.

The **American College of Sports Medicine** recommends 150 minutes of moderate-intensity cardiorespiratory exercise per week. However, patients with OSA often struggle with fatigue and reduced exercise tolerance. Graded, individualised programs are more appropriate and sustainable.

Emerging evidence highlights the role of **oropharyngeal muscle training** in the management of OSA. Strengthening the muscles of the tongue, throat, and soft palate - through targeted exercises, wind instrument use, or even structured vocal training (e.g., daily singing) - has been shown to reduce snoring, daytime somnolence, and sleep fragmentation.

Final Thoughts

As this chapter illustrates, OSA is intricately linked with the broader pathophysiology of metabolic syndrome, forming a vicious cycle of systemic inflammation, insulin resistance, and sympathetic activation. Encouragingly, OSA often responds to a combination of **low-tech lifestyle interventions** and **high-tech medical therapies**.

Additionally, the impact of OSA extends to oral health. Mouth breathing, reduced salivary flow, and bruxism (teeth grinding) are common among OSA patients and can increase the risk of periodontal disease. As research continues to reveal the interconnectivity between sleep, metabolism, and oral health, addressing OSA becomes even more critical. We will explore the relationship between OSA and periodontal disease in the following chapter.

CHAPTER 10

Periodontal Disease: A Local Problem with Systemic Consequences

In clinical practice, I routinely observe patients presenting with symptoms such as tooth pain, bleeding gums, and persistent bad breath. These are hallmark signs of periodontal (gum) disease - a condition often perceived as merely dental but, in fact, with far-reaching systemic consequences. I emphasise to patients the importance of consulting both their dentist and physician. Addressing periodontal disease is not only vital for preserving oral health but also for preventing or mitigating serious metabolic conditions such as hypertension, type 2 diabetes, and cardiovascular disease.

Maintaining Oral Health can Save Lives.
This chapter explores the intricate relationship between periodontal disease and metabolic syndrome. We will examine the stages of gum disease, delve into the mechanisms that connect oral and systemic health, and discuss prevention strategies that target both dental and metabolic conditions.

Healthy Gums: The First Line of Defence

At birth, all individuals have healthy, soft gums - typically pink in colour, though this may vary with ethnicity. These gums form a tight seal around the teeth, shielding the underlying bone and preventing the formation of pockets where bacteria can thrive. When this natural barrier is compromised, the consequences extend well beyond the mouth.

From Leaky Gums to Leaky Systems

Periodontal disease stands as a compelling example of how a local pathology can trigger systemic dysfunction. It illustrates the concept of "leaky borders" - where breakdown in one barrier (e.g., oral epithelium) increases vulnerability in others, such as the intestinal lining or blood-brain barrier. Chronic gum inflammation facilitates the entry of bacterial toxins and inflammatory mediators into circulation, fuelling systemic inflammation and insulin resistance. This interconnectedness highlights the potential of a unified clinical strategy: by managing periodontal disease, we can simultaneously address metabolic dysregulation.

The following case illustrates how neglected gum disease contributed to significant systemic illness.

Case Study:
A Life Unravelling from the Gums Outward

Helen, a 57-year-old woman, presented with a complex medical history that included frequent migraines and a longstanding metabolic disease. Since childhood, she reported a strong craving for sugar and carbohydrate-rich foods, which led to significant weight gain and, eventually, obesity. Despite multiple dieting efforts, Helen was unable to achieve lasting weight loss. Over time, she developed high blood pressure, insulin resistance, and abnormal lipid profile - hallmarks of **metabolic syndrome**.

Her clinical findings included:

- A **BMI** of 31.4 kg/m² (classified as obesity),
- **Blood pressure** of 145/95 mmHg (grade 1 hypertension),
- **Waist circumference** of 44 inches (111 cm),
- **Acanthosis nigricans** in her right armpit, signalling insulin resistance,
- An enlarged, likely **fatty liver**,
- **Dyslipidaemia**: total cholesterol of 5.9 mmol/L, LDL cholesterol of 4.9 mmol/L, and HDL cholesterol of 0.93 mmol/L,
- **Elevated uric acid** at 425 µmol/L,
- **HbA1c** at 39 mmol/mol (5.7%), consistent with prediabetes,
- **hs-CRP** of 2.7 mg/L, indicating chronic low-grade inflammation.

Recently, Helen underwent coronary angioplasty with the placement of **two stents** to treat narrowed coronary arteries - an urgent intervention following the onset of angina. Despite the procedure, her risk for major cardiovascular events remained high due to her persistently abnormal lipid profile and systemic inflammation, both of which promote thrombosis.

The Overlooked Origin: Chronic Gum Disease

Helen had suffered from periodontal disease for most of her adult life. It began with intermittent tooth pain, bleeding gums, and halitosis. Over time, she received 17 mercury (amalgam) fillings, multiple rounds of antibiotics for recurring gum infections, and treatment for repeated dental abscesses. However, she dismissed these symptoms as minor or inevitable - never suspecting a link to her systemic health.

This misconception is common - many view gum disease as a localised dental issue, unaware of its systemic implications.

The Hidden Burden of Gum Disease

Gum disease is highly prevalent, affecting approximately **42% of adults**, and typically begins around **middle age**. Its systemic effects are profound. Research shows that periodontal disease **doubles the risk of cardiovascular events** and is significantly associated with: [2]

- **Obesity**,
- **Hypertension**,
- **Type 2 diabetes**,
- **Non-alcoholic fatty liver disease (NAFLD)**,
- **Dementia**,
- **Colorectal cancer**.

In short, periodontal disease is not merely an oral health issue - it is a chronic inflammatory condition with systemic repercussions.

This case underscores the need for a paradigm shift in how we approach oral health. The mouth is not an isolated system but an integral part of the body. Periodontal care must be viewed as part of comprehensive chronic disease prevention.

In the following sections, we will explore how gum disease progresses, the mechanisms linking it to systemic inflammation, and how early intervention can halt its destructive course - not only in the mouth, but throughout the body.

Plaque: A Gateway to Dental and Systemic Disease

Dental plaque is more than just an unsightly film on the teeth - it is a dynamic, bacteria-laden biofilm that can initiate a cascade of oral and systemic health problems. When plaque accumulates along the gumline, it becomes a fertile ground for bacteria that inflame the gums, leading initially to **gingivitis**, the earliest stage of gum disease. This condition is characterised by redness, swelling, and bleeding of the gums, often occurring during brushing or flossing.

With diligent oral hygiene - regular brushing, flossing, and dental check-ups - gingivitis is reversible. However, if left unaddressed, the disease can advance. Bacteria-laden plaque begins to disrupt the delicate seal between the teeth and gums, forming periodontal "pockets" that allow deeper bacterial infiltration. As the infection penetrates, it damages the connective tissues and bone that support the teeth - a condition known as **periodontitis**.

The Escalating Effects of Gum Disease

As periodontitis progresses, the gums recede, and teeth may begin to feel loose. Tooth sensitivity, pain, persistent halitosis (bad breath), and visible gum recession are common. One major culprit is the fermentation of dietary sugars by oral bacteria, which produces lactic acid. This acid not only erodes tooth enamel but also worsens inflammation, accelerating tissue damage.

Advanced cases of gum disease often require professional intervention. Dentists may perform scaling and root planning to remove hardened plaque, known as **tartar or calculus**, which cannot be removed by brushing alone. Tartar, formed from mineralised plaque, creates a rough surface that harbours further bacterial growth. Over time, if the jawbone is significantly eroded, even tooth replacement via dental implants becomes difficult or impossible, as implants require stable bone for anchorage.

Risk Factors for Periodontal Disease

Multiple factors increase the risk of gum disease:

- Inadequate oral hygiene
- Diets high in sugar and refined carbohydrates
- Dry mouth (xerostomia) due to dehydration, stress, or autoimmune diseases
- Use of medications such as diuretics, anticholinergics, oral contraceptives, and sedatives
- Chronic sleep deprivation
- Tobacco smoking

These factors not only disrupt the oral environment but can also impair immune responses, making it easier for oral infections to become chronic.

The Metabolic Connection:
Periodontitis and Systemic Inflammation

There is now compelling evidence linking **periodontal disease with metabolic syndrome**, a cluster of conditions including obesity, insulin resistance, hypertension, and dyslipidaemia. The common denominator appears to be **chronic systemic inflammation and oxidative stress.**[3]

Periodontal disease contributes to a persistent, low-grade inflammatory state that can worsen insulin resistance, further fuelling the metabolic syndrome. As discussed in previous chapters, insulin resistance plays a pivotal role in weight gain, increased waist circumference, and cardiovascular risk.

Among the metabolic syndrome components, **hyperglycaemia and obesity** show the strongest association with periodontitis. While hypertension and abnormal lipid profiles (dyslipidaemia) also contribute, their impact is less pronounced. Notably, the **risk of periodontitis increases with the number of metabolic syndrome components present**, suggesting a cumulative effect.[4]

Bi-directional Benefits: Treating the Mouth to Heal the Body
Improved oral hygiene and periodontal care have been shown to reduce systemic inflammatory markers, including C-reactive protein (CRP), which are associated with an increased risk of cardiovascular disease.[5] This suggests a potential role for oral care as part of an integrated approach to managing metabolic syndrome.

Physicians should be aware of the oral health status of their patients with metabolic syndrome, and dentists should consider referring patients with signs of systemic inflammation or metabolic dysfunction. Such **interdisciplinary collaboration** could lead to earlier interventions and better health outcomes.

Preventing Plaque: Practical Strategies
Maintaining good gum health goes beyond the toothbrush. Effective plaque control involves:

- Brushing teeth at least twice daily with fluoride toothpaste
- Cleaning interdental spaces using floss or interdental brushes
- Reducing intake of sugary foods and beverages
- Encouraging saliva flow by chewing thoroughly and using sugar-free gum
- Avoiding tobacco
- Staying well-hydrated
- Managing stress and getting sufficient sleep
- Eating a balanced, anti-inflammatory diet rich in whole foods
- Spending time outdoors for sunlight exposure and circadian balance

A Personal Story: Helen's Transformation

Helen's journey illustrates the profound link between oral and systemic health. Diagnosed with early periodontitis and at high risk for cardiovascular disease, she took proactive steps to reverse both. Guided by personalised insights from her genetic and biochemical profile, Helen adopted a targeted lifestyle program. She reduced sugar intake, improved her oral hygiene, and embraced a nutrient-rich, anti-inflammatory diet.

The results were striking. Helen lost significant body fat, normalised her blood glucose levels, improved her lipid profile, and brought her blood pressure under control - all with minimal medication. More importantly, she reported enhanced energy, mental clarity, and emotional well-being. Her story exemplifies how integrative, patient-centred care can transform health from the inside out.

Genetic Testing and Therapeutic Actions in Periodontal Disease

As mentioned earlier, Helen's treatment plan included insights drawn from her genetic profile. While lifestyle factors undeniably play a pivotal role in the development and progression of periodontal disease, genetic predispositions can significantly influence an individual's vulnerability. Recent advances in genetic testing have opened new avenues for personalised care in dentistry and systemic health.

One such innovation is the **DNA Smile** test, developed by Nordic Laboratories. This test examines a broad range of genetic markers that impact oral and systemic health. Specifically, it assesses genetic variants related to both the **innate and adaptive immune systems**, **sugar cravings (often linked to dietary habits)**, **lipid metabolism**, and the **body's ability to detoxify environmental toxins**. This broad scope enables a more comprehensive understanding of why periodontal disease develops in certain individuals, allowing clinicians to tailor interventions accordingly.

For example, the decision to remove **dental amalgam fillings** - which contain mercury - can be informed by a patient's ability to detoxify. Some individuals possess deletions in key genes such as **GSTM1**, **GSTT1**, or **GSTP1**, all of which encode enzymes critical for neutralising and excreting heavy metals. A deficiency in these pathways suggests that the individual may have impaired detoxification and would likely benefit from the removal of mercury-based restorations. Similarly, the presence of **APOE genetic variants** - especially the APOE4 allele - has implications not only for cardiovascular and neurodegenerative disease risk but also offers valuable insights into lipid metabolism dysfunctions, which are relevant in inflammatory and infectious conditions, such as periodontitis.

General therapeutic strategies for managing or preventing periodontal disease include:

- **Cessation of smoking** reduces inflammation and improves healing capacity.
- **Rigorous oral hygiene practices**, such as brushing, flossing, and professional cleanings.
- **Reducing intake of saturated fats**, which are known to exacerbate systemic inflammation.
- **Repopulation of the oral microbiome** with beneficial bacteria, which can suppress pathogenic strains associated with gum disease.

These interventions are not only foundational for dental health but also intersect with broader systemic benefits, particularly in individuals with underlying metabolic disturbances.

Final Reflections: Oral Health and Systemic Implications

Oral health is far more than an aesthetic or localised concern - it is a window into systemic well-being. Although the management of periodontal disease may appear straightforward at first glance, ranging from improved hygiene to more advanced periodontal treatments, its implications reach well beyond the oral cavity.

Helen's case underscores this reality. Despite a serious cardiovascular history - including two coronary stents and an elevated risk of clot formation - she was able to make substantial improvements in her health trajectory through primarily **lifestyle-based interventions**, guided in part by genetic insights. Her story is a testament to the power of personalised, preventative care.

As we draw this chapter to a close, it is worth highlighting one particularly intriguing and emerging connection in medical research: the link between **periodontal disease and benign prostatic hyperplasia (BPH)**. Multiple studies have identified shared risk factors between these two conditions, including **age (especially in men over 50)**, **smoking, obesity**, and **metabolic disorders such as diabetes**. [6] Moreover, periodontal disease not only increases the risk of developing BPH but also appears to exacerbate its progression.

What makes this connection even more compelling is the overlap **in microbes**. In one study, bacteria commonly isolated from dental plaque in the mouth were also found in **prostate secretions**, suggesting a possible microbial bridge between oral infections and prostatic inflammation. [7] These findings emphasise the importance of oral health as a component of systemic disease prevention and will set the stage for our exploration of BPH in the following chapter.

CHAPTER 11

Benign Prostatic Hyperplasia - A Metabolic or Hydraulic Problem?

Benign prostatic hyperplasia (BPH) is a condition characterised by the non-cancerous enlargement of the prostate gland, leading to obstruction of the bladder outlet. Traditionally viewed through a urological lens, BPH is often managed surgically or pharmacologically to relieve obstructive urinary symptoms. However, emerging evidence compels us to ask: Is BPH merely a hydraulic issue best treated with surgical intervention, or is it a metabolic disorder rooted in systemic dysfunction? This chapter examines the nature of BPH and its implications from a holistic, metabolic perspective.

Prevalence and Conventional Approach

BPH is exceedingly common among ageing men. It affects approximately 60% of men over the age of 50 and increases in prevalence to 80% by age 70. It ranks as the fourth most common condition in men over 50, trailing only cardiovascular disease, hypertension, and type 2 diabetes. Symptoms typically include urinary frequency, urgency, nocturia, weak urinary stream, and incomplete bladder emptying - collectively classified as lower urinary tract symptoms (LUTS).

The standard medical approach often centres on pharmacological agents - such as alpha-blockers and 5-alpha-reductase inhibitors - or surgical interventions, particularly transurethral resection of the prostate (TURP). While these treatments offer symptomatic relief, they do not address the root causes of prostatic overgrowth. As a result, patients frequently experience recurrence, ongoing medication dependence, or surgical complications.

Benign Prostatic Hyperplasia

BPH is a benign growth of the prostate obstructing the urethra (urine passage), causing recurrent urinary symptoms.

A Case in Point: Andy's Journey

"I need to start a trouser fund, as my clothes are falling off me."

Andy, a 62-year-old man, was first diagnosed with an enlarged prostate following several months of distressing urinary symptoms. He described frequent daytime urination, multiple nocturnal awakenings to void, and occasional urinary incontinence due to urgency. A weakened stream and the sensation of incomplete emptying further impaired his quality of life.

Imaging revealed a significantly enlarged prostate. A biopsy confirmed the diagnosis of BPH. Like many men, Andy was apprehensive about surgery. He began medical therapy to relax the prostate smooth muscle and improve urinary flow. However, his broader health picture revealed deeper concerns: he had obesity (BMI of 31 kg/m^2), type 2 diabetes, hypertension, and dyslipidaemia - collectively pointing to metabolic syndrome.

Annual prostate monitoring left Andy anxious about the potential cancerous transformation. Dissatisfied with fragmented care, he sought a more integrative approach and enrolled in the Vitality Clinic's lifestyle intervention programme.

Within months of adopting a structured, personalised plan - including a whole-food diet, regular physical activity, stress management, and targeted nutraceuticals - Andy experienced a transformation. He lost over 10 kilograms (more than 10% of his body weight), achieved normal blood glucose, blood pressure, and cholesterol levels, and - most notably - reported significant improvement in urinary function. His sleep was no longer interrupted by frequent urination, and episodes of urgency and incontinence ceased. For the first time in years, Andy felt in control of his health.

Is BPH a Metabolic Disease?

Andy's case is not an anomaly. A growing body of research suggests that BPH is more than just a mechanical problem. Its pathogenesis appears to be closely linked to metabolic dysfunction. Epidemiological studies have demonstrated a strong association between BPH, LUTS, and the components of metabolic syndrome - including insulin resistance, abdominal obesity, and systemic inflammation. Up to 50% of men with LUTS meet the criteria for metabolic syndrome.[2]

The prostate is a hormone-sensitive gland, and its growth is modulated by insulin, insulin-like growth factors, sex hormones, and inflammatory cytokines - all of which are dysregulated in metabolic syndrome. Furthermore, the Western dietary pattern - rich in refined carbohydrates, sugars, and saturated fats - exacerbates this hormonal imbalance and fuels prostatic hypertrophy.

Despite this, BPH continues to be primarily managed in urology clinics, where lifestyle factors are rarely addressed. A paradigm shift is needed: one that integrates metabolic optimisation into the standard care of men with BPH. By doing so, we not only reduce prostate size and relieve urinary symptoms but also mitigate the risk of cardiovascular disease, diabetes, and cancer.

Complications and Cancer Risk

Although BPH is a benign condition, its complications can be severe. Chronic bladder outlet obstruction may lead to recurrent urinary tract infections, bladder stones, and even renal impairment. Moreover, the psychological toll of LUTS - ranging from sleep disturbance to social embarrassment - can significantly impair quality of life.

It is essential to clarify that BPH does not evolve into prostate cancer. However, the two conditions can coexist, and distinguishing between them remains a diagnostic priority. Patients like Andy, who undergo regular monitoring due to concerns about malignancy, often experience ongoing anxiety. Providing holistic care and clear communication can offer reassurance and empower men to take ownership of their health.

Rethinking BPH: A Holistic Model

Benign prostatic hyperplasia, while localised in the urogenital system, may be a sentinel marker of systemic imbalance. A narrow focus on mechanical obstruction misses the broader opportunity to intervene upstream. As we gain a deeper understanding of the metabolic underpinnings of BPH, we are compelled to consider lifestyle medicine not as an adjunct, but as a cornerstone of management. In the chapters ahead, we will continue to explore how metabolic health intersects with seemingly unrelated organ systems - and how a root-cause, patient-centred approach transforms not only lab results but lives.

Prostate Growth and Development

Androgens, a class of steroid hormones, are pivotal in male sexual differentiation and function. Testosterone - the principal androgen - drives the formation of the male genital tract and the growth and maturation of the prostate gland. While the terms "androgen" and "testosterone" are often used interchangeably in clinical discourse, it is testosterone specifically that orchestrates the nuanced stages of prostate development.

At birth, the prostate weighs approximately 1.5 grams. Under the influence of androgens, it expands to about 10 grams during early puberty, reaching around 20 grams by the third decade of life. During this time, growth is uniform and gland-wide. However, from midlife onward, growth becomes selective, occurring predominantly in the periurethral zone - the area surrounding the urethra. This is the anatomical site where benign prostatic hyperplasia (BPH) typically arises.

BPH is characterised by non-malignant enlargement of the prostate, which can progressively encroach upon the urethral lumen. As the urethra becomes compressed, a spectrum of lower urinary tract symptoms (LUTS) may emerge. These include increased urinary frequency and urgency, hesitancy (difficulty initiating urination), weak urinary stream, straining to void, incomplete bladder emptying, nocturia, and, in some cases, urinary incontinence.

Metabolic Syndrome and the Rise of Benign Prostatic Hyperplasia

A growing body of evidence links BPH to metabolic syndrome - a cluster of metabolic abnormalities including central obesity, hypertension, insulin resistance, hyperglycaemia, and dyslipidaemia (particularly elevated triglycerides and low high-density lipoprotein [HDL] cholesterol). Several large-scale epidemiological and clinical studies reinforce this association:

- **Hypertension:** Hypertensive individuals tend to have larger prostate volumes and more rapid prostate growth than normotensive counterparts.[3] In a study of 2,372 men, LUTS were significantly more prevalent among those with elevated blood pressure.[4]
- **Dyslipidaemia:** A Taiwanese cohort demonstrated that men with BPH exhibited significantly higher levels of total and low-density lipoprotein (LDL) cholesterol, coupled with lower HDL levels, compared to controls.[5] Similarly, a U.S.-based study of over 51,000 men aged 40-75 years found that central obesity strongly predicted both the incidence and progression of LUTS.[6]
- **Central Obesity:** In the Baltimore Longitudinal Study of Ageing, obesity was associated with a 3.5-fold increased likelihood of prostate enlargement. Each unit increase in body mass index (BMI) correlated with a 0.41 mL increase in prostate volume.[7] Waist circumference, a more direct marker of visceral fat, has also been implicated. Men with waist measurements over 109 cm (42.9 inches) were 2.4

times more likely to undergo surgical intervention for BPH than those with waistlines under 89 cm (35 inches)[8]. Notably, larger waist circumference was also predictive of post-surgical complications.[9]

Pathophysiological Mechanisms Linking Metabolic Syndrome and BPH

At the cellular level, metabolic syndrome promotes a hormonal environment conducive to prostate enlargement.

Hyperinsulinemia - a hallmark of insulin resistance - stimulates the proliferation of prostatic epithelial and stromal cells. It also disrupts the androgen-oestrogen balance critical for normal prostate homeostasis.

Elevated insulin levels increase hepatic production of sex hormone-binding globulin (SHBG), which binds circulating testosterone, thereby reducing the fraction of bioavailable free testosterone. Concurrently, visceral adiposity enhances the peripheral conversion of androgens to oestrogens via aromatase activity. This excess oestrogen imposes negative feedback on the hypothalamic-pituitary-gonadal axis, suppressing luteinizing hormone (LH) secretion and, consequently, testosterone synthesis - a condition known as hypogonadism.

The net result is a hormonal milieu marked by androgen deficiency and relative oestrogen excess, which favours the development of BPH. This endocrine imbalance may also explain why men who are castrated before puberty do not develop BPH.

BPH and Prostate Cancer: Distinct but Coexisting

It is crucial to differentiate BPH from prostate cancer. BPH is not a precancerous lesion and does not inherently increase the risk of malignancy. Anatomically, BPH originates in the transitional (periurethral) zone of the prostate, whereas prostate cancer predominantly arises in the peripheral zone. However, the two conditions can coexist in the same individual.

Because both BPH and prostate cancer can elevate prostate-specific antigen (PSA) levels, distinguishing between them is critical. PSA elevations due to BPH are generally modest and less diagnostically significant than those associated with malignancy.

Historically, digital rectal examination (DRE) served as a frontline tool for prostate assessment. A benign prostate feels smooth and rubbery, whereas a malignant one is often firm, nodular, or irregular. Although DRE remains a useful clinical tool, its diagnostic value has largely been superseded by advanced imaging and laboratory testing.

Complications of Untreated BPH

BPH can lead to serious complications if not addressed. Progressive enlargement may culminate in acute urinary retention, often necessitating catheterisation. Chronic obstruction increases the risk of urinary tract infections, bladder stone formation, and potentially irreversible kidney damage due to hydronephrosis and chronic kidney disease.

Timely diagnosis and appropriate medical or surgical intervention can prevent these sequelae and significantly improve quality of life.

Metabolic Dysfunction and Related Urogenital Disorders

BPH is not the only urogenital condition influenced by metabolic derangements. Erectile dysfunction (ED) and hypogonadism frequently coexist with insulin resistance. Hyperinsulinemia impairs endothelial function and nitric oxide synthesis - both essential for penile erection and vascular integrity.

Moreover, the reduction in bioavailable testosterone due to increased SHBG and aromatisation contributes to testicular underdevelopment and diminished sexual function. These overlapping pathologies underscore the systemic impact of metabolic syndrome on male reproductive and urologic health.

Addressing insulin resistance through lifestyle intervention, weight loss, and pharmacologic therapy holds promise not only for mitigating BPH progression but also for restoring hormonal balance and improving sexual health.

Management: Treat the Metabolism, Not Just the Symptoms

The conventional medical approach to benign prostatic hyperplasia (BPH) and lower urinary tract symptoms (LUTS) tends to focus on structural interventions - most notably, surgical procedures aimed at relieving urethral obstruction. While such procedures can provide symptomatic relief, they do not address the underlying causes that drive prostate enlargement and urinary dysfunction in the first place.

This symptom-focused paradigm overlooks a critical insight: **BPH and LUTS are often downstream manifestations of broader metabolic dysfunction**. Convincing both clinicians and the public to shift focus from surgical correction to metabolic restoration remains a challenge, but one with considerable reward. The evidence increasingly suggests that metabolic health is a key modifiable factor in the development and progression of BPH and LUTS.

Targeting Modifiable Risk Factors

Lifestyle interventions - improving diet, increasing physical activity, and reducing tobacco and alcohol use - hold remarkable potential for reversing not only LUTS and BPH but also their upstream driver: metabolic syndrome. These modifiable behaviours directly influence insulin sensitivity, systemic inflammation, hormonal balance, and lipid metabolism - all of which intersect with prostatic growth and urinary function.

The Power of Weight Loss and Exercise

Numerous studies support the notion that **sustained weight loss and increased physical activity can significantly improve LUTS and reduce prostate volume**. A consistent finding is that losing more than 10% of body weight correlates with measurable improvements in metabolic parameters and urinary symptoms.

For instance, a large Korean cohort study found that men with sedentary lifestyles were significantly more likely to experience severe LUTS. In contrast, those who engaged in regular physical activity reported fewer symptoms. Another study in men over 45 demonstrated a clear inverse relationship between physical activity levels and LUTS severity.

Diet: Fruits, Vegetables, and Nutritional Compounds

Dietary patterns also exert a measurable influence. **High consumption of fruits and vegetables, particularly those rich in antioxidants and phytonutrients, is associated with a reduced risk of BPH and LUTS severity.** Leafy greens are protective. Nutrients like - carotene, lutein, and vitamin C - when consumed through whole foods rather than supplements - are inversely correlated with BPH progression.

On the flip side, lifestyle factors such as excessive alcohol intake appear detrimental. In Chinese men, the consumption of seven or more alcoholic beverages per week was independently associated with a higher incidence of moderate to severe LUTS. Meanwhile, naturally occurring compounds in **green tea and saw palmetto** have been shown in some studies to exert anti-androgenic and anti-inflammatory effects, potentially shrinking the prostate and alleviating LUTS.

Statins: Metabolic Modulators With Urological Benefits

Interestingly, **statins - primarily prescribed to manage dyslipidaemias - have demonstrated secondary benefits in the context of BPH**. Evidence suggests that these medications can reduce prostate volume, alleviate LUTS, and slow the clinical progression of BPH. These effects are likely mediated through improved lipid profiles and reduced inflammation.

Simvastatin appears to produce a more significant reduction in prostate volume than atorvastatin, especially in men who are obese or have dysregulated lipid profiles. The observed benefits have been linked to reductions in total cholesterol and interleukin-6 (IL-6), a pro-inflammatory cytokine discussed in Chapter 3, alongside increased levels of protective HDL cholesterol.

Diabetes and LUTS: A Compounding Effect

Diabetes represents another major contributor to LUTS. Men with type 2 diabetes experience more frequent and severe urinary symptoms than their non-diabetic counterparts. Moreover, diabetic men receiving treatment still show elevated LUTS prevalence, likely due to persistent metabolic dysregulation. Notably, while treatment may manage glycemia, it does not consistently optimise prostate volume or prostate-specific antigen (PSA) levels.

The Broader Perspective:
Metabolic Health as a Unifying Framework

Surgical treatment of BPH - while sometimes necessary - often bypasses the metabolic roots of the condition. **By failing to address insulin resistance, inflammation, and dyslipidaemias, we miss** the opportunity to resolve not just LUTS but also prevent long-term complications such as cardiovascular disease, stroke, dementia, and type 2 diabetes.

For patients experiencing LUTS or diagnosed with an enlarged prostate, a comprehensive metabolic evaluation is not just prudent - it is essential. Correcting underlying metabolic imbalances may resolve the urological issue while safeguarding long-term health.

A Note on Female Metabolic Equivalents
Although BPH is unique to men, the **metabolic disturbances that drive prostate enlargement have parallels in women**. A prime example is polycystic ovary syndrome (PCOS), a condition characterised by ovarian cysts, hyperandrogenism, insulin resistance, and frequently, obesity. Like BPH, PCOS is rooted in metabolic dysfunction and may manifest with a spectrum of symptoms, including infertility and hirsutism. This condition will be addressed in detail in the following chapter.

CHAPTER 12

Polycystic Ovary Syndrome: A Metabolic Disorder with Far-Reaching Impact

Polycystic ovary syndrome (PCOS) is one of the most common endocrine-metabolic disorders affecting women of reproductive age. Though often underdiagnosed, it is estimated to affect approximately 15% of women in their 20s and 30s, and it remains a leading cause of infertility worldwide. PCOS is far more than a reproductive issue - it is a systemic condition closely tied to insulin resistance, metabolic dysfunction, and cardiovascular risk.

Clinically, PCOS is characterised by a spectrum of signs and symptoms, including menstrual irregularities, chronic anovulation, polycystic ovaries on ultrasound, hyperandrogenism (manifesting as hirsutism, scalp hair thinning, and acne), and central obesity. Many women with PCOS also report persistent fatigue, sleep disturbances, and intense sugar cravings - symptoms rooted in underlying metabolic imbalance.

Crucially, PCOS responds well to lifestyle interventions. Diet, physical activity, and sleep optimisation often lead to significant clinical improvements, even without pharmacological treatment.

A Historical Glimpse

Although the term "polycystic ovary syndrome" gained prominence in the late 20th century, its history dates back several centuries. In 1721, Italian physician Antonio Vallisneri described the case of an infertile woman with large, white, shiny ovaries - likely one of the earliest clinical depictions of PCOS. The condition was later formally characterised by Irving Stein and Michael Leventhal in 1935, hence the historical eponym "Stein-Leventhal syndrome."

Diagnostic clarity has evolved. The National Institutes of Health (NIH) proposed the first formal criteria in 1990, focusing on chronic anovulation and hyperandrogenism. The more inclusive Rotterdam criteria, introduced in 2003 and updated in 2013, allowed for diagnosis with any two of the following: irregular ovulation, hyperandrogenism, or polycystic ovaries - broadening the clinical understanding of PCOS and acknowledging its heterogeneity.

Case Study: Sarah's Journey Through PCOS

To understand the lived experience of PCOS, consider the story of Sarah, a 29-year-old woman who presented with persistent scalp hair thinning and coarse hair growth on her chin - features that undermined her self-esteem and caused her to withdraw from social life.

She and her husband had been trying to conceive for seven years without success. Her menstrual cycles were irregular, often absent for months at a time. She reported mild premenstrual symptoms and a history of benign breast cysts, which she noticed had improved with the addition of broccoli sprouts to her diet - a source of sulforaphane, known for its anti-inflammatory properties.

Sarah's dietary habits, however, were typical of a modern high-glycaemic load lifestyle: frequent consumption of refined carbohydrates, sugary snacks, processed food, and sweetened beverages rich in high-fructose corn syrup. She also drank alcohol in the evenings and reported persistent hunger, fluctuating energy, and an afternoon slump that only resolved in the evening. Her sleep was fragmented and insufficient - she got only six hours of sleep per night - and she awoke feeling unrefreshed.

Physically, Sarah exhibited central obesity, with a body mass index (BMI) of 34.8 kg/m² and a waist-to-hip ratio of 0.95, indicating visceral fat accumulation. Her blood pressure was mildly elevated at 135/85 mmHg. Wearable health data and a subsequent sleep study revealed mild sleep apnoea, a condition frequently associated with insulin resistance.

Laboratory investigations confirmed elevated androgens, and a pelvic ultrasound showed multiple cystic follicles consistent with PCOS. Despite her efforts to exercise - walking, treadmill workouts, resistance training, and Pilates - Sarah was unable to lose weight. In fact, she had recently gained 9 kg (20 lbs). Her concern deepened when she shared that her father had died suddenly of a heart attack in his 50s.

Intervention and Transformation

Following a consultation at the Vitality Clinic, Sarah committed to a comprehensive lifestyle overhaul. She transitioned to a nutrient-dense, whole-food, low-glycaemic index (LGI) diet. She eliminated ultra-processed foods, significantly reduced her sugar intake, and incorporated time-restricted eating and intermittent fasting, eventually extending her fasting duration under the guidance of a clinical expert.

With the support of targeted nutritional supplements and continued physical activity, Sarah experienced a dramatic improvement. She lost a significant amount of weight, regained her confidence, and - most importantly - conceived naturally for the first time.

The Normal Follicle and Ovulation

A follicle is a small, fluid-filled sac located within the ovary, each containing an immature egg (oocyte). At the onset of puberty, a female possesses approximately 500,000 primordial follicles. With each menstrual cycle, a selection process begins, culminating in the maturation of a single dominant follicle that releases an egg around mid-cycle, typically on day 14.

The hypothalamic-pituitary-ovarian axis orchestrates this process. The pituitary gland secretes two key gonadotrophins: luteinising hormone (LH) and follicle-stimulating hormone (FSH). LH stimulates the theca cells in the ovary to produce androgens, primarily testosterone. FSH promotes the conversion of these androgens to oestrogens in the granulosa cells, which in turn drives follicular maturation and the eventual ovulatory release of a fertilisable egg.

Ovarian follicle development can be monitored using ultrasound, particularly during fertility assessments. As women age, both the number of follicles (ovarian reserve) and the quality of oocytes decline, contributing to reduced fertility and irregular ovulation.

The Pathophysiology of Polycystic Ovary Syndrome (PCOS)

Polycystic ovary syndrome is a complex endocrine and metabolic disorder characterised by three principal features: hyperandrogenism (elevated androgens such as testosterone), oligo- or anovulation (infrequent or absent ovulation), and polycystic ovarian morphology.

At the heart of PCOS is a metabolic dysfunction. Most notably, insulin resistance leads to compensatory hyperinsulinaemia. High insulin levels act directly on the ovarian theca cells to stimulate androgen production and suppress hepatic synthesis of sex hormone-binding globulin (SHBG), increasing the proportion of circulating free, biologically active androgens.

This androgen excess disrupts normal follicular development. Oestrogen synthesis becomes impaired, which triggers increased pituitary LH secretion - further amplifying ovarian androgen production in a vicious cycle. Chronic LH stimulation also causes theca cell hyperplasia. Follicular growth stalls at various stages of development, resulting in multiple immature follicles lining the ovarian cortex. This produces the characteristic "string of pearls" appearance seen on ultrasound. Diagnostic criteria include at least one ovary with a volume >10 mL or the presence of ≥10 small antral follicles.

PCOS is strongly associated with metabolic syndrome. Numerous studies confirm that insulin resistance is central to the condition, and interventions that improve insulin sensitivity—such as dietary change, physical activity, or medications like metformin - can substantially reduce androgen levels and restore ovulation.

Contributing Factors in PCOS Diet and the Gut Microbiome
A Western-style diet, high in processed carbohydrates, refined sugars, and industrial seed oils, is a potent driver of metabolic dysfunction and PCOS. Foods such as sugary beverages (especially those sweetened with high-fructose corn syrup), white bread, pizza, and pasta contribute to insulin resistance, weight gain, and hormonal imbalances.

These diets also disrupt the gut microbiome - the complex community of bacteria that inhabits the intestines. In PCOS, microbial diversity is often diminished. Beneficial bacteria, such as *Lactobacillus* and *Bifidobacterium,* are depleted, while potentially pathogenic genera, like *Escherichia* and *Shigella*, proliferate. This dysbiosis increases intestinal permeability, allowing lipopolysaccharides (LPS) - bacterial endotoxins - to enter the bloodstream.

As described in Chapter 3, circulating LPS triggers systemic low-grade inflammation and impairs insulin receptor signalling, thereby exacerbating hyperinsulinaemia and further stimulating androgen production. The result is a reinforcing cycle of metabolic and reproductive dysfunction.

Environmental and Lifestyle Factors

In addition to diet and metabolic factors, several environmental and lifestyle influences have been implicated in PCOS:

- **Vitamin D Deficiency**: Low vitamin D levels are associated with insulin resistance, ovulatory dysfunction, and increased androgen levels.
- **Chronic Stress**: Persistent activation of the hypothalamic-pituitary-adrenal axis leads to elevated cortisol levels, which interfere with gonadotropin signalling and promote insulin resistance.
- **Smoking**: Cigarette smoke contains a variety of harmful substances, including polycyclic aromatic hydrocarbons (PAHs), which induce oxidative stress and disrupt endocrine function. Smoking increases circulating free testosterone and reduces oestrogen levels, promoting ovulatory failure.
- **Exposure to PAHs and Burnt Foods**: PAHs are found in smoke from burning coal or wood, as well as in charred or overcooked foods. These compounds act as endocrine disruptors, increasing the risk of PCOS.

Endocrine Disrupting Chemicals

Emerging evidence also implicates endocrine-disrupting chemicals in the pathogenesis of PCOS. Bisphenol A (BPA), a synthetic compound found in many plastics, exhibits both estrogenic and anti-androgenic properties.[2] Although now regulated in many countries, BPA remains ubiquitous in the environment. Studies consistently show higher BPA levels in women with PCOS, and a positive correlation between BPA concentration and serum testosterone levels has been observed.[3]

Long-Term Health Risks

Although PCOS itself is not classified as a precancerous condition, its underlying hormonal milieu carries significant long-term risks. Persistently elevated androgens and unopposed oestrogen can increase the risk of endometrial hyperplasia and, ultimately, endometrial cancer. Moreover, insulin resistance places affected individuals at heightened risk for developing type 2 diabetes, cardiovascular disease, and non-alcoholic fatty liver disease (NAFLD).

Understanding the multifaceted causes of PCOS - from disrupted folliculogenesis and insulin resistance to environmental exposures - enables targeted lifestyle and medical interventions that can mitigate symptoms, restore ovulation, and reduce long-term health risks.

Treatment

The management of polycystic ovary syndrome (PCOS) hinges on a multifaceted lifestyle approach aimed at addressing its root metabolic causes. Core interventions include adopting a whole-food diet, practising intermittent fasting, engaging in regular physical activity, ensuring adequate sleep, and managing stress. These pillars collectively combat obesity - often a central feature of

PCOS - and help lower insulin levels, support hormonal balance, and restore healthy body weight.

A low glycaemic index (LGI) diet, particularly one rich in unprocessed whole foods, has demonstrated broad metabolic benefits. Clinical evidence shows that such a dietary pattern reduces waist circumference, fasting insulin levels, triglycerides, total cholesterol, low-density lipoprotein (LDL) cholesterol, and androgen levels. When combined with exercise and omega-3 fatty acids, it further elevates high-density lipoprotein (HDL) cholesterol. Moreover, the high fibre content of LGI foods nourishes the gut microbiota, promoting the production of short-chain fatty acids (SCFAs), such as butyrate, which are critical compounds for maintaining gut integrity and systemic metabolic health.

Notably, LGI diets may influence appetite-regulating hormones. In women with PCOS, one study found reductions in ghrelin (a hunger hormone) and increases in glucagon (a hormone that promotes energy expenditure), potentially aiding in long-term weight regulation.[4] A recent meta-analysis confirmed the effectiveness of LGI diets in managing PCOS and recommended routine dietary assessments for all individuals diagnosed with the condition.[5]

Another dietary strategy gaining traction is the ketogenic diet. By severely restricting carbohydrates and increasing fat intake, this approach effectively reduces blood glucose levels, promotes fat loss, and improves menstrual regularity and liver function in women with PCOS, especially those with coexisting obesity or non-alcoholic fatty liver disease. In a 12-week study, participants on a ketogenic diet exhibited significant reductions in body weight, BMI, insulin, triglycerides, total cholesterol, and LDL cholesterol, alongside a rise in HDL cholesterol. Emerging data suggests that ketogenic diets may outperform LGI diets in women with PCOS and advanced metabolic dysfunction.

Exercise

Exercise is a cornerstone intervention for enhancing insulin sensitivity and restoring metabolic homeostasis in PCOS. However, recent findings suggest that the **intensity** of physical activity exerts a more profound effect than duration. A meta-analysis confirmed that vigorous aerobic activity and resistance training significantly improve body composition, insulin responsiveness, and cardiorespiratory fitness in affected women.[6] As such, clinicians should encourage patients with PCOS to engage in high-intensity interval training and resistance-based workouts tailored to individual capabilities.

The Gut Microbiome

An emerging area of interest in PCOS research is the role of the gut microbiome in modulating systemic inflammation, insulin resistance, and androgen excess. Therapeutic strategies targeting the gut include prebiotics, probiotics, and faecal microbiota transplantation (FMT).

Probiotic supplementation with **Lactobacillus acidophilus** for 12 weeks has been shown to reduce body weight and BMI in women with PCOS significantly.[7] Meanwhile, prebiotics - non-digestible fibres that selectively stimulate beneficial gut bacteria - help regulate blood glucose, lower triglycerides and total cholesterol, and increase HDL cholesterol.

FMT represents a more advanced intervention, restoring microbial diversity and increasing SCFA production, especially butyrate. This compound not only enhances gut barrier integrity but also promotes immunoglobulin secretion and reduces systemic inflammation, thereby supporting both gastrointestinal and reproductive health.

Complementary Therapies and Supplements

Acupuncture has shown promise in improving metabolic and reproductive outcomes in PCOS. By modulating neuroendocrine function and increasing β-endorphin levels, acupuncture enhances gonadotropin release, promoting ovulation and menstrual regularity.

Additionally, several nutraceuticals have shown efficacy in managing PCOS. These include:

- **Vitamin D** - for insulin sensitivity and ovarian function
- **Resveratrol** - an antioxidant that reduces androgen levels
- **Alpha-lipoic acid** - for glucose metabolism
- **Omega-3 fatty acids** - for lipid control and inflammation
- **Berberine** - a botanical insulin sensitiser with effects comparable to metformin

Pharmacological Interventions

Pharmacotherapy is often reserved for patients who do not fully respond to lifestyle measures or have specific symptomatic concerns. A typical regimen includes a combination of oral contraceptives, antiandrogens, insulin sensitisers, and ovulation-inducing agents.

- **Oral contraceptives** are considered first-line for managing menstrual irregularities, acne, and hirsutism.
- **Finasteride**, an antiandrogen, is used to alleviate symptoms related to excess androgen activity.
- **Metformin**, an insulin sensitiser, has demonstrated efficacy in reducing insulin resistance, lowering testosterone levels, and improving ovulatory cycles.

In comparative studies, lifestyle interventions and metformin both led to BMI reductions in women with PCOS. However, only metformin significantly decreased serum testosterone levels.[8] Another randomised controlled trial showed that metformin alone, without concurrent lifestyle changes, reduced BMI and improved lipid profiles in women with obesity and PCOS.[9]

For ovulation induction, **clomiphene citrate** remains the first-line agent. It functions by stimulating the release of follicle-stimulating hormone (FSH), enhancing oestrogen production, and initiating follicular growth and ovulation. Alternatively, low-dose gonadotropin therapy using FSH and luteinising hormone (LH) can promote controlled mono-follicular development, offering another viable path to conception.

Final Thoughts

As explored in this chapter, PCOS is a multifaceted condition that can be effectively managed - and in some cases, reversed - through targeted lifestyle interventions. These changes not only address the core metabolic dysfunctions of PCOS but also offer enduring benefits with minimal risk. In contrast, pharmaceutical treatments, while often necessary, carry potential side effects and should be approached with caution.

Chronic low-grade inflammation in PCOS may also extend its impact to the musculoskeletal system. Increasing evidence suggests a higher prevalence of osteoarthritis in women with PCOS, potentially due to shared inflammatory and metabolic pathways. The next chapter will further explore this relationship, focusing on the intersection of metabolic syndrome and osteoarthritic degeneration.

CHAPTER 13

Osteoarthritis: When Joints Reflect Metabolic Distress

Osteoarthritis (OA) holds the unwelcome distinction of being the most prevalent joint disorder in the world, and it is a major contributor to chronic pain and reduced mobility. While OA can strike at any age, it is most seen in middle-aged and older adults, and it tends to worsen progressively over time. It particularly targets joints that bear the load of daily movement, including the knees, hips, and spine. But it doesn't stop there - smaller joints, such as those in the hands, are also frequent victims. OA is a common and often overlooked cause of persistent lower back pain.

For decades, OA was attributed to mechanical "wear and tear" - an inevitable consequence of ageing or overuse. This explanation, although intuitive, is now considered incomplete. Mounting evidence reveals that osteoarthritis isn't just about grinding cartilage and creaky joints - it's deeply intertwined with metabolic health. This new understanding reshapes OA not simply because of time and movement, but as a metabolically influenced degenerative condition driven by inflammation, oxidative stress, and cellular dysfunction.

How Metabolism Meets the Musculoskeletal System

The bridge between osteoarthritis and metabolic syndrome is now well-recognised in the medical literature. Metabolic syndrome - characterised by abdominal obesity, insulin resistance, high blood pressure, and abnormal lipid levels - creates a pro-inflammatory internal state that promotes cartilage breakdown and joint degeneration. Far from being isolated to joints, OA is increasingly understood as one piece of a broader metabolic puzzle.

While structural changes in joints may seem irreversible once established, that assumption is being challenged by real-world observations. Improving underlying metabolic dysfunction has been shown to alleviate pain, restore function, and, in some cases, delay or even prevent the need for surgery.

A Road Back: The Cyclist Who Reclaimed Movement

Consider the story of a former competitive cyclist in his 60s, whose active lifestyle had been derailed by a suite of chronic conditions. He struggled with uncontrolled type 2 diabetes (HbA1c: 9.2%), elevated blood pressure (160/100 mmHg), high cholesterol (6.7 mmol/L), and recurrent gout. His body mass index (BMI) was 31.5 kg/m^2 - technically obese - and his spine was so affected by arthritis that he could no longer lie flat in bed, instead relying on a reclining chair to sleep.

He embarked on a comprehensive, personalised metabolic program that included a whole-food diet, carefully chosen supplements, intermittent fasting, and regular movement adapted to his capacity. Within six months, he had shed 13 kilograms, brought his blood sugar and blood pressure under control, and significantly reduced his dependence on medication.

But perhaps the most dramatic transformation came from the joints themselves. His back pain and stiffness diminished to the point where he could resume once-abandoned routines

- gardening, cycling, even household chores. This wasn't just symptomatic relief; it was a testament to the regenerative potential of the body when inflammation and metabolic overload are lifted.

Rethinking the Surgery Script

In another robust case, a 62-year-old man of Asian heritage was living with chronic knee pain stemming from an injury sustained decades earlier. Over time, this trauma evolved into severe osteoarthritis. His metabolic profile was similarly concerning; he was overweight (BMI: 29.4 kg/m^2), hypertensive, and diabetic, and he was managing all of this with an expanding list of medications. His dietary habits - rich in animal fats, white rice, and industrial seed oils - were fuelling a metabolic fire.

A targeted nutritional overhaul was initiated. White rice was swapped for fibre-rich legumes; processed oils were replaced with heat-stable fats like coconut and avocado oil; and the man's intake of anti-inflammatory fruits, vegetables, and omega-3s was dramatically increased.

The results were striking. Within months, he lost weight, his metabolic indicators returned to healthy ranges, and his need for medication diminished. Most remarkably, his knee pain fell by 50%, and then continued to improve. Eventually, he regained full, pain-free mobility and was officially taken off the knee replacement waiting list following an orthopaedic review. His case is a striking example of how addressing inflammation and metabolic imbalance can turn what seems like an orthopaedic inevitability into a non-surgical success.

Understanding Osteoarthritis: More Than Just a Joint Problem

Osteoarthritis (OA) is the most common form of arthritis, but it's far from a simple consequence of ageing or overuse. Clinicians categorise OA into two broad types. Primary OA arises seemingly out of the blue in joints that were previously healthy. Secondary OA, on the other hand, develops in response to pre-existing joint insults - whether from injury, congenital anomalies, or previous infections.

OA can range from a subtle nuisance to a debilitating condition, classified by severity from grade 1 (mild) through grade 4 (severe). It tends to target the body's weight-bearing joints - the knees, hips, and lower spine - as well as the small joints of the hands.

The hallmark symptoms of OA typically unfold gradually:

- Stiffness in the morning that eases within 30 minutes
- Joint pain that intensifies with activity and improves with rest
- A diminishing range of movement
- Muscle weakness surrounding affected joints
- Altered posture or gait due to compensatory movement patterns

As the disease progresses, symptoms can become more intrusive. Pain may persist even at rest or during the night. Muscles may begin to atrophy, joints might emit audible clicks or grinding noises (crepitus), and visible deformities - such as the knobby Heberden's and Bouchard's nodes in the fingers - can develop.

Hand signs of osteoarthritis

Osteoarthritis (OA) begins with pain and stiffness and can affect the small joints of the hand. It progresses to the development of bony prominences known as Heberden's and Bouchard's nodules. OA symptoms and signs should prompt individuals to seek medical advice.

More Than Just Wear and Tear

OA is often oversimplified as a wear-and-tear condition - an inevitable result of ageing joints. However, this view falls short of explaining why OA also occurs in non-weight-bearing joints, such as those in the hands. Mechanical stress isn't the only culprit.

There's growing evidence that systemic factors - including metabolic and inflammatory pathways - play a central role. In fact, individuals with sedentary lifestyles appear more vulnerable to OA than their more active counterparts. This may seem counterintuitive at first glance, but it makes sense when considering muscle physiology. Strong muscles, particularly in the quadriceps and core, help stabilise joints and distribute forces evenly during movement. Weak muscles, conversely, disrupt joint mechanics and hasten cartilage degradation.

Also striking is the fact that many elderly people retain remarkably healthy joints. Age alone, therefore, is not destiny. What truly matters is the body's internal environment - its metabolic resilience and capacity for repair. Identifying these metabolic vulnerabilities early opens the door to preventive strategies before irreversible joint damage takes hold.

Who's at Risk?

While OA becomes more prevalent with advancing age, affecting around 80% of those over 75, age is just one piece of the puzzle.[1] Several other risk factors significantly influence susceptibility:

- Excess body weight, which increases joint loading and systemic inflammation
- Misaligned joints, often the legacy of old injuries
- Muscle imbalances or joint hypermobility
- Gout and other crystal-related joint disorders
- Metabolic syndrome, which brings with it a cascade of damaging biochemical effects

Interestingly, long-distance marathon runners - once thought to be prime candidates for OA - are no more at risk than the general population.[2] Regular, moderate exercise appears to fortify joint structures and delay degeneration.

A Metabolic Disorder in Disguise

The connection between osteoarthritis and metabolic health is now undeniable. While the mechanical burden of excess weight does damage joint surfaces, fat tissue itself is a biochemical troublemaker. Visceral fat - especially around the abdomen - acts like a rogue endocrine organ, releasing inflammatory mediators such as interleukin-6 (IL-6) and tumour necrosis factor-alpha (TNF-α). These compounds promote inflammation both systemically and within the joint environment.

Moreover, metabolic byproducts like uric acid - which tend to accumulate in individuals with insulin resistance - can crystallise in joints and trigger inflammation, contributing to the pathology not just of gout, but also of OA.

Research consistently shows that osteoarthritis often clusters with the other hallmarks of metabolic syndrome: abdominal obesity, elevated blood glucose, high blood pressure, and dyslipidaemia. A comprehensive meta-analysis found that OA patients were far more likely to have elevated triglycerides, reduced HDL cholesterol, and impaired glucose metabolism. The risk increases with the number of metabolic risk factors.[3] In fact, each 1 mmol/L increase in triglycerides corresponded with a 9% rise in OA risk.[4]

Even more compelling, low HDL and high blood pressure were linked with increased OA severity, particularly in advanced grade 4 cases.[5] And OA doesn't exist in a vacuum - it often co-occurs with type 2 diabetes and cardiovascular disease, both of which are known to accelerate joint degeneration.

On the flip side, individuals who maintain a metabolically healthy profile - with balanced blood sugar, normal blood pressure, and healthy lipid levels - appear to enjoy greater joint longevity. This suggests that managing one's metabolic health may be just as crucial for joint preservation as managing mechanical strain.

Understanding Joints:
From Harmony to Disrepair
The Architecture of a Healthy Joint

Imagine the joint as a finely tuned piece of biological engineering. It's not just where bones meet - it's where movement becomes possible. At the heart of this dynamic system lies the **articular cartilage**, a silky-smooth, rubbery tissue that acts like nature's shock absorber. This cartilage blankets the ends of bones within synovial joints (such as the knees, hips, and shoulders), ensuring that bones glide over each other with minimal friction and maximum ease.

What makes cartilage especially unique is its composition. It's made up of specialised cells called **chondrocytes**, which are embedded within a dense extracellular matrix rich in collagen and proteoglycans. This matrix is what gives cartilage its resilience and compressive strength. Unlike most tissues in the body, cartilage doesn't have its own blood vessels. Instead, it relies on nutrients diffusing in from the surrounding **synovial fluid** - a slippery, viscous liquid that lubricates the joint capsule. This lack of direct blood supply means that cartilage repairs itself at a glacial pace, especially when compared to bone or muscle.

This delicate equilibrium of nourishment, structure, and movement keeps the joint agile and pain-free - until, that is, the system begins to falter.

When Things Go Wrong: The Spiral of Osteoarthritis

Osteoarthritis (OA) is not a sudden invader - it's a slow-burning fire that takes root when the joint's resilience is repeatedly tested and eventually compromised. The usual culprits: A combination of **mechanical overload, metabolic imbalance, and chronic inflammation**.

At the earliest stages, the cartilage begins to thin - not uniformly, but in patches - due to the gradual loss of chondrocytes, the cells responsible for maintaining cartilage health. Once these cells begin to die off or malfunction, the integrity of the matrix weakens. Pro-inflammatory molecules, such as cytokines, infiltrate the joint space, accelerating this breakdown and disturbing the natural repair mechanisms.

As cartilage deteriorates, the underlying **subchondral bone** steps in - overcompensating by becoming denser and forming **osteophytes** or bone spurs. These bony protrusions may be the body's way of trying to stabilise the joint, but they end up further limiting movement and irritating nearby tissues. It's a bit like laying down bricks on a warped foundation - well-intentioned, but ultimately counterproductive.

Muscle plays a vital role here as well. When the muscles surrounding a joint are weak, poorly coordinated, or imbalanced, the forces across the joint become uneven. This mechanical misalignment hastens cartilage wear and alters joint motion. Over time, the joint capsule - the fibrous outer sleeve - may thicken, and supporting ligaments can lose their elasticity or orientation.

In individuals with elevated blood sugar or insulin resistance - conditions explored in depth earlier in this book - the progression of joint damage is more aggressive. Oxidative stress and mitochondrial dysfunction impair cellular energy production, not only in the cartilage but also in the supporting tissues, thereby compounding the degenerative cycle.

As the joint becomes a battlefield of inflammation, fragments of broken cartilage or bone may float freely in the synovial fluid. These "loose bodies" further irritate the joint's lining, triggering swelling and pain. And with **sarcopenia** - the age-related or metabolic loss of muscle mass - the scaffolding that holds the joint in place weakens, making every movement feel like a laborious effort.

How Osteoarthritis Shows Up on an X-Ray

While we can't directly see cartilage on a standard X-ray, the damage it leaves behind is unmistakable. Radiologists look for telltale signs that hint at the underlying pathology. These include:

- **Narrowed joint spaces**, which indicate that the protective cartilage cushion has thinned or vanished.
- **Subchondral sclerosis**, where the bone just beneath the cartilage becomes abnormally dense due to stress and microfractures.
- **Osteophytes**, or bone spurs, that project outward along joint margins - often a giveaway of chronic OA.
- **Subchondral cysts**, fluid-filled sacs that develop within the bone, add another layer of complexity to joint function.

These visual clues are not just academic - they correlate strongly with symptoms such as stiffness, swelling, and reduced range of motion. However, it's worth noting that some individuals can have radiological evidence of OA without experiencing significant pain, while others with minor X-ray changes might suffer considerably. This mismatch is part of what makes osteoarthritis such a perplexing and personalised condition.

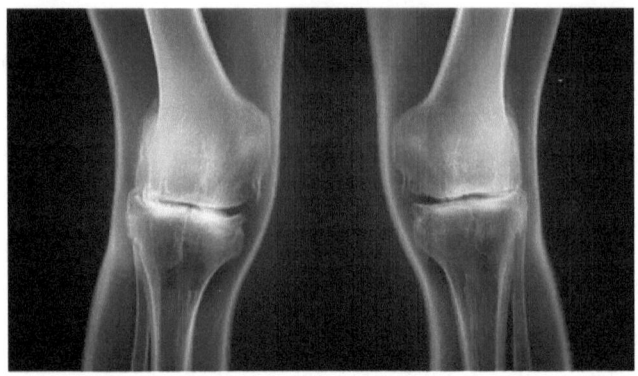

Radiological appearance of knee osteoarthritis

Throughout this chapter, we've seen how deeply interconnected metabolic health is with the structural and functional integrity of our joints. The case studies presented serve as vivid reminders that when the body's internal environment improves - when inflammation is reduced, insulin sensitivity is restored, and weight is brought under control - joints often respond with surprising resilience.

Rather than accepting joint degeneration as a foregone conclusion, particularly in conditions like osteoarthritis (OA), we now understand that the health of cartilage, synovial fluid, and supportive musculature can be preserved - and in some cases, partially restored - through thoughtful lifestyle intervention. The most promising strategies include:

- Embracing a nutrient-rich, anti-inflammatory dietary pattern
- Engaging in regular, joint-conscious movement
- Maintaining a body weight that minimises mechanical stress
- Prioritising deep, restorative sleep to enhance tissue repair and hormonal balance

Clinical evidence suggests that even a modest reduction in body weight - as little as 10% - can significantly alleviate joint discomfort, enhance mobility, and improve overall joint function in individuals with OA. This underscores the idea that progress doesn't always require perfection. Small, consistent lifestyle changes can yield meaningful relief.

Food as Joint Medicine

What we eat plays a fundamental role not only in nourishing our tissues but in influencing the biological pathways that drive joint inflammation and repair. Dietary approaches that calm systemic inflammation also tend to support joint integrity.

An anti-inflammatory eating pattern is built around whole, minimally processed foods. Omega-3 fatty acids - abundant in oily fish like salmon, sardines, and mackerel - have a well-documented ability to temper inflammation and support joint lubrication. Antioxidant-rich fruits and vegetables, particularly colourful varieties such as berries, bell peppers, citrus fruits, and tomatoes, deliver critical vitamins like A, C, and E, along with phytonutrients like lycopene and flavonoids that combat oxidative stress.

Key components to include regularly:

- **Nuts, seeds, legumes** - excellent sources of vitamin E and magnesium, which help regulate inflammation
- **Ginger, turmeric, green tea, and dark chocolate** - potent natural compounds with anti-inflammatory and antioxidant properties
- **Avocados, olives, and raw nuts** - healthy monounsaturated fats that support cellular health and reduce joint stress

Conversely, it's important to limit:

- **Highly processed seed oils** (e.g., soybean, corn, sunflower) that are high in omega-6 fatty acids and may exacerbate inflammatory pathways
- **Refined carbohydrates, added sugars, and excessive saturated fats**, which promote insulin resistance and increase systemic inflammation

Emerging research is now pinpointing specific nutrients and compounds that appear to support joint structure and function directly:

- **Collagen, hyaluronic acid, and proteoglycans** - key components of cartilage matrix
- **Vitamin C** - essential for collagen synthesis and protection against oxidative damage
- **Vitamin K2** - helps prevent inappropriate calcification within cartilage and contributes to bone remodelling

Movement: The Forgotten Elixir for Joints
For individuals living with osteoarthritis, pain and stiffness can make physical activity feel daunting. Yet ironically, avoiding movement tends to accelerate joint degeneration. Inactivity leads to muscle atrophy, reduced circulation, and declining joint lubrication - all of which worsen the condition.

The right kind of exercise, however, can be profoundly therapeutic. It encourages cartilage repair through mechanical stimulation, enhances flexibility, reduces pain, and restores function

Benefits of targeted physical activity include:

- Improved range of motion and flexibility
- Reinforcement of stabilising muscles
- Enhanced joint alignment and load distribution
- Reduction in stiffness and swelling

A structured rehabilitation program tailored to the individual's needs - ideally developed in collaboration with a physiotherapist - can make a significant difference. Techniques such as manual therapy, posture correction, and muscle rebalancing can realign joints and relieve excess strain. Some patients also benefit from chiropractic care aimed at optimising joint mechanics, or adjunct therapies such as heat application to promote blood flow and relax tight tissues.

Importantly, consistent movement doesn't just help the joints - it also improves insulin sensitivity, reduces visceral fat, and lowers systemic inflammation. The benefits ripple outward, reinforcing the body's metabolic resilience.

A Systems-Based Approach to Osteoarthritis

Managing osteoarthritis effectively requires more than symptomatic treatment. It calls for an integrative strategy that addresses the root causes - both mechanical and metabolic.

Core pillars of an integrative OA management plan include:

- Reducing joint load and inflammation
- Strengthening surrounding muscles for stability
- Improving joint mobility and neuromuscular coordination
- Tackling systemic issues like insulin resistance and oxidative stress

While conservative measures should be the first line of defence, advanced joint degeneration may eventually require surgical options such as total joint replacement. When indicated, such interventions can dramatically restore function and quality of life - but ideally, they are a last resort, not a first response.

Rethinking Osteoarthritis

The prevailing narrative around osteoarthritis - as an unavoidable byproduct of age or wear and tear - deserves to be retired. OA is not merely the result of "old joints," but a reflection of broader physiological imbalances. Chronic low-grade inflammation, poor glycaemic control, mitochondrial dysfunction, and mechanical strain all converge to erode joint health.

Encouragingly, these are modifiable factors.

By improving metabolic health through a whole-food, anti-inflammatory diet, regular joint-friendly movement, and other lifestyle upgrades, we can often slow - sometimes even reverse-the trajectory - of osteoarthritis. Pain levels drop, function returns, and patients frequently report feeling younger, lighter, and more agile.

Even in cases where the disease has advanced, improvements in systemic health can produce substantial benefits in joint performance and day-to-day comfort. This reframes OA from a degenerative inevitability into a manageable, and in many cases, improvable, condition.

Finally, it's worth noting that OA often coexists with other signs of metabolic dysfunction. One example is the surprisingly frequent link between knee osteoarthritis and **varicose veins** - a connection likely rooted in shared risk factors such as chronic inflammation, vascular dysfunction, and impaired circulation. This intriguing overlap will be explored in depth in the next chapter.

CHAPTER 14

Varicose Veins — Metabolic, Ubiquitous, and Unsightly

A Personal Prelude

As noted in the introduction, I experienced a life-threatening haemorrhage in my thyroid gland 25 years ago. Emergency surgery was required to evacuate the blood and remove one thyroid lobe. A second operation soon followed, removing half of the remaining lobe. I was left with a mere quarter of my thyroid gland and remained unconscious in intensive care for seven days - one of the hospital's most critical cases at the time. This event was a turning point, compelling me to examine and improve my overall health.

But the challenges did not end there. Years later, a vascular surgeon and friend from King's College London identified prominent varicose veins in my left leg. At his recommendation, I underwent a procedure described as routine - a vein ligation behind the knee. Initially, the results were promising, but within months, deterioration resumed. This clinical setback prompted me to re-evaluate my medical history for clues.

Metabolic Foundations

Since childhood, I had carried a slight stomach bulge despite maintaining a normal weight. Eventually, I was diagnosed with insulin resistance, which impaired my ability to metabolise carbohydrates and sugars efficiently. I often experienced hypoglycaemic episodes - severe shaking and near-fainting - particularly before meals. Over time, it became apparent that excess fat had accumulated in my liver, a condition known as non-alcoholic fatty liver disease (NAFLD). This gave me a disproportionately distended abdomen despite an otherwise lean appearance.

Fatty liver is closely associated with hyperinsulinaemia - elevated levels of insulin in the blood - which I now believe was a significant contributor to the formation of my thyroid cyst and subsequent haemorrhage. The metabolic derangement, marked by chronic insulin elevation, likely laid the groundwork for both endocrine and vascular complications.

The Link to Varicosity

Retrospective analysis suggests that hepatomegaly - enlargement of the liver - led to congestion in the portal venous system, which carries nutrient-rich blood from the gastrointestinal tract to the liver. Portal hypertension can cause retrograde pressure into connected venous networks, including the oesophagus, stomach, rectum, and lower extremities. Indeed, haemorrhoids (rectal varices) and varicose veins in the legs may be different manifestations of the same underlying issue: chronic venous congestion due to metabolic stress.

This hepatic pressure likely impaired venous return from the lower limbs, resulting in extensive varicosity in my left leg. Compounding this was a strong family history - two of my brothers underwent surgery for haemorrhoids. Epidemiological data support this hereditary link: a Japanese study found that 42% of patients with varicose veins reported a family history, compared with only 14% among those without.[1]

Varicose veins are not rare. Approximately one-third of individuals in Western societies are affected. This chapter seeks to explore several questions: What causes varicose veins? Are they merely cosmetic, or do they pose medical risks? Can they be prevented or reversed? Are surgical options the only recourse, or do lifestyle interventions and natural remedies offer viable alternatives? And finally, why do varicose veins represent such a deeply personal subject for me?

The Physiology of Venous Drainage

Two interconnected systems facilitate venous return from the lower limbs:

- **Superficial veins**, which drain the skin and subcutaneous tissues, account for approximately 10% of venous return.
- **Deep veins**, located within the muscle compartments and supported by connective fascia, account for the remaining 90%.

These systems are equipped with one-way valves that maintain unidirectional blood flow - upward, against gravity - toward the heart. Valves open to allow blood to pass and then close to prevent reflux. The muscular pump mechanism, especially involving the calf muscles, aids this process.

When valve function deteriorates - due to ageing, inflammation, or structural weakness of the vein wall - blood can pool in the lower limbs, resulting in **venous hypertension**. This leads to vein dilation, valve incompetence, and ultimately, the tortuous and swollen vessels that define varicose veins.

Varicosity is most observed in the **great and small saphenous veins**, which are part of the superficial system and lack the supportive fascia that protects deep veins from excessive dilation. Additionally, thrombi formed in the deep venous system can obstruct normal blood flow and contribute to the development of secondary varicosity.

A Deteriorating Course

Years after my initial vein ligation, I noticed a precipitous decline in my marathon performance - my times had slowed by over 30 minutes, with no obvious explanation. I also suffered from instability and occasional falls. A chiropractic assessment revealed a right-sided pelvic tilt, and spinal X-rays confirmed early degenerative changes in the vertebrae.

Symptoms intensified after my son's wedding, a period marked by dietary indulgence and increased sugar intake. The swelling in my left leg worsened, and I developed a chronic ulcer that resisted healing - likely the result of glycaemic spikes affecting vascular integrity.

Following a Thai massage, I experienced severe lower leg pain that disrupted sleep and mobility. Despite normal blood tests and no evidence of thrombosis on imaging, an X-ray revealed a calcified segment in the central vein, 10 cm above the medial malleolus. The likely cause was post-phlebitis calcification - possibly from a previous, unrecognised vein infection. The massage likely fractured this calcified vein, resulting in sharp, stabbing pain with movement.

Radiofrequency ablation was proposed to eliminate the damaged vein. However, I was startled to learn the plan included stripping the entire great and small saphenous veins. Unconvinced this radical approach was justified, I chose to forgo the procedure.

Causes and Risk Factors

Several physiological and lifestyle factors contribute to the development of varicose veins:

- **Ageing**: Prevalence increases with age - 25% in people aged 55-64 versus 10% in those aged 18-24.[2] Age-related muscle weakening, valve deterioration, and vein wall thinning are key contributors.
- **Pregnancy and Hormones**: In late pregnancy, the expanding uterus can compress pelvic veins, impeding venous return. Oestrogen and progesterone, whether from pregnancy or contraceptive pills, further reduce vein tone. Progesterone appears particularly detrimental to venous integrity.
- **Obesity and Sedentary Lifestyle**: Excess weight increases intra-abdominal pressure and impairs venous return. Prolonged sitting or standing, as well as habits like leg-crossing, exacerbate venous pooling.
- **Metabolic Syndrome,** characterised by hypertension, insulin resistance, and type 2 diabetes, impairs venous function through increased pressure, inflammation, and endothelial dysfunction. Elevated blood glucose increases blood viscosity, slows flow, promotes glycation of vascular structures, and damages endothelial cells.

Symptoms and Complications

Common symptoms include:

- Heavy, aching legs
- Swelling of ankles and feet
- Burning, itching, and darkened skin over affected veins
- Night cramps and restlessness

In advanced cases, complications may include:

- Skin ulceration
- Recurrent bleeding (often difficult to control)
- Superficial thrombophlebitis
- Deep vein thrombosis (more common in diabetic patients)

This intensely personal journey with varicose veins reflects the complex interplay between metabolism, vascular health, and lifestyle. In the following sections, we will explore diagnostic strategies, preventive measures, conservative treatments, and when - and whether - intervention is truly necessary.

What Can You Do?

Managing and preventing varicose veins requires a multifaceted approach that targets lifestyle, diet, and, when necessary, medical intervention. While genetics and hormonal influences are significant, numerous modifiable factors can also impact the onset and progression of this condition. Below are practical strategies you can adopt.

Lifestyle Strategies for Prevention and Management

- **Achieve and maintain a healthy weight.** Excess body weight increases venous pressure and impairs circulation, accelerating the development of varicose veins.
- **Avoid smoking.** Smoking significantly raises the risk - by as much as 2.5 times - by damaging blood vessels and impairing circulation.

- **Stay hydrated.** Adequate water intake improves blood viscosity and reduces the likelihood of venous congestion. Limit dehydrating substances like caffeine found in tea, coffee, and energy drinks.
- **Use compression therapy.** Wearing knee-high compression stockings during the day helps support venous return and alleviate symptoms. They should be removed at night.
- **Reduce prolonged immobility.** Avoid sitting, standing, or crossing your legs for extended periods. Incorporate regular movement throughout your day to promote venous flow.
- **Elevate your legs.** When sitting or resting, elevate your legs to reduce venous pressure and improve circulation.
- **Monitor blood glucose levels.** Keep fasting glucose and glycated haemoglobin (HbA1c) within the normal range to protect vascular integrity.
- **Maintain foot health.** Regular podiatry visits (every six months) ensure early identification of foot or nail issues that may indirectly affect circulation.
- **Exercise regularly.** Physical activity enhances venous return, reduces symptoms, and slows the progression of varicose veins.
- **Review contraceptive options.** Women prone to varicose veins may benefit from non-hormonal methods, as oestrogen-containing birth control pills can exacerbate vascular issues.

Dietary Recommendations to Support Vein Health

- **Fibre-rich foods.** A diet abundant in fibre from fruits, vegetables, legumes, whole grains, nuts, and seeds helps prevent constipation - a key contributor to increased intra-abdominal pressure and venous insufficiency.

- **Eat a rainbow of vegetables.** Different pigments signal diverse antioxidants, which protect vein walls from oxidative stress and "rusting."
- **Vitamin C intake.** Essential for collagen and elastin synthesis - key components of vascular integrity - vitamin C is found in bell peppers, kiwis, and citrus fruits.
- **Omega-3 fatty acids.** Found in oily fish such as salmon, mackerel, and herring, omega-3 fatty acids reduce inflammation and support vascular flexibility. Garlic, another anti-inflammatory agent, possesses antimicrobial properties that aid detoxification.
- **Cruciferous vegetables.** Members of the Brassica family (broccoli, cabbage, cauliflower, kale) are high in vitamin K1, which supports blood flow by assisting coagulation regulation.
- **Healthy fats.** Avocados and olive oil provide vitamin E and vital phytonutrients that maintain vessel elasticity and cellular health.
- **Hydrophilic vegetables.** Foods like cucumber, celery, and fennel reduce fluid retention and ease leg swelling (oedema), particularly helpful in the later stages of venous disease.

Supplements with Vascular Benefits

- **Vitamins A, B complex, C, E, and K** support the repair and maintenance of vascular tissues.
- **Omega-3 supplements and turmeric (specifically,**

curcumin) offer anti-inflammatory effects that help mitigate vascular injury.
- **Horse chestnut extract,** a natural compound with anti-inflammatory and venotonic properties, strengthens vein walls and improves circulation.
- **Probiotics and prebiotics** enhance gut microbiota, which may indirectly support vascular health by reducing systemic inflammation.

Surgical Options: When Natural Strategies Are Not Enough

For some individuals, surgical intervention becomes necessary - often driven by discomfort or cosmetic concerns. Women may seek treatment for aesthetic reasons.

- **Ligation and stripping** are traditional surgical options for larger varicose veins.
- **Minimally invasive procedures** - such as laser ablation, radiofrequency ablation, or sclerotherapy - are commonly used to treat smaller or medium-sized veins.
- **Microphlebectomy** is a precise technique that removes varicose veins using a small, hooked instrument.

Although effective, surgery is not without risks. Complications may include bruising, infection, bleeding, nerve damage (which can occasionally lead to foot drop), or deep vein thrombosis. In rare cases, a dislodged clot may result in **pulmonary embolism**, a life-threatening emergency.

Drawing from personal experience, while surgery may be life-saving or necessary in some cases, it should be a last resort. Always exhaust non-invasive, lifestyle-based interventions first. Once a vein or body part is removed, there is no going back.

A Personal Reflection

As highlighted in Chapter 13, a patient of mine with severe osteoarthritis successfully reversed his metabolic dysfunction and postponed surgery through disciplined lifestyle changes. With improved blood sugar control and weight loss, his joint pain eased, and he voluntarily withdrew from the knee replacement waiting list. This example highlights the body's remarkable capacity for self-repair when provided with the right conditions.

I, too, narrowly avoided surgery at a critical point and remain committed to maintaining a lifestyle that keeps me off the operating table. Varicose veins are not merely cosmetic - they are a **metabolic manifestation**. The comprehensive approach outlined in Section 3 of this book - emphasising a whole-food diet, consistent physical activity, restorative sleep, stress management, and meaningful relationships - provides a sustainable, long-term strategy to prevent and manage this condition.

SECTION 3

THE NATURAL SOLUTION

CHAPTER 15

Health Goal Setting: A Personal Turning Point

Following surgical procedures and a period in intensive care, I was discharged on extended medical leave. The physical ordeal was profound, but the emotional impact proved equally challenging. Initially, I grappled with denial, directing blame toward my medical team for failing to shield me from such an outcome. Yet, as the dust settled, I came to a crucial realisation: responsibility for my health ultimately rested with me. Rather than simply adhering to a regimen of prescribed medications, I resolved to understand the root causes of my illness better.

This shift in perspective marked the beginning of a transformational journey - one that hinged on several pivotal lifestyle changes. Determined to reclaim my health, I returned to the basics of life's necessities: diet and regular physical activity. Gradually, my stamina improved. To my surprise, the new simple habits I gained evolved into something extraordinary: by my 60s, I had completed over 120 marathons. What had begun as rehabilitation became a source of profound strength and renewal.

With this background, let's explore how you can also start your journey towards better health.

Rethinking the Patient-Doctor Relationship

Traditionally, the patient-doctor dynamic has cast the patient as a passive recipient of expert advice, largely centred around pharmacological solutions. However, in functional and integrative medicine, this paradigm is turned on its head. Patients are no longer mere bystanders in their health journey; they are empowered to take the wheel - armed with knowledge, agency, and a renewed sense of purpose.

Let us examine this shift in the context of metabolic syndrome - a condition that emerges from a constellation of metabolic imbalances. It typically begins with a decrease in energy production. Feeling fatigued, individuals often reach for quick sources of energy - foods high in sugars and unhealthy fats. Rather than fuelling the body, these foods are stored as visceral fat, particularly around the abdomen. Central obesity soon gives rise to a cascade of other risk factors: elevated blood pressure, impaired glucose tolerance, increased triglycerides, and reduced levels of HDL ("good") cholesterol.

In contrast to conventional medicine, which tends to isolate and treat each symptom independently, a holistic approach seeks to uncover and correct the underlying drivers - many of which stem from deeply held, yet flawed, beliefs.

Real Stories, Real Lessons

Take, for instance, a bus driver I once treated. He suffered from morbid obesity and routinely consumed large quantities of sweets, chocolate, sugary beverages, and fizzy drinks. His rationale was rooted in a sincere, albeit mistaken, belief. Because he bore the immense responsibility of safely transporting dozens of passengers, he believed he needed an equally tremendous supply of energy. Unfortunately, this misunderstanding contributed directly to the development of metabolic syndrome.

Another patient, also struggling with obesity, adhered to minimal physical activity in an attempt to "preserve" his body and avoid depreciation, while consuming excess calories for "nourishment." This strategy, while well-intentioned, led him down a path of chronic disease.

A third case was more severe. After buying a car, a previously active and healthy man ceased his daily walks and adopted a sedentary lifestyle. Warning signs - weight gain, hypertension, elevated blood glucose - were ignored. This series of seemingly minor changes culminated in chronic kidney disease, leaving him dependent on dialysis and significantly diminishing his quality of life.

Andy's Journey: From Crisis to Commitment

Consider Andy. Two years ago, he underwent emergency surgery for an aortic dissection, complicated by a left-sided stroke. In its aftermath, he was diagnosed with hypertension and prescribed several medications.

At his initial assessment, Andy's BMI was within normal limits (22.7 kg/m^2), and he had a resting pulse of 47 beats per minute - suppressed by beta blockers. However, his blood pressure remained elevated at 168/85 mmHg (grade 2 hypertension), and his waist-to-hip ratio of 0.97 signalled excessive visceral fat. His liver was enlarged, and neurologically, he exhibited reduced sensation in both feet, mild left-sided weakness, and required both a walking stick and his wife's support for mobility.

Determined to reclaim his independence, Andy committed to a structured lifestyle intervention. Over the course of a year, he adopted an anti-inflammatory diet and gradually increased his physical activity, boosting his daily walk from one kilometre to three. The results were remarkable: his neurological deficits nearly resolved, and his quality of life improved dramatically.

At times, Andy questioned whether the occasional indulgence - a slice of chocolate cake or a glass of wine - was justifiable. The key to his success lay not in rigid restriction but in reframing his goals. Together, we shifted the focus to what truly mattered: being present for his grandchildren, dancing at his granddaughter's wedding, and living a full, active life. With this clarity, long-term health became more meaningful than short-term gratification.

Let this serve as both inspiration and invitation: the path to better health begins not with perfection, but with commitment and knowledge - one step, one meal, and one choice at a time.

Your Vision and Roadmap to Achieve Health Goals

Improving your health is not a mystery reserved for the lucky or the genetically gifted - it is a structured process available to anyone willing to commit. But like all worthwhile pursuits, it begins with clarity. You need a **vision** of where you want to go and a **roadmap** to get there.

Imagine planning an overseas holiday without choosing a destination, booking a flight, or checking the weather. That trip would never take off. Yet many of us approach our health in a vague and unstructured way. We want to "feel better", or "lose weight", or "be healthy," but we rarely define what that means. Vague desires lead to ambiguous results.

Step One: Clarify Your Vision

Start by asking yourself: **What do I want my health to look like in 12 months? Five years? Twenty years?** Don't settle for generalisations. Think about how you want to feel, move, sleep, and live. Do you want to reduce joint pain, restore your energy, or play football with your grandchildren without getting out of breath? Do you want to reverse type 2 diabetes or lower your blood pressure naturally?

To bring this vision to life, **write it down**. Use sensory details: describe your energy levels, daily routines, physical appearance, and emotional state. Keep it somewhere you can revisit often - it will serve as your compass.

Action prompt: Take ten minutes right now. Write a paragraph describing the healthiest version of yourself. Where are you? What are you doing? How do you feel?

Step Two: Turn Your Vision Into SMART Goals

Goal setting demands time and reflection. Ask yourself: Is it meaningful? Is it a stretch that will inspire growth? Recall the story of Roger Bannister, who broke the "impossible" four-minute mile in 1954 - only to be followed by others within weeks. The impossible became achievable once someone proved it could be done.

Once you've clarified your vision, it's time to break it into **SMART goals**: Specific, Measurable, Achievable, Relevant, and Time-bound.

Instead of "I want to get fit," say: "I will walk briskly for 30 minutes, five days a week, for the next three months. Instead of "I want to lose weight," say: "I will reduce my waist circumference to 32 inches (81 cm) within six months by following a Mediterranean-style diet and exercising regularly."

Goals must be measurable so you can track progress. They must be achievable - not easy, but within reach. They should be relevant to your deeper values, and they need a deadline to provide urgency.

Action prompt: Write down 2-3 SMART goals related to your health. Be specific and set a realistic timeline for yourself.

Step Three: Map Out Milestones and Barriers

With SMART goals in hand, the next step is to design your **personal roadmap**. Start with small, sustainable actions. Identify the **first**

steps that move you toward your goals. Then anticipate the likely **barriers**: time constraints, energy dips, cravings, and lack of support.

Create a plan for how you will respond when obstacles arise. For instance, if evenings are too chaotic for exercise, mornings or lunch breaks may be better options. If late-night snacking is your downfall, consider setting a kitchen curfew to help you stay on track.

Teaching point: Planning for obstacles is not pessimism - it's wisdom. People don't fail because they lack willpower; they fail because they didn't plan for the dips in willpower.

Action prompt: Choose one SMART goal. Now write down:

- The first three actions you can take this week.
- The top three obstacles you expect.
- One solution for each obstacle.

Your goals should be personal, positive, and inspiring. You must fall in love with your vision to stay committed.

Step Four: Assess Your Readiness

It's essential to understand your **stage of readiness**. Behavioural scientists describe five key stages of change:

- **Pre-contemplation:** You don't yet see a problem or have no intention to change.
- **Contemplation:** You recognise the issue but are uncertain about the solution.
- **Preparation:** You're researching, planning, and getting ready.
- **Action:** You're actively making changes.
- **Maintenance:** You're sustaining your progress and preventing relapse.

- **Termination**: The new habit becomes part of your identity, with no temptation to relapse.

Where are you right now? Be honest. There's no shame in starting from the beginning - what matters is your willingness to move forward.

Action prompt: Which stage are you currently in? Write it down. What would help you move to the next stage?

Begin With the End in Mind

As Stephen Covey famously said, *"Begin with the end in mind."* Create a mental image - or better yet, a photo - of your health goals achieved. If you once had a period of robust health, use that memory. If not, create a compelling vision of what's possible.

Let that image be your fuel. Motivation fluctuates, but vision anchors you when challenges arise.

The Psychology of Willpower and Motivation

Willpower is not endless. Think of it as a battery - it drains throughout the day. That's why **your reasons matter**. Why do you want to change? Your answer must be personal, powerful, and emotionally charged. It may be your children, your career, your longevity, your spiritual mission, or a desire to escape pain and suffering.

The more closely aligned your goals are with your values and identity, the stronger your persistence will be.

Action prompt: List 3-5 reasons why achieving your health goal matters deeply to you.

Replace negative inner dialogue with affirming beliefs. Tell yourself:

- "I am becoming stronger every day."

- "I choose health and vitality."
- "I have done hard things before—I can do this too."

Understand your **inner performer and inner critic**. The critic will speak first, often loudly. And present all the reasons you might fail; the **performer** knows what you're capable of.

Action: Silence the critic - release the performer.

The Role of Habits and the Subconscious Mind

Real change doesn't just happen through conscious decision-making - it involves reprogramming your subconscious mind, where 90% of your daily actions are formed.

A habit forms when three elements converge:

- **Knowledge** - You understand what to do.
- **Skill** - You know how to do it.
- **Desire** - You want to do it.

To establish new habits:

- Start small.
- Repeat often.
- Tie the habit to an existing routine (e.g., "After brushing my teeth, I'll do 10 squats").

Teaching tip: Don't try to erase bad habits - **replace** them. Every habit fills a need. Find a healthier way to meet that need.

Action prompt: Identify one unhelpful habit. What reward does it give you? Now create a new habit that offers the same reward in a healthier way.

Why Do People Do What They Do?

Human behaviour is often less about deliberate choice and more about ingrained patterns. Much of what we do each day is driven by habit, unconscious routines, or even addictive tendencies. These actions often occur without our full awareness, operating on what might be called "autopilot."

Consider a familiar morning routine: you wake up, light your first cigarette, and pick up a large pastry and coffee from the café near the train station. These actions feel automatic, almost inevitable - not the result of a conscious decision, but a series of impulses playing out beneath the surface.

Habits work by creating a kind of mental 'itch' - a subtle discomfort or urge that builds until it is relieved by performing the routine. This cycle, once established, reinforces itself, making the behaviour feel natural and necessary. The key to changing these patterns lies in bringing them into conscious awareness.

When you recognise the impulse behind a habit, you create space between the trigger and your response. That awareness is powerful. It allows you to choose differently - to replace an unconscious reaction with a conscious decision. Lasting change begins not with willpower alone, but with understanding the hidden drivers of our behaviour.

Social Support: Your Secret Weapon

One of the most powerful tools for change is the community. We are social beings. Behaviour spreads through groups - just as unhealthy habits can be contagious, so can healthy ones.

In my own experience leading a lifestyle programme in a local church, the community dynamic was transformative. Initial reluctance gave way to motivation when one participant shared his early success. This sparked a ripple effect of encouragement, accountability, and collective momentum - outcomes rarely seen in clinical settings.

Action prompt: Who can support you on this journey? A friend, spouse, coworker, or a walking group? Reach out and invite them to join you in your health goals.

Visualising Long-Term Success

The further out the goal, the harder it is to visualise - but that's where deep transformation happens. Consider the story of Andy, who struggled to imagine playing with his future grandchildren. Once he embraced that image, his motivation soared. Your vision must be emotionally alive.

Take baby steps toward that future, and you'll begin to live it sooner than you think.

Reflect, Adjust, and Persist

Review your progress regularly. What's working? What's not? Adjust your schedule, strategies, and support systems accordingly.

Failure is not the end - it's feedback. Learn from it. Thomas Edison, after thousands of failed lightbulb prototypes, famously said, *"I have not failed. I've just found 10,000 ways that won't work."* Each setback is part of the process.

Then, he concluded, *"Our greatest weakness lies in giving up. The most certain way to succeed is always to try just one more time."*

Action prompt: At the end of each week, reflect:

- What did I do well?
- What challenged me?
- What will I try differently next week?

Final Thoughts

We meticulously plan our holidays - yet often overlook the importance of planning for our health. It's time to reverse that trend.

Pick up a pen. Reflect on the habits that are undermining your well-being. List them and consider how you might replace them with life-enhancing alternatives. Define your long-term goals. What smaller goals will lead you there? Who will support you - your spouse, a friend, or a coach?

Refine your goals until they become irresistible.

Then act: buy a T-shirt and a pair of running shoes. Clear your kitchen of unhealthy foods. Draft your first healthy shopping list.

In the next chapter, we'll build on this foundation by introducing the diet prescription that will transform your health and energise your life.

The journey to lifelong health begins here - with clarity, commitment, and courage.

CHAPTER 16

The Metabolic Diet Prescription

After a severe health crisis - ironically, as the most seriously ill patient in my own hospital - I finally reached a turning point. Something had to change. I emerged from that low with a renewed sense of purpose. Wearing my holistic medicine hat, I asked myself the most fundamental question in medicine: What was the root cause?

Two key changes in my life stood out: my diet and physical activity. Since leaving Africa, these pillars of health had undergone drastic shifts. Yes, I was also under immense stress, constantly on call, working antisocial hours, and chronically sleep-deprived - but those factors weren't immediately modifiable. My diet and lifestyle, however, were. My goal was clear: to shed the 30 kilograms (66 pounds) I had gained in just two years of living in the United Kingdom and reclaim my health. The solution seemed obvious: return to the way I used to eat and live back in Africa.

In this chapter, I'll explore how different dietary patterns influence metabolism and outline what I call the ultimate metabolic diet prescription.

Why the African Diet Was the Solution

The diet I grew up with in Africa was natural, unprocessed, and rich in nutrients. Food came from farms, not factories. It was grown, picked, prepared, and eaten without the use of additives or refining. In contrast, the Western diet is characterised by ultra-processed foods engineered for shelf life, taste, and convenience - at the cost of nutrition.

Whole foods are the optimal fuel for the human body. They provide energy in the form of carbohydrates and fats, fibre to regulate absorption, and micronutrients essential for processing that energy. As I explained in Chapter 4, fibre plays a key role in slowing the absorption of sugar and fat, preventing the sharp spikes and crashes in blood sugar that drain energy and destabilise appetite. Micronutrients - though required in tiny amounts - are critical. They act as metabolic cofactors, allowing the body to convert calories into usable energy.

Food processing strips these essential components away. Fibre is removed for texture and preservation. Nutrients are lost through refinement. The result: A calorie-dense product made primarily of starches with a high glycaemic index - essentially, sugar in disguise. These products enter the bloodstream rapidly, causing blood sugar spikes followed by crashes. Over time, this disrupts insulin function, impairs energy use, and drives fat storage. This is how a corrupted metabolism takes root.

While living in Africa and eating whole foods, I enjoyed consistent energy, mental clarity, and a stable, healthy weight. That diet was humanity's original menu - what we thrived on for millennia. We typically ate two or three meals per day, and snacking was virtually non-existent. Snacks, as we know them today, only became commonplace in the 1980s, following the industrialisation of the food supply.

The rise of the modern Western diet, often referred to as the Standard American Diet (SAD), brought a surge of sugar-laden beverages, refined carbohydrates, and fast food. And with it came a tidal wave of obesity and metabolic disease.

The metabolic diet prescription

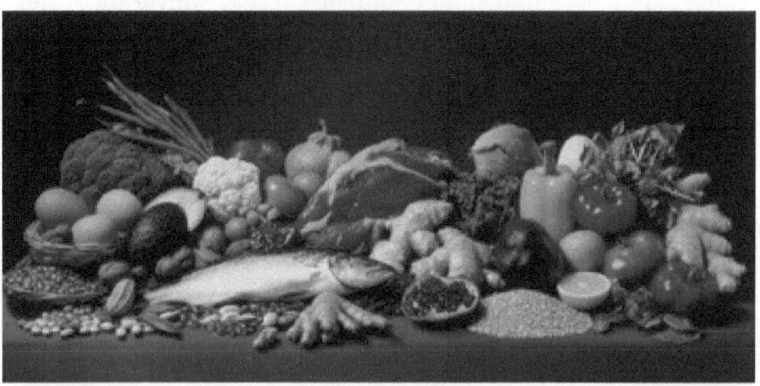

The metabolic diet prescription includes whole foods such as fruits, vegetables, beans, nuts, and seeds, as well as organic eggs and poultry, grass-fed meat, and wild small oily fish. Whole Food: The Ideal Fuel for the Human Engine

Don't just take my word for it - let the data speak

In the 1960s, the obesity rate in the United States hovered around 15%. Today, it exceeds 42%. This rise coincided with the mass industrialisation of food that began in the 1970s. Over the same period, daily calorie intake has ballooned - by some estimates, up to 1,000 calories more per person per day. Predictably, this has been mirrored by an explosion in obesity, type 2 diabetes, fatty liver disease, and other metabolic disorders.

An unintentional "experiment" in Cuba confirmed my convictions. In 1990, US trade sanctions disrupted the import of processed foods.[2] Cubans had to rely on their local, traditional whole foods. The result: Weight loss, improved health, and a dramatic drop in chronic disease rates and mortality.[3] Once again, Mother Nature proved to be the best pharmacist.

The whole-food diet I advocate isn't new or revolutionary - it's ancestral, intuitive, and profoundly effective. It naturally intersects with other evidence-based approaches, such as low-carb and low-calorie diets. Dr David Unwin has used a low-carbohydrate diet to reverse type 2 diabetes.[4] Professor Roy Taylor at Newcastle University has demonstrated similar success with a low-calorie approach.[5] All these methods align with the principle of consuming low calories and reducing metabolic strain.

The paleo diet, which eliminates processed foods and mimics ancestral eating, shares a similar ethos. It isn't about labels - it's about nourishing the body with the foods it was designed to handle.

Challenging Conventional Dietary Wisdom

For decades, conventional dietary advice promoted low-fat, low-cholesterol diets in the name of heart health. But this guidance overlooked one critical truth: cholesterol is essential to life. Every cell membrane in your body contains cholesterol. It's the building block of hormones and brain tissue. Demonising cholesterol without addressing the real culprits - refined carbs, added sugars, and ultra-processed foods - was a major misstep.

A diet low in fat but high in processed carbohydrates is a recipe for metabolic disaster. It may reduce cholesterol intake but accelerate fat storage, insulin resistance, and systemic inflammation.

Modern life moves fast, and many people turn to processed food because it's quick, cheap, and palatable. But these short-term gains come with long-term costs: weight gain, low energy, metabolic syndrome, and chronic illness. Highly processed foods override the body's natural satiety mechanisms. They're designed to stimulate appetite and promote overconsumption.

Processed Carbs and the Rising Body Weight 'Set Point'

Let's delve into a fascinating concept: **the body weight set point**.

In nature, systems seek balance. Animals breathe in oxygen and exhale carbon dioxide. Plants absorb carbon dioxide and release oxygen. No waste accumulates. Energy flows through a closed-loop cycle.

Humans are no different. Our bodies regulate energy intake and expenditure through a sophisticated hormonal network. But processed foods hijack this balance.

The human body requires approximately **75 to 125 grams of carbohydrates** per day. Yet the typical Western diet delivers over 300 grams daily, often from refined sources. This excess not only leads to fat accumulation - it **raises the body's weight set point**, meaning your body begins to defend a higher baseline weight, making weight loss more difficult over time.

When you consume whole foods - nutrient-dense and fibre-rich but lower in calories - your set point gradually resets. Your body naturally returns to a weight that matches your energy needs and activity level.

For most people, this "ideal" weight is reached in early adulthood - around age 20 - when physical activity is high and diets are less distorted. That's where I was 30 years ago, before I moved to the UK and transitioned to a Western diet of bread, pasta, pizza, crisps, biscuits, fast food, fizzy drinks, and fruit juice. The result was a 30-kilogram weight gain and full-blown metabolic syndrome.

But when I returned to a whole-food diet, my metabolism recovered. My weight dropped. My energy returned. The transformation was complete.

Healing Through Real Food

Whole food is not just about nutrition - it's about restoration. It brings your metabolism back online, stabilises energy levels, and helps regulate appetite naturally. Whether it's through a low-carbohydrate, low-calorie, or ancestral (paleo-style) approach, the goal remains the same: to correct energy imbalance and heal the metabolic system.

Other methods, like **bariatric surgery**, also aim to achieve this by physically reducing calorie intake. Such surgeries can reverse diabetes in just weeks - but they come with risks and aren't always sustainable. The stomach can adapt, stretch, and regain volume. Surgery doesn't address the root cause: the food itself.

Real healing starts with real food. Whole food is not a trend or a temporary fix. It is the original, time-tested diet of humankind. It provides the perfect balance of energy, fibre, and nutrients - designed not by laboratories but by nature herself.

A Wealth of Dietary Choices

Navigating the world of nutrition can feel like wandering through a maze of competing claims and trendy diets. One moment it's all about cutting carbs; the next, fat is the enemy - or the saviour. The truth is, while many of these diets may help with weight loss in the short term, few are designed with long-term metabolic health in mind. Before we explore my recommendations, let's take a thoughtful look at what science has to say about some of the most popular approaches.

The Plant-Based Diet: Healthy, But Not Entirely Self-Sufficient

Plant-based eating has earned its place at the table when it comes to reducing the risk of disease. Numerous studies have shown that individuals who primarily eat plants tend to have a lower BMI, healthier cholesterol and triglyceride levels, and better blood sugar control than those who consume a mix of both animal and plant foods.[6] People who follow vegetarian or vegan diets often show a significantly reduced risk of developing metabolic syndrome and certain types of cancer.

However, there's a nutritional catch. While plants offer fibre, antioxidants, and phytonutrients in abundance, they may fall short on essential nutrients like vitamin B12, iron, iodine, omega-3 fatty acids, and high-quality protein. These gaps don't make the diet ineffective - but they do require attention. When properly supplemented or strategically planned, a plant-based diet can even reverse metabolic dysfunction if deficiencies are avoided.[7]

Interestingly, getting enough vegetables is a common hurdle. Many of my patients struggle to meet the recommended intake, despite their best intentions. For those individuals, incorporating fresh vegetable juices or smoothies can be a practical and enjoyable solution. One study even found that this simple strategy improved adherence to the DASH diet's vegetable targets and led to measurable weight loss in individuals with metabolic syndrome.[8]

Fat: Not the Enemy

It's time to bust the long-standing myth that fat makes you fat. Quite the opposite: healthy fats play a crucial role in metabolic regulation. Unlike sugar, dietary fat doesn't cause significant insulin spikes, which means your body can stay in fat-burning mode longer. This not only supports weight loss but also provides more stable energy levels throughout the day.

Fats from whole foods - think avocados, seeds, nuts, and their oils - offer more than just calories. They're rich in fibre, which nourishes your gut microbiota and supports the production of short-chain fatty acids like butyrate. This compound has been demonstrated to enhance gut barrier integrity, mitigate inflammation, and support brain and liver health. In essence, good fats do far more than fill you up - they help heal and protect.

The Ketogenic Diet: Fat-Fuelled and Fibre-Friendly

For those who prefer not to count every calorie or constantly feel hungry, the ketogenic diet offers a compelling alternative. This high-fat, moderate-protein, and very low-carbohydrate approach trains the body to burn fat for energy - a state known as ketosis.

The classic keto plate typically includes foods such as eggs, fish, poultry, cheese, avocado, olive oil, nuts, seeds, and non-starchy vegetables. While fruit and grains are largely off-limits, fibrous vegetables like leafy greens and cruciferous varieties are encouraged. These help slow sugar absorption, regulate digestion, and keep you full without spiking insulin levels.

A daily carbohydrate limit of around 30 to 50 grams is usually required to maintain ketosis, and tracking ketone levels can help you stay on target. Many people report a reduction in appetite, improved mental clarity, and accelerated weight loss. However, it's essential to balance this approach with a focus on nutrient density - avoiding processed meats and favouring whole, unrefined fats.

The Atkins Diet: A High-Protein Cautionary Tale

Long before keto went mainstream, Dr. Robert Atkins popularised the low-carb lifestyle with his eponymous diet. Emphasising animal protein and fat, the Atkins diet restricts carbohydrates to just 5%–10% of total intake, while fat makes up 60%–70% and protein about 20%–30%.

In theory, this approach induces ketosis and leads to rapid weight loss by reducing insulin levels and increasing energy expenditure. However, the high protein content comes with its own concerns. Unlike fat and carbohydrates, the body cannot store excess protein. Surplus amino acids are converted into glucose via a process called gluconeogenesis, which can raise insulin levels and disrupt the intended metabolic benefits of the diet.

Even more concerning, high protein intake can elevate insulin-like growth factor 1 (IGF-1), a hormone linked to accelerated ageing, cardiovascular disease, and certain cancers. Lower levels of IGF-1 are consistently associated with improved longevity and a reduced risk of metabolic diseases.

Tragically, Dr. Atkins himself struggled with obesity and cardiovascular complications later in life, passing away at the age of 72 with a body weight suggestive of metabolic imbalance. His story serves as a cautionary reminder: weight loss alone is not a reliable marker of health.

The Ultimate Metabolic Prescription

Food, at its core, should heal - not harm. It's the cornerstone of true metabolic health, and in most cases, the most potent "medicine" we can offer our bodies. While we often seek complex solutions to manage weight and chronic illness, the truth is far simpler: long-term health begins on the plate.

Rather than offering yet another trendy diet, the metabolic approach advocates a return to our roots - eating as our ancestors once did, when food came from the earth, not a factory. When we favour natural, whole foods and strip away modern ultra-processing, remarkable things happen. Waistlines shrink, insulin levels drop, cholesterol and triglycerides fall into line, and energy returns. Whole foods nourish not only the body but also the trillions of microbes in our gut, which ferment plant fibres into powerful compounds like butyrate - short-chain fatty acids (SCFAs) that reduce inflammation and support everything from digestion to brain health.

A remarkable feature of this way of eating is how self-regulating it becomes. There's little need to count calories or measure portions obsessively. Instead, learning to stop eating when you feel about

80% full - what the Japanese call *hara hachi bu* - can accelerate your journey to health without restriction or deprivation. Even when we do overeat whole foods, the body tends to store the excess as subcutaneous fat rather than the more dangerous visceral fat that drives disease.

If you prefer a less strict approach, you'll find harmony in the Mediterranean diet—a time-tested and culturally rich way of eating that blends tradition with powerful metabolic benefits. With its generous servings of olive oil, legumes, vegetables, seafood, fermented dairy, and moderate wine, the Mediterranean diet has repeatedly been shown to reduce abdominal fat, improve cholesterol balance, lower blood pressure, and stabilise blood sugar. With about 50% of calories from complex carbohydrates, 30% from healthy fats, and 20% from lean protein, it achieves a balanced nutrient profile that promotes longevity - especially when paired with regular physical activity and stress reduction.

The science is clear: eating this way lowers insulin resistance and improves nearly every marker associated with metabolic dysfunction. By reducing LDL particle size, increasing HDL, and lowering triglycerides, this dietary strategy not only manages symptoms - it also rewires your metabolism.

Habits That Heal

Over the years, I've found that small, practical habits often make the biggest difference in my patients' lives. The first step is always the same: helping people reframe food as medicine and encouraging them to choose "living" food from farms, rather than the "dead" food produced by factories.

Nutrition isn't just about macronutrients and calories. It's also about how we eat. Even those who consume organic, nutrient-rich meals can experience deficiencies - often because of rushed, distracted eating. I've had countless conversations that begin with advice as simple as: "Chew your food at least 25 times," "Don't eat in front of the TV," and "Take 30-45 minutes to enjoy your meal." Eating slowly and mindfully helps unlock the full nutritional value of food and reconnects us with the social joy of shared meals.

Stress is a major disruptor of digestion. If you've ever felt bloated, fatigued, or nutrient-depleted despite a healthy diet, stress may be the underlying cause. When we're anxious, our bodies divert blood away from the digestive system, prioritising survival over digestion. In this state, nutrient absorption suffers. That's why taking a few deep breaths and relaxing before meals can be more powerful than the most expensive supplement.

Why Vitamin B12 Matters

One essential nutrient that deserves special attention is vitamin B12. It's found only in animal products, particularly organ meat and red meat, and its absorption begins in the stomach with the help of digestive acids and enzymes. When digestion falters - often due to stress, low stomach acid, or rushed meals - B12 absorption drops.

I once met a vibrant, professional woman in her mid-fifties who was plagued by fatigue, memory issues, and numbness in her feet. Despite eating well, she had developed a significant B12 deficiency. Her rapid eating habits, high stress levels, and poor digestion were the culprits. With proper supplementation and mindful eating, including magnesium and stress-reducing practices such as deep breathing, her symptoms improved dramatically.

Timing Fluids Wisely

Hydration is critical, but **when** you drink matters. Drinking large amounts of water during meals dilutes digestive enzymes, reducing their effectiveness. To optimise digestion, it's better to hydrate 30 minutes before meals or at least 2 hours afterwards. This small change can significantly improve symptoms such as bloating, reflux, and indigestion.

Plants as the Foundation

The metabolic diet is deeply rooted in plants - comprising 80-90% of your daily intake. That means a colourful spectrum of vegetables, legumes, fruits (in moderation), nuts, and seeds. Home-pressure-cooked beans, organic produce, and raw, unsalted seeds are at the heart of this approach.

I encourage patients to shift away from factory-farmed meats and instead choose small oily fish such as sardines, herring, mackerel, and wild salmon. These are rich in anti-inflammatory omega-3 and carry a lower risk of mercury contamination than larger species, such as tuna. Avoid canned baked beans, which are often laced with added sugar and packaged in BPA-lined tins with preservative chemicals.

Some fruits, such as grapes and bananas, as well as honey, can spike blood sugar and contribute to metabolic dysfunction due to their high fructose content. Berries and pomegranates, on the other hand, are lower in sugar and rich in antioxidants - ideal choices for those with insulin resistance.

Vegetables can be grouped to understand their benefits better:

- **Leafy greens**: Spinach, kale, rocket, Swiss chard - rich in folate and ideal for those with methylation issues.
- **Cruciferous vegetables:** Broccoli, cabbage, cauliflower - contain sulforaphane, a detoxifying compound with anti-cancer benefits.
- **Rainbow vegetables**: Carrots, beets, bell peppers, tomatoes - each colour represents a different antioxidant profile.

- **Alliums and roots:** Garlic, onions, turmeric, ginger - anti-inflammatory and immune-supporting.

Fat: Friend, Not Foe

It's time to debunk the myth that fat is the enemy. The right fats are essential to hormone production, cellular health, and brain function.

Nuts and seeds provide plant-based omega-3, fibre, and micronutrients. Chia seeds, rich in quercetin and protein, are excellent for gut health and satiety. Macadamias, Brazil nuts, and cashews nourish the microbiome and support bowel regularity.

Animal-based omega-3 from fish are even more potent, especially EPA and DHA, which help combat inflammation. The modern Western diet is heavy in omega-6 fat - found in seed oils and grain-fed meat - which can tip the balance toward inflammation. Our ancestors consumed omega-6 and omega-3 in a 1:1 ratio. The Mediterranean diet averages 4:1. The Western diet is closer to a 20:1 ratio. Restoring this balance is crucial for preventing metabolic disorders and promoting overall well-being and longevity.

Protein: Quality Counts

Protein is more than just a building block for muscle - it's also essential for neurotransmitter production, immune function, and blood sugar stability. Tyrosine supports dopamine and thyroid hormones; tryptophan leads to serotonin; BCAAs prevent muscle loss with age.

Aim for 100 to 200 grams of protein daily, ideally with 30-50 grams per meal. Animal proteins tend to be more complete, with all essential amino acids, but well-planned plant-based diets can suffice - with supplementation of B12 and BCAAs.

Protein quality matters. Eggs rank highest in biological value, followed by fish and red meat. Be cautious with commercial meats due to antibiotic residues, which have been linked to weight gain and metabolic disturbances, especially in children.[9]

Carbohydrates: Not All Created Equal

Carbs often get a bad rap, but they come in many forms. Beans, for instance, are nutrient-dense and surprisingly protein-rich. In the world's healthiest regions - known as Blue Zones - beans are a daily staple. They provide resistant starch and fibre that feed the gut microbiome and slow down sugar absorption, stabilising energy and appetite.

Fibre, though indigestible to us, is a feast for gut bacteria. These microbes ferment fibre into SCFAs, particularly butyrate, which nourishes the intestinal lining, supports kidney and brain health, and offers anti-inflammatory and anti-cancer effects.

Think Organic, Think Clean

Choosing organic foods whenever possible limits exposure to persistent organic pollutants (POPs), pesticides, and chemicals such as bisphenol A (BPA), which is found in plastics. These toxins disrupt hormone function, impair insulin sensitivity, and damage the gut microbiome - contributing to the very conditions we're trying to prevent.

Let this be your food philosophy: Eat simply, eat naturally, eat with intention. Nourish your body, honour your biology, and trust that the food we evolved to eat is the food that will heal us.

How to Implement the Metabolic Diet

Begin with a Gentle Transition

Changing how you eat isn't just a decision - it's a physiological shift. The body, especially if accustomed to sugar-heavy or ultra-processed foods, may initially resist the change. In the first few days, you might experience fatigue, headaches, or cravings - this is your internal ecosystem adjusting. Harmful gut bacteria thrive on sugar and protest when it's removed, much like an addict being cut off from a fix.

To ease this transition, start by gradually reducing your intake of refined sugars and processed carbohydrates. Transition from simple sugars to fruit sugars, and then shift towards low-glycaemic, high-fibre vegetables such as celery, cucumbers, green beans, and leafy greens. To sustain your energy and reduce cravings, incorporate healthy fats from avocados, coconut oil, nuts, and seeds into your diet. Pair these with high-quality proteins at every meal to support satiety and stabilise blood sugar.

Natural compounds like cinnamon, chromium, Brahmi, and Ashwagandha can also help buffer withdrawal symptoms by calming the nervous system and improving glucose regulation.

Support Your Body's Detox Process

Fat cells don't just store energy - they also harbour toxins. As your body begins to burn fat, those toxins are released into circulation. This is a critical phase that requires active detox support.

Incorporate foods that promote natural detoxification. Herbs and spices such as coriander, fennel, black pepper, garlic, and cinnamon support liver function and aid in the elimination process. Cruciferous vegetables - like broccoli, cauliflower, kale, cabbage, and Brussels sprouts - contain sulforaphane, a compound known to boost detox enzyme activity.

Soluble fibres found in psyllium husk and flaxseeds can help bind toxins in the gut and prevent reabsorption. Reduce your toxic burden further by choosing organic produce, avoiding plastic food containers, and filtering your water. Additional practices like sauna sessions and regular physical activity enhance sweat-based detoxification.

For moments when cravings hit hard, try low-glycaemic snacks - like celery sticks dipped in hummus or cucumber slices with guacamole. These provide nourishment without triggering a blood sugar spike.

Embracing Intermittent Fasting

The traditional model of three meals and three snacks daily keeps your digestive system on overdrive. This constant grazing doesn't allow time for cellular repair or metabolic recalibration. Instead, ease into a lighter eating pattern by gradually removing snacks - perhaps starting with the mid-morning or post-dinner nibble.

The goal is to establish a sustainable rhythm, such as eating two to three meals per day. Let lunch be your most substantial meal to support daytime energy needs. One of the most accessible and effective fasting methods is the 16/8 approach, which involves stopping eating by 6 p.m. and resuming by 10 a.m. the next day. This gives your body 16 hours to rest, reset, and repair.

Intermittent fasting stimulates fat burning and activates hundreds of genes involved in healing and longevity. Fat loss can average between 0.25 and 0.7 kilograms (0.5 and 1.5 pounds) per week. Under professional guidance, longer fasts - such as 24, 36, or even 72 hours or more - can offer deeper metabolic benefits.

The key is to nourish your body with whole, unprocessed foods during your eating window. This is not about calorie restriction - it's about aligning with your body's natural rhythms.

Daily Nutritional Blueprint

Use the following as a foundation for meal planning, aiming to meet your body's needs while promoting healing and resilience:

- **Vegetables and fruits**: 5-10 servings daily, prioritising low-sugar and richly coloured options.
- **Leafy greens**: A natural source of folate and fibre.
- **Cruciferous vegetables**: Enhance detoxification through compounds like sulforaphane.
- **Rainbow vegetables**: Supply a wide range of antioxidants.
- **Seeds**, such as flax, chia, pumpkin, and sunflower seeds, support gut health and promote detoxification.
- **Healthy fats**: 3-4 servings daily from avocados, olive oil, nuts, and seeds.
- **Fibre-rich legumes and nuts**: Help regulate blood sugar and feed beneficial gut bacteria.
- **Cooking oils**: Use stable saturated fats like coconut oil and avocado oil. While butter may suit some, others may need to avoid it.
- **Fermented foods**, such as yoghurt, sauerkraut, and kombucha, help repopulate your microbiome.
- **Bitter foods**: Lemons and bitter melon promote bile flow and support liver detoxification.
- **Healing broths**, such as bone broth and cabbage soup, aid in restoring gut integrity and reducing inflammation.
- **Salt**: Choose sea salt or Himalayan salt over processed table salt.
- **Protein**: Opt for grass-fed meats, organic poultry, and small wild-caught fish such as sardines, herring, and salmon.

A Metabolic Reset Is Within Reach

The good news is that metabolic dysfunction is not destiny. It is almost always reversible. Even modest weight loss - approximately 10% of your body weight - can significantly improve insulin sensitivity, reduce inflammation, and boost energy levels.

This is not about deprivation. Unlike rigid fad diets, a metabolic diet encourages abundance: abundant nutrients, abundant health, and, eventually, an abundant life. By focusing on whole, plant-rich foods with healthy fats and quality protein, you teach your body to burn fat efficiently and reset your hormonal environment.

Don't overlook hydration. Cellular function relies on it. Aim for 2 to 3 litres of water daily. Begin each morning by rehydrating: mix one teaspoon of organic apple cider vinegar with one teaspoon of lemon or lime juice in 500 ml of warm water. This simple practice helps restore electrolytes, stimulates bile production, and gently activates your detox pathways.

Targeted Support

In addition to food, several natural supplements may assist your metabolic transition:

- **Mulberry leaf extract:** slows the digestion of complex carbohydrates into simple sugars, thereby improving insulin sensitivity.
- **Lemon (containing Aeriocepine):** lowers the glycaemic index of starchy foods taken along with it by slowing the conversion of starch into simple sugar.
- **Berberine**: Helps lower blood sugar and improve lipid profiles.
- **Mixed-strain probiotics**: Support gut health and reduce inflammation.
- **Prebiotic fibre**: Feeds beneficial microbes.
- **Chromium and cinnamon:** Help stabilise glucose levels.
- **Psyllium husk**: Promotes satiety and supports bowel regularity.
- For added insight, consider using a **continuous glucose**

monitor (CGM). This technology enables you to see how specific foods affect your blood sugar in real-time, helping you fine-tune your diet with precision and confidence.

Before You Begin: Set Yourself Up for Success
Preparation is your most powerful ally. Start by decluttering your kitchen - clear out ultra-processed, sugary, and packaged foods. Write your first healthy grocery list and stock your pantry with staples. Map out meals for the week ahead. Set fixed mealtimes. Develop strategies to navigate cravings and manage detox symptoms.

Record your starting health metrics: weight, height, BMI, waist and hip circumference, and waist-to-hip ratio. These numbers are not just data - they're benchmarks of your transformation.

Finally, make walking a post-meal ritual. This simple practice helps stabilise blood sugar and supports digestion. In the next chapter, we'll explore how structured movement - including resistance and cardiovascular training - further amplifies your metabolic power.

CHAPTER 17

The Metabolic Exercise Prescription

During my time working in Dundee, I developed the habit of going for a morning run before heading into the hospital. I'd often return, sweaty and breathless, entering through the staff entrance just in time to start my day. Almost every morning, I would encounter a rather portly gentleman, likely part of the administrative staff. His reaction to my dishevelled post-run state was consistent - visible discomfort, perhaps even mild disdain. We frequently crossed paths again on the upper floors: I had taken the stairs, and he the lift. His expression didn't change.

But then, something shifted. After months of these silent, awkward encounters, he suddenly greeted me with a bright, "Good morning!" - a noticeable change from his usual reserved glare. A few weeks later, I noticed him on the stairs beside me. It turned out he had started parking his car a mile away and walking the rest of the distance to work. Over time, I saw a visible transformation: he looked healthier, more energised. Eventually, he started talking about running. To my quiet satisfaction, I learned he had taken it up himself. It was a rewarding reminder that health leadership can come from simply modelling behaviour - no formal consultation necessary.

There's truth in the adage: "Use it or lose it." Sadly, I learned this the hard way through personal experience. But that difficult lesson became the motivation behind a turning point in my own health journey. Physical activity has become a cornerstone of my recovery and continues to be the foundation of my well-being. Exercise, as I came to appreciate more deeply, isn't just about fitness - it's a powerful metabolic regulator. It boosts mood by releasing endorphins, relieves stress and anxiety, and strengthens confidence and self-esteem. It's also one of the most accessible, affordable, and effective interventions we have at our disposal.

In contrast, sedentary living is a silent saboteur of health - arguably more harmful than smoking, excessive alcohol intake, or high cholesterol. The evidence is compelling: physical inactivity raises the risk of type 2 diabetes, cardiovascular disease, depression, certain cancers, and even premature death. Yet so many of us struggle to fit movement into our busy lives.

This chapter focuses on how to integrate exercise into your lifestyle, particularly if you're over 50. We'll explore how regular physical activity rewires your metabolism, helps preserve your muscle mass and vitality, and supports healthy ageing. You'll also learn how to build a realistic, sustainable routine - no matter how hectic your schedule might be.

How Age Alters Your Metabolism and Body Composition

As we move through our 40s and beyond, the body's metabolic machinery begins to change. One of the earliest shifts is a slowdown in insulin sensitivity. You might recall from earlier in the book that insulin acts like a key, allowing glucose to enter cells to be used for energy. When cells become resistant to this hormone, glucose lingers in the bloodstream, contributing to fat gain and metabolic sluggishness.

Simultaneously, the natural ageing process chips away at our muscle mass - about 5% each decade after 30. This shift increases fat-to-muscle ratio, raising the risk of conditions like type 2 diabetes, heart disease, and sarcopenia (age-related muscle loss). For women, menopause introduces further challenges: declining oestrogen levels contribute to bone thinning, heightening the risk of osteoporosis and fractures.

Weight-bearing exercises, like walking, resistance training, or dancing, can help counteract these changes. They allow you to burn fat, maintain lean muscle, and strengthen bones - essential factors for preserving mobility and independence in later years.

And there's more. By the time we reach our 70s, we've lost up to 75% of the mitochondria - the tiny power plants inside our cells responsible for producing energy. However, the good news is that exercise, especially at moderate to high intensity, can stimulate the regeneration of these mitochondria. This process occurs through autophagy, where cells break down and recycle their old, worn-out components. Think of it as cellular spring cleaning, a metabolic reboot triggered by stressors such as fasting, heat exposure, or a brisk uphill walk. Our ancestors relied on this very mechanism to survive famines, hunt game, and maintain physical resilience under extreme conditions.

Hormonal shifts also shape the ageing metabolism. As "feel-good" hormones like testosterone and oestrogen decline, and stress hormones such as cortisol and insulin become more dominant, energy levels dip, body composition changes, and mood may suffer. But again, exercise is a potent hormonal modulator. It stimulates the release of youth-preserving hormones and helps recalibrate the hormonal imbalances that often accompany ageing.

Perhaps one of the most startling demonstrations of inactivity's toll comes from the 1966 Dallas Bed Rest and Training Study. In this landmark experiment, five healthy young men underwent three weeks of strict bed rest. Their physical capacity was measured before and after the rest period - and again 30 years later. Astonishingly, the three weeks of complete inactivity led to a more significant decline in cardiovascular fitness than three decades of natural ageing.[2] It was a sobering revelation: doing nothing can age the body faster than time itself.

In the sections that follow, we'll examine how to harness movement as a strategic tool for longevity, not just in years, but in quality as well. Exercise isn't a punishment for indulgence or a means to aesthetic perfection - it's an essential, life-giving practice. Whether you're rediscovering your fitness after decades or just beginning the journey, it's never too late to take that first step - perhaps even up the stairs.

How Exercise Works – And Why It Matters So Much

Exercise, at its core, is the purposeful repetition of movement designed to improve or maintain one or more components of physical fitness. But not all movement is created equal. There's a broad spectrum - from the simple act of walking to structured high-intensity workouts - and each type offers unique metabolic and physiological benefits.

Let's begin by clarifying a distinction that's often overlooked: **exercise versus physical activity**. Physical activity includes all the unplanned movements that fill your day—climbing stairs, carrying groceries, cleaning the house, or gardening. These actions are vital; they represent the natural ways we use our muscles in everyday life. Exercise, on the other hand, is intentional, focused, and typically goal-oriented - like going for a jog, doing resistance training, or attending a dance class.

Powering Movement: Where the Energy Comes From

Your body is a marvel of engineering, and movement - whether planned or spontaneous - it requires fuel. Surprisingly, only about **5% of your total energy expenditure** comes from formal exercise. Another **10% is used in digesting and processing food**, known as the thermic effect of food. However, a significant **20% of your energy** is devoted to physical activity and movement throughout the day, whether you're walking the dog or pacing during a phone call. The bulk - roughly **70% of your daily calorie burn** - is dedicated to keeping your body alive at rest: maintaining your heartbeat, brain activity, temperature, breathing, and cellular housekeeping. This is known as your **basal metabolic rate (BMR)**.

The implication: You don't need to run marathons to boost your metabolism - though that certainly helps. Even simple efforts like increasing your daily steps or doing a few bodyweight exercises can add up, especially when supported by activities that increase your **resting metabolic rate (RMR)**, such as strength training.

Choosing Your Exercise: Match Movement With Meaning

There's no one-size-fits-all approach to fitness. Whether it's walking, swimming, cycling, dancing, or lifting weights, the best exercise is the one you enjoy and can stick with. But your goals should guide your choices.

For many, especially those in midlife or beyond, the goal isn't to sculpt an athletic physique, but to maintain independence, confidence, and vitality. Think of it this way: **Can you comfortably carry shopping bags? Climb stairs without breathlessness? Play with your grandchildren? Dance at your granddaughter's wedding?** If so, your fitness is working in your favour.

After age 50, your exercise priorities may need a shift in emphasis - from sheer muscle or cardio endurance to elements that preserve functionality: **balance, agility, flexibility, coordination, and reaction time**. These are the silent protectors against falls and fractures. Incorporating **resistance training twice a week** alongside **30 minutes of moderate-intensity exercise on most days** is the gold standard. And while more can be better, excessive training without rest can lead to burnout or injury - so more is not always more.

Set Your Sights: Personalising Your Goals

Generic goals like "get fit" or "lose weight" often fail to achieve their objectives. Instead, go specific and meaningful: *Run 10 km in under an hour. Reduce waist circumference by 5 cm. Reach a BMI in the healthy range within four months.* These targets turn vague hopes into actionable commitments.

More importantly, your goals should connect with what truly matters to you. When your "why" is clear, staying motivated becomes far easier.

Metabolism in Motion: What Exercise Really Does

One of exercise's underrated benefits is how it shifts your metabolic gears. Activity of any kind - especially that which engages large muscle groups - increases your calorie burn not just during the activity but often for hours, sometimes days, afterwards.

A walk after a meal, for instance, helps blunt blood sugar spikes without relying on insulin. It works because **muscles can directly absorb glucose from the bloodstream during contraction**, sparing the pancreas from overworking. This can have dramatic long-term benefits. A relative of mine, shocked by a diagnosis of type 2 diabetes, adopted a whole-food diet, began daily 60-minute walks, and practised intermittent fasting. Just two months later, her HbA1c - a measure of average blood sugar

- dropped from a worrisome 7.4% to a pristine 4.5%, without medications.

More intense forms of exercise, such as resistance training or **High-Intensity Interval Training (HIIT)**, offer additional metabolic benefits. Muscle tissue is metabolically active; it burns calories even while you sleep. By increasing your **muscle-to-fat ratio**, you enhance your BMR, making it easier to maintain or lose weight and stave off chronic disease.

HIIT: Small Investment, Big Return

If you're pressed for time, **HIIT** is an efficient powerhouse. A simple protocol - such as 10 cycles of 30 seconds of effort followed by 90 seconds of recovery - can stimulate muscle growth, burn fat, and maintain an elevated metabolism for up to 48 hours. Studies show that just 12 weeks of HIIT can significantly boost **VO$_2$ max** (a measure of aerobic capacity), improve insulin sensitivity, and reduce belly fat by nearly 20%.[3] And because it's so efficient, it's ideal for those who struggle to find long stretches of time for traditional workouts.

Why Exercise Is a Multisystem Healer

It's hard to think of a body system that doesn't benefit from regular movement. Exercise is like a multipurpose tonic:

- **Brain health:** Cardiovascular workouts trigger the release of **brain-derived neurotrophic factor (BDNF)**, a protein that promotes the growth and development of new neural connections.[4] This not only enhances memory and focus but also reduces the risk of dementia. That old saying, "move it or lose it," holds true for your brain as well as your body.

- **Mood and mental resilience**: Physical activity releases endorphins, those natural mood enhancers. For many, exercise becomes a reliable antidote to stress, anxiety, and even mild depression.
- **Bone and muscle strength**: Weight-bearing exercise stimulates both bones and muscles. This is crucial for preventing **osteoporosis** and the dangerous falls that accompany it. Incredibly, even women in their 90s, living in nursing homes, gained significant strength and muscle mass after just eight weeks of resistance training - some were even able to regain independence.[5]
- **Detoxification and circulation**: Through sweat and muscle contraction, exercise helps your body eliminate metabolic waste and environmental toxins, such as BPA, pesticides, and heavy metals. It also promotes **lymphatic circulation**, enhancing immune function.
- **Gut function**: Exercise stimulates the digestive system. You may notice increased bowel movements or less bloating after a walk - that's your gut saying thanks.
- **Fat-burning and weight regulation**: A wider waistline has been linked to a smaller brain and increased risk of cognitive decline.[6] Exercise, particularly when combined with a nutritious diet such as the Mediterranean diet, helps reverse metabolic syndrome and encourages fat loss, especially around the abdomen.[7]

In Summary

Exercise is more than just a lifestyle choice - it's an essential component of vibrant, long-term health. And while the sheer number of benefits can be overwhelming, the takeaway is simple: **move more, more often, and with purpose.** Whether it's a brisk walk after lunch or a challenging strength session, every bit counts - and every bit adds up to a stronger, sharper, more resilient you.

Exercise Alone Is Not the Magic Bullet for Weight Loss
It's a familiar scene: someone laces up their trainers, hits the gym with gusto, and expects the scale to reward their efforts. When that doesn't happen, frustration sets in. I've encountered many such individuals - motivated, consistent, and bewildered that their weight isn't dropping despite all the sweat. The issue: Exercise, while powerful, isn't a stand-alone solution for shedding pounds.

Let's dispel a common myth: the primary purpose of exercise isn't weight loss. Yes, it contributes, but not in the way most people expect. Regular activity improves strength, stamina, heart health, and insulin sensitivity. But when it comes to shifting body fat, especially visceral fat around the abdomen, it needs to be part of a broader strategy.

Why doesn't exercise alone cause dramatic weight loss? First, physical activity stimulates appetite. Your body, detecting a caloric deficit, ramps up hunger signals. If you're not careful, you may eat more than you've burned - especially if you're following old advice to 'refuel' immediately post-workout with energy bars or sugary sports drinks. The irony: You might end up consuming more calories than you've just expended.

Consider the maths: walking 10 miles (around 16 kilometres) burns roughly 500 calories. To burn off 1,000 calories, you'd need to run that same distance at a brisk pace. It's achievable - but time-consuming and exhausting. Realistically, most people can't rely on physical activity alone to create the calorie deficit required for meaningful weight loss.

Moreover, exercise-induced weight changes can be deceptive. You might burn fat and simultaneously build muscle, which is denser than fat. The scale won't budge, even though your body is changing for the better. That's why weight alone is a poor proxy for progress.

Beyond the BMI: Focus on What Really Matters

BMI (Body Mass Index) is often used as a quick measure of health, but it's a blunt instrument. It doesn't distinguish between muscle and fat, nor does it reflect where fat is stored. A muscular athlete and someone with excess abdominal fat can have the same BMI. What truly matters is your **body composition** - the proportion of fat, muscle, and lean tissue.

Even if your BMI is "normal," fat stored around your internal organs (visceral fat) can significantly raise your risk of metabolic diseases. That's why using a bioimpedance scale or another body composition tool can be so empowering. It gives a more nuanced picture and shows the benefits of increasing lean mass and reducing fat.

As a general goal, men should aim for a body fat percentage of under 20%, and women under 30%. Tracking these metrics over time helps you stay focused on what counts: not your weight, but your metabolic health and strength.

Making Exercise a Natural Part of Your Life

To sustain an active lifestyle, you need to find what works for *you*. Not everyone enjoys running, and that's perfectly fine. Some people flourish when they discover activities such as cycling, swimming, rowing, dancing, or strength training. Others thrive in group settings or clubs, where social connection reinforces the habit.

Select an activity that suits your physical abilities and preferences. Identify your best time of day for movement - some find morning energising, others prefer unwinding in the evening. Build your exercise sessions into your weekly schedule just as you would any important appointment.

Consistency is key. Partnering with a friend, setting goals, and gradually increasing your activity level will help cement the habit. You don't need expensive gear - a yoga mat, a pair of dumbbells, or simply your own body weight can be enough to get started. Resistance bands, park benches, or even stairs at home can serve as your home gym.

Look for ways to integrate physical activity into your daily life:

- Park further from entrances or choose the longest walking route.
- Skip the elevator - take the stairs.
- Turn housework and gardening into mini workouts.
- Opt for a standing desk and take movement breaks every hour.
- Schedule 'walking meetings' instead of sit-downs.
- Use your phone's step counter as a daily accountability tool - aim for 10,000 steps, including a brisk 15-minute walk after lunch.
- Spend your weekends in nature, hiking on trails or exploring local parks.

A Practical Roadmap for Active Living

All movement counts. Even everyday tasks like carrying groceries, vacuuming, or walking the dog contribute to maintaining a healthy metabolism. These "non-exercise" activities burn calories, enhance insulin sensitivity, and boost energy expenditure.

Structured workouts have their place as well. Cardiovascular exercises - such as brisk walking, cycling, or swimming - raise your heart rate and enhance insulin function. Over time, this lowers your baseline insulin levels, allowing your body to burn stored fat more effectively. This is especially helpful in tackling belly fat, the epicentre of metabolic dysfunction.

Strength training - whether it's bodyweight exercises like squats and push-ups or gym-based resistance training - builds lean muscle. More muscle means a higher basal metabolic rate (BMR), which means you burn more energy even at rest. High-Intensity Interval Training (HIIT) combines cardiovascular and strength elements, offering powerful benefits in short timeframes.

Crucially, certain types of physical stress, like intense exercise or varied movement patterns, help your cells generate more **mitochondria** - the energy powerhouses within your cells. These improve your energy production, enhance fat-burning capacity, and contribute to longevity.

Equally important are movements that improve **agility, flexibility, balance, and coordination**. These qualities become especially vital as we age, supporting independence, preventing falls, and improving quality of life. Whether it's yoga, tai chi, or functional strength training, integrating such practices helps you move better, live longer, and feel younger.

Remember: progress is best measured not just in pounds lost but in muscle gained, energy restored, and vitality regained.

Final Thoughts: The Metabolic Power of Movement

Daily movement doesn't just shape your body - it tunes your metabolism, boosts your mood, and enhances your sleep. Physical activity helps deplete your energy molecule, ATP (adenosine triphosphate), during the day. As ATP is used, it releases adenosine, which accumulates and builds a sense of sleep pressure, making you naturally drowsy at night. This is one reason why physically active people tend to sleep better.

During restful sleep, your body replenishes energy stores and resets for the day ahead. We'll explore this metabolic rhythm - and how to optimise it through sleep - in the next chapter.

But for now, remember this: exercise is not merely a tool for burning calories. It's a profound signal to your body - a reminder to grow stronger, build resilience, and stay metabolically young. When combined with wise nutrition, restorative sleep, and stress management, physical activity becomes a cornerstone of lifelong health.

CHAPTER 18

The Metabolic Sleep Prescription

Shakespeare once wrote, *"Sleep…knits up the ravelled sleeve of care."* In those few words, he captured what modern science confirms: sleep is a process of repair, restoration, and renewal. And in a world that prizes productivity and busyness, it's worth revisiting the timeless wisdom: *"Early to bed and early to rise makes you healthy, wealthy, and wise."*

But this isn't just a quaint saying - it's a metabolic truth.

Your nightly slumber is not a passive shutdown. It is a finely orchestrated physiological reset, influencing everything from appetite regulation and fat storage to immune resilience and brain function. When sleep is disrupted or insufficient, a cascade of metabolic disturbances follows: cravings for high-calorie foods, impaired calorie burning, and systemic inflammation - all leading to weight gain, insulin resistance, and chronic diseases like type 2 diabetes and heart disease.

Poor sleep also weakens the immune system, making you more susceptible to infections and illnesses, while simultaneously raising the risk of mood disorders and cognitive decline.

This chapter delves into the fascinating biology of sleep,

exploring what triggers sleep, how your body cycles through different stages each night, and the crucial role of your internal biological clock, known as your circadian rhythm. You'll learn how to craft a personalised sleep strategy to support your metabolic health, restore your energy, and protect against disease.

What Drives Sleep?

Two key biological processes govern when and how you sleep: the gradual accumulation of adenosine - a metabolic signal of cellular fatigue - and your circadian rhythm, the master clock that aligns your body with the day-night cycle.

Adenosine: Your Brain's Sleep Switch

As discussed earlier in the book, ATP (adenosine triphosphate) is the energy currency used by every cell. Throughout the day, as ATP is spent to power your muscles, brain, and organs, adenosine - the "spent" byproduct - builds up. High levels of adenosine dampen neural activity, nudging you toward drowsiness. Think of it as your brain's gentle nudge that it's time to power down.

During sleep, the body rebuilds ATP and clears adenosine. By morning, adenosine levels are low, your energy stores are replenished, and you're ready to face the day. Physical activity during the day helps accelerate this process, resulting in more restful sleep at night.

The Circadian Rhythm: Nature's Timekeeper

Layered atop the adenosine system is your circadian rhythm - a 24-hour internal clock housed in a region of the brain called the suprachiasmatic nucleus (SCN). This clock synchronises with natural light-dark cycles. Bright light in the morning and during the day signals alertness. As evening falls and darkness sets in, the SCN cues the pineal gland to release melatonin - the sleep hormone.

But melatonin is far more than a sleep trigger. It's also a master antioxidant that bathes your tissues nightly, neutralising harmful oxidants that accumulate throughout the day. This is crucial for protecting your mitochondria, the energy generators in your cells. When mitochondria are damaged by oxidative stress, your metabolism suffers.

Disruptions to the circadian rhythm - whether caused by shift work, late-night screen exposure, or travel - can disrupt these finely tuned processes. The result: Poor blood sugar control, increased fat storage, hormonal imbalances, and mood disturbances.

For example, night shift workers often struggle with metabolic health. Studies consistently show that those working overnight hours tend to have slower metabolisms, greater fat retention, and higher rates of obesity than their daytime counterparts. This is no coincidence - their circadian rhythms are out of sync with their behaviour.

Jet lag, too, is more than just travel fatigue. Crossing time zones throws off your internal clock, impairing sugar metabolism and increasing stress hormone (cortisol) levels. The body, unsure whether it's day or night, struggles to regulate mood, appetite, and energy levels.

When Breathing Interrupts Sleep: Obstructive Sleep Apnoea
Another major disruptor of restorative sleep is obstructive sleep apnoea (OSA), a condition characterised by repeated episodes of blocked airflow during sleep, often accompanied by loud snoring and gasping. These interruptions fragment sleep and plunge oxygen levels, with severe consequences for metabolic health.

OSA is strongly associated with insulin resistance and weight gain. Up to 60% of people with type 2 diabetes also suffer from OSA

- many without knowing it.² The good news is that treatment with continuous positive airway pressure (CPAP) has been shown to improve blood sugar levels, reduce insulin resistance, and even rival the effects of common diabetes medications, such as metformin.³

Circadian Rhythms and Mental Health

Your internal clock doesn't just manage metabolism - it also governs mental wellbeing. Seasonal affective disorder (SAD), commonly known as winter depression, emerges when diminished daylight disrupts circadian rhythms. People with dementia often show a similar disruption - sleeping by day and staying awake at night - highlighting how fundamental the sleep-wake cycle is to brain health.

Circadian alignment is also crucial for DNA repair, a vital process in cancer prevention. Skimping on sleep or sleeping at irregular hours compromises the body's ability to repair genetic damage.

When Digestion Interferes with Sleep

Late-night meals, especially those that are heavy or spicy, can lead to acid reflux and disrupt your sleep. This is particularly common in individuals with overweight or obesity. If you find yourself waking with a sour taste or a burning sensation in your throat, your stomach contents may be rising due to gravity and pressure.

To avoid this, aim to finish your evening meal at least 2 to 4 hours before bedtime, and consider elevating the head of your bed slightly. This simple change can make a big difference.

The Four Stages of Sleep

Every night, your brain cycles through a rhythm of non-REM and REM sleep - about four to six times per night, in roughly 90-minute intervals:

- **Stage 1 (non-REM):** The lightest sleep, a transition from wakefulness that lasts just a few minutes.
- **Stage 2 (non-REM):** A deeper sleep where body temperature drops, heart rate slows, and muscles relax. This phase can last up to 25 minutes.
- **Stage 3 (non-REM):** Also known as slow-wave sleep (SWS), this is the deepest and most restorative stage. Here, the body repairs tissues, builds bone and muscle, strengthens the immune system, and restores metabolic balance.
- **Stage 4 (REM):** Brain activity ramps up and dreaming occurs. While your brain is active, your muscles are largely paralysed to prevent you from acting out your dreams.

The deep, slow-wave sleep of stage 3 is particularly crucial for maintaining metabolic health. Most of it occurs early in the night - between 10 p.m. and 2 a.m. - reinforcing the value of an early bedtime. Missing this window means missing the most rejuvenating part of your sleep cycle.

One study found that cutting sleep over just three nights reduced slow-wave sleep by 25%, mimicking the sleep patterns of older adults or those with OSA.[2] This reduction was enough to impair insulin sensitivity and increase the risk of diabetes.

The Role of Growth Hormone

Growth hormone isn't just for kids - it plays a central role in adult repair and metabolic renewal. Seventy percent of growth hormone is released during early night-time sleep, particularly during stage 3 slow-wave sleep. If you delay bedtime, you miss the hormonal wave that helps repair your muscles, regulate fat, and stabilise blood sugar.

Your Sleep Prescription

To harness the full metabolic power of sleep, follow these guidelines:

- **Aim for consistency.** Go to bed and wake up at the same time every day, even on weekends.
- **Get sunlight early.** Morning light exposure helps set your circadian rhythm, making you feel sleepy at night.
- **Move your body.** Regular physical activity helps increase the production of adenosine and promotes restful sleep.
- **Eat early.** Finish your evening meal 2 to 4 hours before bed.
- **Limit screens.** Blue light from phones and laptops can delay melatonin release - dim your lights and unplug 60-90 minutes before bedtime.
- **Create a sleep sanctuary.** Cool, dark, quiet bedrooms help enhance melatonin and signal to the body that it's time to rest.

With these habits, you can transform sleep from a neglected necessity into a powerful metabolic ally - one that sharpens your mind, protects your body, and restores your energy for the life you want to lead.

Sleep and the Gut Hormones: More Than Just Rest

We've often been told that managing weight is as simple as eating less and moving more. But that advice only scratches the surface. One decisive, frequently overlooked factor in metabolic health is **sleep** - not just its duration, but also its quality. The quality and quantity of your sleep have a profound influence on your hunger, satiety, energy levels, and fat storage patterns. How does this happen? The answer lies in two key gut-derived hormones: **ghrelin** and **leptin**.

Ghrelin and Leptin: The Yin and Yang of Appetite

Ghrelin is often referred to as the "hunger hormone." Produced primarily in the stomach, it signals your brain that it's time to eat. In contrast, leptin, produced by fat cells, sends the opposite message: you're full, you've eaten enough, and it's time to stop. These two hormones work together in a delicate balance to regulate food intake and energy expenditure.

However, poor sleep disrupts this harmony. When you're sleep-deprived, ghrelin levels rise, and leptin levels fall. The result? You feel hungrier and less satisfied after meals. Even a single night of restricted sleep - approximately 4.5 hours - can significantly shift these hormone levels, leading to increased hunger the next day.

Sleep Deprivation Skews Your Cravings

Lack of sleep doesn't just make you hungry - it changes what you crave. You're more likely to reach for energy-dense, ultra-processed foods loaded with sugar, fat, and salt. These "comfort" foods are not only hard to resist when you're tired but also prime drivers of weight gain and metabolic disease. On the flip side, getting high-quality, uninterrupted sleep helps regulate these hormones, supporting better food choices and promoting metabolic balance.

Energy, Activity, and Fat Storage

Sleep is when your body recharges its energy stores for the next day. Without enough of it, your energy levels plummet. Fatigue makes physical activity feel harder or less appealing. In this depleted state, the body becomes more inclined to store calories as fat rather than burn them. In effect, your metabolism slows, and the risk of weight gain rises.

Blood Sugar, Stress Hormones, and Night-Time Wakefulness

But the story doesn't end with appetite. Sleep deprivation also interferes with **glucose metabolism** and **insulin sensitivity**, increasing the risk of developing type 2 diabetes. Poor sleep raises cortisol, the body's primary stress hormone, which is notorious for impairing insulin function and raising blood glucose levels. Cortisol also disrupts your natural sleep-wake cycle, particularly when elevated at night due to stress, alcohol, caffeine, or erratic blood sugar.

People who struggle with unstable blood sugar - especially those who consume high-glycaemic meals late in the day - often wake up between 1 and 2 a.m. and find it difficult to fall back asleep. One practical strategy to avoid this glucose crash is to include **resistant carbohydrates** in your evening meal. Foods like beans release glucose gradually, helping to maintain stable blood sugar throughout the night and reducing early waking.

The Metabolic Cost of Poor Sleep

Studies confirm what many of us experience: inadequate sleep wreaks havoc on your metabolism. In one striking experiment, healthy young men were restricted to just four hours of sleep for six nights. When given a high-carb breakfast, their ability to process glucose dropped by a staggering 40% - a level of dysfunction seen in prediabetes.[5]

Another study showed that even short-term sleep loss leads the body to store more fat from meals.[6] Trying to "catch up" on weekends only partially restored fat-burning efficiency. A 2020 study from Spain found that middle-aged, sedentary individuals who reported poor sleep had markedly lower fat oxidation,[7] regardless of whether they followed a Mediterranean diet.[8] In other words, even a healthy diet may not be enough to overcome the metabolic damage caused by consistently poor sleep.

How to Know If You're Sleeping Well

It's possible to spend eight hours in bed and still wake up groggy. True **restorative sleep** means more than just clocking time. High-quality sleep is characterised by:

- Falling asleep within 30 minutes of lying down
- Sleeping through the night or waking up only once
- Falling back asleep within 20 minutes if awakened
- Feeling refreshed, energised, and focused the next morning

Signs that your sleep may be compromised include daytime fatigue, needing caffeine to stay alert, mood swings, poor concentration, and even forgetfulness. Irregular sleep schedules, excessive evening screen time, mental stress, and dietary factors like alcohol or sugar can all impair your sleep quality.

The Sleep Protocol: A Practical Guide

Improving sleep doesn't require expensive gadgets or complicated rituals. The following protocol supports both falling asleep and staying asleep - and is essential for metabolic repair.

- **Stick to a consistent sleep schedule**: Aim to go to bed around 10 p.m., even on weekends. This anchors your circadian rhythm.
- **Get enough sleep**: Adults should target 7-8 hours of restful, uninterrupted sleep each night.
- **Eat wisely in the evening**: Incorporate resistant carbs, such as lentils, chickpeas, or beans, with dinner. These foods digest slowly and help maintain blood sugar stability throughout the night.

- **Limit screen time before bed**: Avoid using screens for at least one hour before going to sleep. If needed, use blue-light-blocking glasses.
- **Light matters**: Daylight exposure in the morning and afternoon helps reinforce your sleep-wake cycle. Conversely, sleeping in a completely dark room can help support the production of melatonin.
- **Stay active**: Physical movement during the day boosts adenosine, a compound that builds up in the brain and promotes sleepiness at night.

Final Thoughts

Sleep is where healing begins. It's when your brain resets, your hormones recalibrate, and your metabolism repairs itself. Cortisol is the hormone of action and wakefulness, while melatonin is the hormone of rest and recovery. When these two are in sync, your body runs like a well-oiled machine. When they're not, you feel it - mentally, emotionally, and physically.

Stress, emotional tension, and poor relationships raise cortisol and disrupt sleep, fuelling a vicious cycle. In the next chapter, we'll explore strategies to manage stress, enhance emotional well-being, and cultivate an inner environment that fosters restful, rejuvenating sleep.

CHAPTER 19

The Metabolic Stress and Relationship Prescription

You've probably said it yourself or heard a colleague exclaim, "This job is killing me!" While usually said in jest, there's more truth to this than we might think. Mounting evidence suggests that persistent stress plays a central role in the development of metabolic syndrome - and the connection runs deeper than just "feeling worn out." It's intricately tied to how our bodies handle fat, sugar, hormones, and even relationships.

Stress is one of the unavoidable costs of modern life. But not all stress is created equal. Some forms galvanise us into action, giving us clarity and purpose. Others quietly erode our health over time. So, how do we differentiate between the helpful and the harmful? What mechanisms link stress to weight gain and metabolic dysfunction? And perhaps most intriguingly, why do some people lose weight under pressure while others gain it?

Understanding Stress:
From Sabre-toothed Tigers to Corporate Deadlines

Stress is not inherently bad. It's a deeply embedded biological process designed to keep us safe. Our ancestors relied on the "fight-or-flight" response to escape predators or hunt for food. But in the modern world, the predators are more abstract: overdue deadlines, unresolved conflicts, financial worries, or the emotional strain of a strained marriage. Unlike acute threats that come and go, many of these stressors are constant, or at least frequent, leading to a state of chronic stress.

When the body detects a potential threat - whether real or perceived - it activates a cascade of responses to prepare for action. The sympathetic nervous system kicks in, flooding the bloodstream with adrenaline, sharpening focus, and boosting energy. This is acute stress in action: fast, intense, but ideally short-lived.

Chronic stress, however, triggers a different hormonal pathway. Instead of a surge of adrenaline, the body shifts into a more insidious mode of preparation. This involves activating the hypothalamic-pituitary-adrenal (HPA) axis, which results in the sustained release of cortisol, a hormone that, while vital in the short term, can be profoundly damaging when elevated over time.

Acute vs. Chronic Stress: Opposite Effects on the Body

Acute stress is your body's emergency toolkit. It sharpens the mind, fuels physical readiness, and often suppresses hunger. This is why people under sudden duress - exams, public speaking, trauma, or surgery - usually experience temporary weight loss. During this state, adrenaline dominates, placing the body in a catabolic (breakdown) mode to mobilise energy reserves. The result: A short-term increase in alertness and physical capacity, often accompanied by a dip in appetite and even rapid weight loss.

Chronic stress, on the other hand, is like a dripping tap. It may not seem dangerous at first, but over time, the constant exposure to cortisol can alter key metabolic processes. Appetite increases, cravings for high-calorie foods intensify, and fat begins to accumulate - especially around the abdomen. This pattern is neither random nor accidental. Under chronic stress, the body is biologically primed to store energy in anticipation of an ongoing threat, even when that threat never materialises.

Metabolism Under Pressure: When Stress Fuels Fat
One of the body's most fascinating (and frustrating) quirks is how it stores fat during stress. Under prolonged cortisol exposure, fat distribution shifts toward the abdomen, resulting in visceral adiposity - belly fat that surrounds the organs and contributes to insulin resistance, high blood pressure - and lipid abnormalities. This classic "apple shape" or android obesity is a hallmark of metabolic syndrome.

More surprisingly, stress-related fat accumulation doesn't always align with increased food intake. In a notable animal study, rats exposed to early acute stress experienced weight loss.[2] Still, with continued exposure (shifting from acute to chronic stress), they began gaining weight - even while eating less. In other words, stress alone can rewire metabolism to prioritise fat storage, independent of diet.

Human studies have reinforced this. In one University College London study, hair samples from 2,500 people revealed that those with higher cortisol levels were far more likely to have a BMI over 30 kg/m^2, qualifying them as obese.[1] Chronic stress not only promotes overeating but also alters where and how the body stores fat.

Stress, Relationships, and the Emotional Web of Metabolic Health
Relationships - whether personal or professional - are among the most significant sources of both support and stress. Emotional

conflicts, loss, unresolved tension, or lack of connection can amplify cortisol output. For example, research shows that women who report dissatisfaction in their marriage are up to three times more likely to develop metabolic syndrome over time.[2] Similarly, workplace stress, especially in roles with low control and high demands, more than doubles the risk of developing metabolic disease.[3]

Even day-to-day emotional turbulence - feeling unsupported, socially isolated, or misunderstood - can quietly influence metabolic health.[4] When stress is persistent, the adrenal glands may struggle to function properly over time, resulting in symptoms such as burnout, fatigue, and poor stress tolerance. These are often overlooked but can be critical early warnings of HPA axis dysregulation.

What complicates matters further is that not all stress is external. Internal stressors, such as poor blood sugar control, nutrient deficiencies, chronic inflammation, and dehydration, can mimic or exacerbate emotional stress. You might feel "wired but tired" without any apparent external trigger. The stress is real, but it's coming from within.

Eustress vs. Distress: The Mind's Role in the Metabolic Equation
Interestingly, not all stress leads to dysfunction. In fact, how we interpret stress plays a major role in its physiological impact. When a challenge is perceived as manageable or an opportunity for growth - what psychologists call *eustress* - the body may respond positively, with increased resilience and motivation. Think of the performer energised before a big show or the athlete pushing through training.

But when stress is perceived as overwhelming, inescapable, or threatening, it becomes *distress*. This type of stress not only saps emotional resources but also derails metabolic regulation, contributing to depression, anxiety, and the progression of chronic illness.

Chronic Stress = Obesity = Metabolic Syndrome

The complete metabolic picture of stress isn't just about cortisol - it's about what cortisol does to our behaviour and biochemistry. Cortisol doesn't just signal a threat; it alters our hunger cues, food preferences, and energy expenditure. It makes high-fat, high-sugar foods more appealing, downregulates satiety signals, and promotes fat storage even when caloric intake hasn't increased. Over time, this leads to weight gain, particularly in the abdomen - a key feature of metabolic syndrome.

Moreover, stress also interferes with reproductive hormones. In women, chronic stress is linked to the development or worsening of polycystic ovary syndrome (PCOS), a condition marked by insulin resistance, central obesity, and increased androgen levels. Many women with PCOS show signs of increased HPA axis activity and elevated insulin levels - yet another example of how deeply stress can embed itself into our metabolic architecture.[5]

Reclaiming Balance:
Healing the Metabolism by Addressing Stress

Managing chronic stress is not just about feeling better - it's about preventing disease. Whether it stems from relationships, the workplace, internal imbalances, or unresolved trauma, chronic stress must be addressed both externally and internally. Supporting adrenal health, improving sleep, resolving emotional conflicts, and reducing internal metabolic stressors (such as blood sugar swings and inflammation) are all vital strategies.

The goal isn't to eliminate stress - that's neither possible nor desirable - but to develop the tools to process it effectively and recover more swiftly. In doing so, we protect not only our minds but also our metabolic health, waistlines, and overall longevity.

The Many Faces of Stress

We often think of stress as a psychological state - an emotional response to life's pressures - but its impact is far more profound. Chronic stress imprints itself on our biology from the very beginning, shaping our metabolic destiny in ways we're only beginning to understand fully.

Stress Before Birth: Low Birth Weight and Early Life Adversity

The story may start as early as the womb. When a pregnant mother experiences high levels of stress, her body produces more cortisol - a hormone that, in excess, can impair foetal growth. The result? Babies are born smaller than expected for their gestational age.

But a low birth weight isn't just a perinatal concern. Numerous studies have shown that it sets the stage for the development of adult diseases. For instance, one large-scale investigation linked low birth weight with a significantly increased risk of adult obesity.[6] Another highlighted its association with elevated blood pressure and type 2 diabetes later in life.[7] Some data even suggest a possible predictive role in the development of polycystic ovary syndrome (PCOS), indicating that metabolic programming begins in utero.[8]

Childhood, too, plays a pivotal role. Research shows that individuals exposed to multiple adverse experiences - whether emotional neglect, abuse, or extreme poverty - face a substantially higher risk of developing severe obesity as adults. One study reported a 1.4 to 1.6-fold increase in risk. Harsh early environments don't just affect physical health; they engrave themselves into the body's stress-response system, predisposing individuals to hypertension, metabolic dysregulation, and other health issues.[9]

Relationships and Stress: The Hidden Weight of Marital Strain

While early life shapes our foundation, adult relationships can continue to influence our health, especially in close partnerships. The MIDUS (Midlife in the United States) study, which followed over 1,300 participants for nearly a decade, found that women who experienced high levels of family-related stress were more likely to gain significant weight.[10] For men, the picture was more nuanced. Middle-aged men who reported high daily stress - not necessarily from family matters - were prone to weight gain exceeding 10 kilograms, while this pattern didn't hold in younger or older men.

This suggests that the impact of stress may not only depend on its source but also gender and life stage. Women may internalise relational discord, which can affect their metabolic health, whereas men may be more sensitive to daily performance-related pressures.

The Workplace: Where Chronic Stress Breeds Chronic Disease

For many, the workplace is an unrelenting source of stress. Jobs that demand high responsibility with low control - common in fields like law enforcement - are strongly associated with metabolic syndrome and cardiovascular disease. Employees with persistent work stress have been found to be more than twice as likely to develop metabolic syndrome than those in lower-stress roles, even after accounting for lifestyle factors.[11]

Interestingly, how we perceive our jobs also matters. A sense of purpose and satisfaction at work protects men from the health consequences of stress. Conversely, job strain disproportionately affects women, increasing their risk of metabolic disorders. Gender differences again appear to play a role - while both sexes might gain weight under pressure, men tend to accumulate fat around the waist, a riskier fat distribution associated with insulin resistance and cardiovascular risk.[12]

Moreover, chronic work stress has been linked to lipid

abnormalities, including higher LDL ('bad') cholesterol, lower HDL ('good') cholesterol, and other patterns characteristic of metabolic syndrome.[13]

How Can You Tell If You're Stressed?

Chronic stress doesn't always feel dramatic. It can be a slow, corrosive force that gradually undermines your well-being. If you find yourself perpetually anxious, tense, or irritable - often without a clear reason - this could be a red flag. Other telltale signs include brain fog, chronic fatigue, mood swings, difficulty sleeping, and even gastrointestinal issues like reflux or stomach pain.

Physically, you might notice recurring neck or back pain, frequent headaches, a weakened immune response (i.e., more frequent colds), or shifts in weight and appetite. Behaviourally, stress can manifest as increased reliance on caffeine, alcohol, or cigarettes - and even as aggression or withdrawal. Over time, these symptoms can evolve into more serious conditions such as depression or even cognitive decline, as chronic stress shrinks the hippocampus, the brain's memory centre.

Understanding the Stress Response: Three Stages

Stress progresses through three main stages:

- **Stage 1: The Awareness Phase**
  You notice the stress but still feel in control. You can actively decide how to respond, using tools to defuse it early.
- **Stage 2: The Resistance Phase**
  The stress response has kicked in, but you're managing. You might feel tense, but you're keeping it together - barely.

- **Stage 3: The Overload Phase**
  Your coping capacity is overwhelmed. You may lash out, shut down, or act impulsively. This is the point of burnout, often followed by exhaustion and regret.

The Stress Playbook of the Successful

Success isn't about having no stress - it's about managing it intelligently. Effective people don't wait until stage 3 to act. They build their day around their natural cortisol rhythm, using the morning energy peak to tackle demanding tasks. They also prioritise recovery and use short- and long-term strategies to manage stress proactively.

Short-term strategies - such as deep breathing, meditation, prayer, or calming movement practices like yoga and Tai Chi - can provide rapid relief. Journaling or listening to music can also help bring clarity and emotional release. The most effective approaches are often combinations - for example, repeating a calming mantra while engaging in mindful breathing.

Long-term strategies include setting boundaries, cultivating healthy relationships, prioritising sleep and physical activity, and ensuring that one's work and lifestyle align with personal values.

Measuring Stress: Going Beyond the Obvious

You might assume that measuring cortisol or adrenaline levels would give an accurate picture of chronic stress. While these can be useful in acute situations, they fluctuate widely and aren't reliable markers of long-term stress exposure.

Instead, **heart rate variability (HRV)** has emerged as a powerful and practical tool. A relaxed, healthy nervous system produces natural variability in the time between heartbeats. When this variability is reduced, it's a strong signal that the body is under persistent stress.

Another marker is **high-sensitivity C-reactive protein (hs-CRP)**, a molecule associated with chronic inflammation. While not specific to stress alone, it reflects the type of low-grade, systemic inflammation that is a common feature of metabolic syndrome.

What Can I Do?

By now, many of the strategies for preventing metabolic syndrome may seem familiar, but there's a good reason for that. The fundamentals work, and at the heart of it all lies one critical theme: stress. More specifically, chronic, unresolved stress.

Stress isn't always dramatic or sudden. Often, it's quiet, persistent, and deeply embedded in our daily lives - shaped by unresolved conflicts, emotional baggage from childhood, workplace frustrations, or recurring tension in our relationships. These aren't just emotional burdens; they can subtly disrupt our physiology, contributing to weight gain, insulin resistance, poor sleep, and eventually, metabolic dysfunction.

Consider the case of a 42-year-old mother I once treated. She had battled her weight for years, following multiple diet programs without long-term success. Her BMI was 31 kg/m² - technically obese - and her waist measured 97 cm, a sign of high visceral fat. Yet, medical tests revealed no genetic or metabolic abnormalities that could explain her condition. The deeper issue turned out to be far more personal.

She described daily morning tension with her 12-year-old daughter, whose disorganised habits were causing constant friction at home. Despite her best intentions, the persistent conflict created a stressful environment that undermined her health and happiness. I encouraged her to try a subtle shift in parenting - she began to praise her younger son, who kept his room tidy, in front of his sister. Motivated by sibling rivalry, the daughter eventually joined in. This small, thoughtful change improved the mother-daughter dynamic and, over time, helped the mother regain control over her health and weight.

The lesson is simple but powerful: identify and defuse the true source of your chronic stress. Whether it stems from a strained marriage, an unfulfilling job, or long-standing emotional patterns, addressing it directly is far more effective than simply treating the symptoms.

Alongside this deeper work, integrating practical, daily techniques to manage stress can provide lasting relief and resilience.

Simple Daily Practices to Soothe Stress

- **Walking** is a gentle yet powerful way to relax. It combines the benefits of light exercise with exposure to fresh air and the calming rhythms of nature.
- **Physical affection** - such as hugging a loved one - stimulates the release of oxytocin, which lowers stress hormones and boosts your sense of connection and happiness.
- **Mindfulness** anchors you in the present. When you consciously tune into your senses - what you hear, feel, smell - you pull yourself out of anxious loops that dwell on the past or anticipate the future.
- **Savasana** (or progressive muscle relaxation) is especially useful before sleep. Slowly tightening and releasing each muscle group, from head to toe, promotes deep physical and mental relaxation.
- **Cognitive Behavioural Therapy (CBT)** can help you recognise the hidden thoughts and beliefs that ignite your stress responses, empowering you to reframe them and take back control.

Long-Term Stress-Proofing Strategies

Preventing chronic stress requires more than short-term fixes. These long-term lifestyle upgrades support emotional stability and physiological health:

- Eat fresh, whole foods instead of processed options.
- Stay hydrated with clean, filtered water.
- Prioritise deep, restorative sleep.
- Exercise regularly and aim to spend weekends outdoors - hiking, walking, or simply exploring.
- Soak in sunlight – safely - to boost mood and vitamin D levels.
- Avoid smoking and limit alcohol and caffeine.
- Invest in meaningful relationships.
- Reconnect with your hobbies and creative outlets.
- Reduce screen time and remove electronics from your bedroom.
- Offer love without conditions.
- Cultivate a sense of purpose.

Self-Care: Your Oxygen Mask First

Self-care is not selfish - it's strategic. When you care for yourself, you improve your capacity to care for others. Here are powerful ways to build a self-nourishing routine:

- Stay optimistic and set a positive vision for yourself.
- Make time for connection with friends, family, and yourself.
- Practice acceptance by focusing on your circle of influence (what you *can* control).
- Rediscover joy through hobbies, humour, and time with pets or grandchildren.

- Connect with your spirituality, whether through prayer, meditation, or visiting places of worship.
- Use massage and aromatherapy with relaxing oils, such as lavender.
- Be mindful of destructive coping habits such as emotional eating, binge drinking, or drug use.
- Balance work and life. Use your time wisely, and permit yourself to say no.
- Set SMART goals - Specific, Measurable, Achievable, Relevant, Time-bound (see Chapter 15).
- Create a movement-friendly workspace - stand periodically, stretch, or use a standing desk.
- Take breaks, plan vacations, and incorporate recovery time into your schedule.
- Find a mentor or coach to guide and support you.
- Embrace your faith or philosophy. Studies have shown that individuals who remain spiritually connected and attend services regularly tend to experience healthier cortisol levels over time.[14]

Stress-Soothing Foods

What's on your plate can either fuel your stress or fight it. The right foods nourish your nervous system, balance your hormones, and ease inflammation.

- **Almonds** and **chamomile** have calming properties that promote the production of GABA and serotonin.
- **Citrus fruits, kiwis, and bell peppers** are rich in vitamin C, which supports adrenal function.
- **Blueberries** and **dark chocolate** contain flavonoids that protect the brain and elevate mood.

- **Green tea** is rich in L-theanine, which boosts calming neurotransmitters.
- **Eggs** provide tryptophan, a precursor to serotonin.
- **Chia** and **flaxseeds** are rich in protein and omega-3 fatty acids, which support brain health.
- **Atlantic salmon**, when eaten three times a week, has been shown to lower stress more effectively than other meats.[15]
- A diet rich in **nuts** is also associated with lower perceived stress levels.[16]

Nutritional Support for the Adrenals

Your adrenal glands regulate your stress response, immune system, and energy levels. Support them with:

- **B-complex vitamins**, especially B5 and B6.
- **Vitamin C** is crucial for cortisol production and immune resilience.
- **Omega-3 fatty acids** for reducing inflammation and stabilising mood.
- **Adaptogenic herbs,** such as Rhodiola, Ashwagandha, passionflower, valerian root, and St. John's wort, help buffer your body against stress and promote recovery.

Final Thoughts

Acute stress can sharpen your focus and motivate you to perform at your best. But when stress becomes chronic, it erodes both physical and mental well-being. I truly believe that low levels of chronic stress are one of the key reasons why residents of Blue Zones - those long-lived communities around the world - consistently outperform modern populations in terms of health and longevity.

In the next chapter, we'll explore what these communities have in common—and what they can teach us about living better, not just longer.

CHAPTER 20

Baby Boomers Got It Wrong - Blue Zoners Got It Right!

The generation known as the Baby Boomers - those born between 1946 and 1964 - are living longer than any previous generation. But there's a critical question worth asking: Are they living better?

Across the globe, there are pockets of people residing in so-called *Blue Zones* who consistently live longer and healthier lives. These communities, located in regions such as Okinawa (Japan), Ikaria (Greece), and Sardinia (Italy), are not just beating the longevity odds - they're redefining them. When we compare these populations with the Baby Boomers in developed nations, a striking contrast emerges. While boomers have benefited from remarkable medical advancements and welfare systems, many are arriving at old age with multiple chronic diseases and a dwindling quality of life.[1]

In essence, while Baby Boomers have added more years to their lives, the Blue Zoners have mastered the art of making the most of their years.

Not So Booming After All

Following the end of World War II, a wave of optimism swept across the Western world. Soldiers returned, economies recovered, and families began to grow rapidly. Between 1946 and 1964, a dramatic rise in birth rates occurred. In the United States alone, 76.4 million people were born during this period, forming what became the largest generational cohort in American history at the time.

Many assumed that this generation, raised with access to better healthcare, nutrition, and education, would age with strength and grace. But reality has been less kind.

Data from a University College London study using the Medical Research Council National Survey of Health and Development found that by ages 60 to 64, the average Baby Boomer in the UK was already managing two chronic health conditions. Hypertension affects about half, obesity affects a third, high cholesterol affects a quarter, and prediabetes or diabetes affects a quarter each.[2] Government statistics reveal that the average person in the UK now spends the final 14 years of life in poor health.

So, what happened?

A Generation Caught in the Middle

Baby Boomers came of age during a time of rising prosperity, increased social mobility, and consumerism. But now, many are caught in the "sandwich generation" - caring for ageing parents while still supporting their children, often while holding down jobs or managing financial stress. This dual responsibility takes a significant toll on health.

Research shows that Baby Boomer caregivers experience higher rates of chronic disease and disability than their non-caregiving peers. Arthritis, asthma, chronic obstructive pulmonary disease (COPD), and frequent mental distress are common.[3] Osteoporosis, particularly in women, and vulnerability to seasonal illnesses like influenza further burden this group. And the challenge is twofold: as more people require care, there are fewer individuals available to provide it. The healthcare system is bracing for a double strain.

Retirement: A Window of Opportunity

Contrary to the traditional image of retirement as a time to slow down, today's longer lifespans open a door to reinvention. In its 2023 annual report, the UK's Chief Medical Officer encouraged older adults to view retirement not as a time to retreat, but as an opportunity to engage - to become more active, socially, and physically.

Indeed, a third of the UK workforce is now over 50, and many choose to continue working past pension age, either out of necessity or desire. Volunteering, mentoring, and joining community groups are all powerful ways to stay mentally alert and physically active - both of which are crucial for long-term well-being.

But living longer comes with financial complexity. While previous generations may have needed to fund 10 years of retirement, today's retirees may need to prepare for 30 years or more. Without adequate savings or robust health, these extra years can become a burden rather than a blessing.

Health by Prescription?

Baby Boomers are often portrayed as ambitious and achievement-oriented, traits that have propelled them through education, careers, and homeownership. But that same drive may have fuelled a culture of consumerism over contentment - luxury cars over lifestyle changes, cosmetic fixes over consistent exercise.

Even with greater financial resources, many Baby Boomers are not investing in the foundational pillars of health: whole foods, physical activity, meaningful relationships, and purposeful living. Instead, there's a reliance on pills over prevention. They're more likely to consult a specialist than a nutritionist, and more attuned to fixing problems than preventing them.

This reactive model of healthcare, driven by medication and medical procedures, creates the illusion of managing disease while failing to promote real health. A stent can open a blocked artery, but it won't undo decades of inactivity or a lifetime of processed food.

Public Health's Frustrating Paradox

It's easy to wonder why improved public health campaigns haven't made a bigger dent. The answer lies in the overpowering influence of modern life. For every campaign promoting exercise or fruits and vegetables, there are hundreds of advertisements for ultra-processed foods, alcohol, or quick fixes. Medical breakthroughs have saved lives - but they've also enabled unhealthy habits to persist.

Compare Baby Boomers with their parents - the so-called "Greatest Generation." Only 13% of Baby Boomers rate their health as excellent, compared to 32% in the preceding generation. More Boomers rely on mobility aids, experience daily limitations, and live with high blood pressure. In the US, 75% of Baby Boomers are hypertensive - more than double the rate seen in their parents' generation.[4]

This isn't just a healthcare problem - it's a cultural one.

We have extended life without extending vitality. We have more treatments but fewer cures. And perhaps most dangerously, we've become passive recipients of healthcare instead of active participants in our well-being.

Looking Elsewhere for Answers

The contrast with Blue Zone populations is instructive. These people don't live longer because they have better access to hospitals or the latest pharmaceuticals. They live longer because their lives are embedded in daily movement, plant-rich diets, tight-knit communities, and a sense of purpose.

The truth is inconvenient but straightforward: the formula for a long and healthy life isn't locked away in a laboratory. It's already being lived - quietly, consistently, and without fanfare - in places we rarely look.

So yes, Baby Boomers may have gotten it wrong. But the story doesn't have to end there. With awareness, action, and perhaps a bit of inspiration from the Blue Zones, it's not too late to add not just years to our life - but more life to our years.

The Five Blue Zones: Lessons from the World's Healthiest Elders
Scattered across the globe are five unique regions - Ikaria (Greece), Sardinia (Italy), Okinawa (Japan), Nicoya (Costa Rica), and Loma Linda (California) - where an unusually high number of people live into their 90s and beyond, often reaching 100 in remarkably good health. These individuals aren't just surviving; they're thriving, often with minimal reliance on medication or invasive procedures. What makes these "blue zones" so special is not a miracle cure or genetic quirk, but a collection of everyday habits that promote longevity.

Each region has its distinctive lifestyle, shaped by local culture, climate, and tradition. On the Greek island of Ikaria, residents enjoy a Mediterranean diet rich in olive oil, vegetables, and herbs, often gathered from their own gardens. Sardinians lead physically active lives in mountainous terrain, tending livestock and enjoying local red wine. In Okinawa, a plant-based diet rich in soy foods is paired with tai chi, and there is a deep cultural emphasis on mindfulness and community. On Costa Rica's Nicoya Peninsula, people remain physically active into old age, eat nutrient-dense staples like beans and squash, and often speak of their "plan de Vida," or life purpose.

Meanwhile, in Loma Linda, a tight-knit community of Seventh-day Adventists follows a biblically inspired vegetarian diet, prioritising spiritual well-being, rest, and family.

A Diet Rooted in Simplicity: Whole Foods and Water

Despite cultural differences, one common thread unites the blue zones: diets grounded in whole, minimally processed foods. Meals are typically prepared from scratch using ingredients grown or sourced within walking distance. These foods - leafy greens, whole grains, legumes, nuts, seasonal fruits, and vegetables - form the cornerstone of daily meals. Processed and packaged products are rare, and sugary soft drinks are virtually non-existent. Instead, water, herbal teas, coffee, and - occasionally - wine are the beverages of choice.

Meals are usually nutrient-dense yet simple. A typical dish might be based on no more than five or six whole ingredients. Leafy greens such as spinach, kale, and turnip tops are frequently consumed, while olive oil - rich in polyphenols and healthy fats - is used generously. In fact, middle-aged residents of blue zones often consume up to six teaspoons of olive oil a day. Research shows this not only boosts HDL ("good") cholesterol but also helps lower LDL ("bad") cholesterol.

Food preparation methods favour health: vegetables are often eaten raw or lightly cooked, grains are soaked or fermented, and bread is made from whole, sprouted grains or sourdough, which improves digestibility and nutrient absorption. Fermented soy products, such as tofu and miso, are staples in Okinawa, while sourdough bread and pickled vegetables are typical in Europe's blue zones.

Hydration and Daily Rituals

Hydration is another subtle but powerful health practice in these regions. People sip water throughout the day rather than relying on sugary drinks. Studies consistently show that proper hydration supports vascular health, reduces the risk of clots, and improves circulation. Coffee, green tea, and herbal infusions are also part of daily routines. In Sardinia and Ikaria, coffee is enjoyed regularly and may contribute to cognitive health, with studies suggesting it can help stave off dementia and Parkinson's disease.[5] Okinawans sip green tea infused with jasmine and turmeric, while herbal brews made from rosemary, sage, and dandelion are prized for their anti-inflammatory benefits.[6]

Beans, Bread, and Nuts: Humble Staples with Powerful Benefits

In all five zones, beans are the unsung heroes of the diet. Lentils, black beans, chickpeas, and soybeans supply steady, slow-burning energy and are rich in both fibre and protein. A half-cup serving per day is the typical amount, and these legumes often serve as the primary source of protein.[7]

Bread is still a dietary staple - but it's not your average store-bought loaf. Traditional breads in Blue Zones are made from whole grains, such as barley, rye, and wheat, often fermented with natural bacteria like Lactobacillus. These methods reduce gluten content, lower the glycaemic index, and create a satisfying texture and taste that commercial white bread lacks.

Nuts also play a central role. A daily handful or two - whether almonds, pistachios, walnuts, or Brazil nuts - provides essential fats, protein, and micronutrients. Studies suggest that nut eaters tend to live two to three years longer than non-nut eaters, with benefits attributed to nutrients like vitamin E, selenium, and plant-based omega-3s.

Animal Products in Moderation

Though predominantly plant-based, the blue zone diets include modest portions of animal products. Free-range eggs are consumed a few times a week, often from chickens fed natural, unmedicated diets. Dairy, when included, comes from goats or sheep and is usually fermented into yoghurt or cheese. Goat's milk is better tolerated by many due to the presence of lactase, which aids digestion.[8]

Fish is eaten sparingly - usually two to three small portions per week - of low-mercury varieties like sardines and anchovies, which are rich in omega-3 fatty acids. Meat consumption is rare, often limited to celebratory meals, with average intakes as low as two ounces five times a month. In Loma Linda, many residents follow a vegan or pescatarian lifestyle, with strong evidence linking these diets to increased longevity and a lower risk of disease.[9]

Eating Patterns: When and How Matters Too

Blue zoners don't just eat better - they eat differently. Meals are savoured slowly, often in the company of family or friends.[11] Okinawans follow the practice of "Hara Hachi Bu," stopping when they're 80% full to avoid overeating. In Nicoya and Okinawa, a slight daily calorie deficit appears to be the norm. Research in humans and animals has shown that moderate caloric restriction can improve metabolic health and extend lifespan.[10]

Moderate red wine consumption - typically 1 to 2 small glasses with meals - is typical in Ikaria and Sardinia. While some evidence supports the cardiovascular benefits of moderate alcohol intake,[12] this likely hinges on context: wine is enjoyed with food, not in isolation, and usually in convivial social settings. Excessive alcohol consumption, by contrast, is consistently associated with increased health risks.

A Life Beyond the Plate

What people in blue zones do when they're not eating is just as vital. Physical activity isn't scheduled - it's woven into daily life. Whether it's tending to a garden, walking to a neighbour's home, or climbing hills with livestock, movement is frequent, natural, and purposeful. Even small habits - like taking the stairs or standing while talking - add up over time. [13]

Sleep is also taken seriously. Blue zoners generally go to bed early, rise with the sun, and follow a consistent sleep-wake rhythm. Seven hours of sleep is considered ideal, while short daytime naps (under 30 minutes) are common and appear to lower stress and the risk of heart disease.[15] Longer naps, however, may be counterproductive.

Spirituality, social ties, and a sense of purpose also play significant roles. Most blue zoners are part of close-knit communities and extended families, and many engage in religious or spiritual practices that provide comfort, a sense of belonging, and meaning. Grandparents often live with or near their children and grandchildren, and those who help care for younger family members tend to live longer.

Final Thoughts: Learning from the World's Healthiest Populations

The lessons of the blue zones aren't mysterious - they're practical, accessible, and profoundly human. Unlike modern lifestyles that prioritise convenience and instant gratification, the blue zone model is based on simplicity, patience, and connection. While many people today are living longer, few are doing so in good health. Blue zoners demonstrate that it's possible to do both.

Their secret: A primarily plant-based, whole food diet; regular, moderate physical activity; restful sleep; strong social bonds; and a clear sense of purpose. And while not everyone can relocate to a sunny island or mountain village, we can all adopt aspects of the blue zone lifestyle - one daily habit at a time.

The Final Word: Your Journey to Health and Vitality

Let's take a moment to look back on everything we've explored together. You started this journey because something didn't feel right. Maybe it was your energy, your weight, your blood pressure - or perhaps it was a deeper sense that your body wasn't working the way it should. And what you've discovered is that you're not broken. Your body isn't the problem. The real issue is that you're living in a world your biology wasn't designed for.

Modern life asks your body to handle far more than it was ever meant to. Constant snacking, consumption of processed foods, stress, poor sleep, and prolonged periods of sitting disrupt the delicate systems that regulate energy, weight, and overall vitality. Over time, your body stops responding to insulin the way it should, and this "insulin resistance" starts a chain reaction: blood sugar rises, belly fat accumulates, cholesterol worsens, and blood pressure climbs. What appears to be five separate diagnoses is actually one underlying issue - your body's energy management system is out of balance.

But here's the powerful part: your body wants to heal. It's wired for recovery. When you stop fighting biology with anti-agents and start working with it, healing begins naturally. You don't need perfection. You don't need a prescription for every symptom. What you need is a return to the rhythm your body understands.

And that rhythm is simple.

You start by eating real food - food that your great-grandparents would recognise. Vegetables, healthy fats, quality proteins, nuts, seeds, and the occasional fruit. No counting calories. No complicated diets. Just nourishment your body knows how to use.

Then, you give your body space to rest. Instead of eating from morning to night, you tighten your eating window. Maybe you eat between 10 a.m. and 6 p.m. - enough time to enjoy two nourishing meals without overloading your system. This time-restricted eating allows your body to reset, lower insulin levels, burn fat, and repair itself.

And finally, you move. Not by punishing workouts, but through natural daily activity. Walking, stretching, dancing, playing - this kind of movement improves insulin sensitivity, reduces stress, and keeps your body strong and agile.

Now, implementation matters. The key is not a one-time sprint, but a steady rhythm. In the morning, hydrate and move gently. Delay your first meal. When you eat, make it work for you. Start with protein and healthy fats. Keep your biggest meal at midday and keep dinner light and early. In the evening, trade snacks and screens for conversation, books, or rest.

You'll face challenges. The first week may be uncomfortable, with cravings, hunger, and fatigue. That's your body letting go of old habits. Then comes the shift: steadier energy, clearer thinking, better sleep. You start feeling like yourself again - maybe for the first time in years.

And it doesn't stop there. As weeks turn to months, your health markers improve, your habits become automatic, and what once felt hard now feels natural. This isn't a crash diet. It's not a temporary fix. This is a return to how your body was meant to live and thrive.

You'll still have off days. Life happens. But now you have a compass. You know how to reset. You know how to get back into rhythm.

And the most important part: You're not alone. This is a shared journey, with others walking beside you, encouraging, learning, growing. You have a Facebook community. You have tools. You have hope.

So, as we close this chapter, remember: the goal isn't just to avoid disease. It's to wake up with energy, clarity, and purpose. To feel alive in your own skin. To live a life that's not just longer, but better.

You were designed to thrive. And you still can.

Start where you are. Use what you have. Begin today.

Your future self will thank you.

SECTION 4

NATURAL RECIPES AND MEALS

The Art of Clean Eating: Simple recipes, Big Flavour

Breakfast Recipes

Overnight Protein & Fibre Oats
Serves: 2

Ingredients
- 1 ½ cups organic jumbo oats
- 2 tbsp ground flaxseed
- 1 tbsp sunflower seeds
- 1 tbsp chia seeds
- ¼ tsp ground cinnamon
- 1 cup kefir (milk or coconut)
- 1 ½ cups milk or plant milk of choice
- 3 kiwifruits, peeled and chopped
- A handful of blueberries

Method
1. In a bowl, combine oats, flaxseed, chia seeds, sunflower seeds, and cinnamon.
2. Add kefir and milk, then mix thoroughly.
3. Cover and refrigerate overnight.
4. To serve, divide into two bowls and top with kiwi and blueberries.

Overnight Chocolate Chia Pudding
Serves: 2

Ingredients
- 40g chia seeds
- 200ml milk or plant milk
- 1 tbsp kefir (dairy or coconut)
- 1 tbsp mixed seeds (flax, sunflower, pumpkin)
- 1 tsp dark cacao powder
- 1 tbsp desiccated coconut
- 1 tsp stevia (optional)
- A handful of berries
- 1 glass jar with a lid

Method
1. Add all ingredients (except berries) to a jar.
2. Seal and shake vigorously for 2–3 minutes or mix well in a bowl.
3. Refrigerate overnight (or at least 4 hours).
4. Serve topped with berries.

Yoghurt Salad

Ingredients:
- Greek or coconut yoghurt
- 1 cucumber, finely chopped or grated
- Himalayan salt and black pepper, to taste
- 1 carrot, grated (for garnish)

Method:
1. Drain excess water from the cucumber.
2. Mix the cucumber with yoghurt, salt, and pepper.
3. Garnish with grated carrot before serving.

Green Smoothie

Ingredients:
- 1 cucumber
- 2 celery sticks
- ½ avocado
- 1 green apple, cored
- 1 kiwi, peeled
- A small piece of fresh ginger
- A handful of kale or spinach
- A few berries (optional)
- Juice of ½ lemon
- Water, as needed for blending

Method:
1. Place all ingredients in a blender.
2. Add water gradually until the desired consistency is reached.
3. Blend until smooth. Serve immediately for maximum freshness.

Almond Banana Avocado Smoothie
Serves: 2

Ingredients
- 1 ripe banana
- 2 tbsp almond butter
- 1 avocado, pitted
- 1 tbsp natural yoghurt
- 1 cup spinach
- 1 cup almond milk
- ½ cup filtered water

Method
1. Add all ingredients to a blender.
2. Blend until smooth (approx. 20 seconds).
3. Serve immediately in two glasses.

Cinnamon Apple Smoothie
Serves: 2

Ingredients
- 1 ripe banana
- 1 medium apple, cored
- A handful of fresh spinach
- 2 tbsp pumpkin seeds
- 2 tbsp sunflower seeds
- 10 walnuts
- 2 tbsp ground cinnamon
- 1 tbsp natural yoghurt or kefir
- 1 cup filtered water

Method
1. Chop the apple and banana into small pieces.
2. Blend all ingredients until smooth (10–15 seconds).
3. Serve immediately.

Beetroot Coconut Smoothie
Serves: 2

Ingredients
- 1 cup boiled, chopped beetroot (approx. 4 medium)
- 1 cup organic coconut milk
- 1 tbsp pine nuts
- 1 tbsp walnut butter

- 1 tbsp almond butter
- 1 cup raspberries
- Ice cubes

Method

1. Pre-boil the beetroot until it is fork-tender (45–60 minutes), then cool.
2. Add all ingredients to a blender and blend for 1–3 minutes.
3. Add ice and blend for an additional 30 seconds. Add water if too thick.
4. Serve immediately in two glasses.

Hearty Chocolate Chia Smoothie
Serves: 2

Ingredients

- 1 ripe banana
- 2 tbsp chia seeds (pre-soaked for 4 hours)
- 2 tbsp almond butter
- 2 tbsp cocoa powder or melted 90% dark chocolate
- 1 cup almond milk
- ½ cup filtered water
- 2 pitted dates
- A few ice cubes

Method

1. Soak chia seeds in water for at least 4 hours.
2. Add soaked chia and all other ingredients to a blender.
3. Blend until smooth (approx. 20 seconds).
4. Serve immediately in two glasses.

Breakfast: Protein and Whole Food Smoothie
Serves: 2

Ingredients

- 1 tbsp natural organic yoghurt or 50 ml kefir
- 1 small cup mixed berries (fresh or frozen)
- 2 tbsp plain grass-fed whey protein or plant-based protein powder
- 1 cup milk or plant milk (e.g., oat, almond)
- 1 tbsp ground flaxseeds
- 2 tbsp whole oats
- 1 tbsp almond butter

Method

1. Add all ingredients to a blender.
2. Blend for about 20 seconds or until smooth.
3. Pour into two glasses and serve immediately.

Apple, Pear & Carrot Bircher Muesli
Serves: 4

Ingredients

- 250g kefir or plain yoghurt
- 200g organic porridge oats
- 1 cup filtered water
- 300g fresh mixed berries
- 1 tsp ground ginger
- 1 tbsp ground cinnamon
- ½ cup chopped raw almonds
- 1 apple, grated (core/seeds removed)
- 1 cup grated carrot
- 1 pear, grated (core/seeds removed)
- 2 tsp stevia (optional)

Method
1. In a bowl, mix oats, ginger, cinnamon, carrot, pear, almonds, kefir, and water.
2. Cover and refrigerate overnight.
3. Serve with berries and stevia drizzle.
4. Store in an airtight container for up to 3 days.

Homemade Granola Mix
Makes: 15–20 servings (store in a jar)

Ingredients
- 3 tbsp coconut oil
- 3 tbsp of pure honey
- 2 tsp ground cinnamon
- 2 cups quinoa flakes
- 2 cups buckwheat groats
- 1 cup sunflower seeds
- 1 cup pumpkin seeds
- ½ cup goji berries
- ½ cup raisins
- ½ cup toasted pecans and walnuts

Method
1. Preheat oven to 180°C (200°C fan).
2. Melt the coconut oil in a large baking tray in the oven.
3. In a bowl, mix quinoa flakes, buckwheat, cinnamon, and honey.
4. Spread onto the baking tray and bake for 40 minutes, stirring occasionally.
5. Let cool, then mix in seeds, berries, raisins, and nuts.
6. Store in an airtight jar. Serve with yoghurt, milk, and fresh berries.

High-Protein Blueberry Pancakes
Serves: 4 (Makes 8 small pancakes)

Ingredients
- 1 cup ground almonds
- ½ cup gluten-free self-raising flour
- 1 tsp ground flaxseeds
- 1 tsp ground sesame seeds
- 1 tsp baking powder
- 1 cup almond milk
- 4 tbsp kefir
- 2 organic eggs
- Zest of 1 lemon
- 150g blueberries
- 3 tbsp coconut oil (for cooking)
- Stevia, to taste (optional)

Method
1. In a mixing bowl, combine all ingredients except the blueberries and coconut oil. Blend until smooth and medium-thick.
2. Gently fold in the blueberries.
3. Heat a skillet over medium heat and add 1 tbsp coconut oil.
4. Pour in spoonfuls of batter to make 3 pancakes (about 10 cm each) per batch.
5. Cook for 2 minutes per side until golden. Repeat with the remaining batter.
6. Serve two pancakes per person, topped with a spoonful of kefir or yoghurt and a drizzle of pure honey.

Anti-inflammatory Spanish Omelette

Serves: 1-2

Ingredients
- 3 eggs, whisked
- 2 tbsp chopped red bell pepper
- A handful of button mushrooms
- 1 garlic clove, minced
- 1 medium tomato, diced
- 1 medium new potato, cooked and chopped
- 2 chopped spring onions
- ¼ tsp cumin seeds
- ½ tsp turmeric
- Feta cheese (matchbox size)
- 5 tbsp extra virgin olive oil

Method
1. Preheat the grill.
2. Chop vegetables into small chunks.
3. In a frying pan, heat olive oil and sauté vegetables, garlic, and cumin seeds for 3-5 minutes.
4. In a bowl, whisk eggs with turmeric for 30 seconds.
5. Pour eggs over vegetables and cook on low heat for 5 minutes.
6. Remove from the hob, top with feta, and grill until the feta is set.
7. Serve with fresh parsley or coriander on a bed of rocket or spinach.

Middle Eastern Fava Beans (Ful Medames)
Serves: 2

Ingredients

- 800g fava beans (pre-soaked and pressure-cooked)
- 1 medium onion, finely chopped
- 4 garlic cloves, crushed
- 100ml extra virgin olive oil
- 1 red chilli, chopped (optional)
- 2 ripe tomatoes, chopped
- 1 tbsp tomato purée
- 1 shredded carrot
- Juice of ½ lemon
- 2 tsp ground cumin
- 2 tbsp tahini
- A handful of rocket or coriander leaves
- ¼ tsp sea salt

Method

1. Heat fava beans in a saucepan with a splash of water.
2. In a separate pan, sauté the onion and garlic in 50 mL of olive oil for 5 minutes.
3. Add salt, cumin, chilli, tomatoes, and carrot.
4. Stir in beans and tomato purée. Simmer for 15 minutes, adding water as needed.
5. Mash with remaining olive oil, lemon juice, and tahini until chunky.
6. Serve on a bed of rocket or coriander leaves.

North African Shakshuka with Spinach
Serves: 4

Ingredients
- 3 tbsp extra virgin olive oil
- 1 large onion, thinly sliced
- 2 red peppers, thinly sliced
- 1 tsp cumin seeds
- 1 tsp smoked paprika
- 1 red chilli, chopped (optional)
- 2 × 400g tins chopped tomatoes
- 150g baby spinach
- 4 medium eggs
- 100g natural yoghurt
- Fresh coriander or parsley
- ¼ tsp sea salt
- Black pepper, to taste

Method
1. Heat oil in a pan over medium heat. Sauté the onion and peppers for 5 minutes.
2. Add cumin, paprika, and chilli. Cook for 1 minute.
3. Add tomatoes, salt, and pepper. Simmer for 15–20 minutes.
4. Add spinach and cook until wilted.
5. Make 4 wells in the sauce and crack in the eggs.
6. Cover and cook for 4–5 minutes, or until eggs are done to your liking.
7. Serve with herbs, a dollop of yoghurt, and a sprinkle of black pepper.

Smoky Beans with Eggs
Serves: 2

Ingredients
- 400g cannellini beans (jar or tin)
- 2 garlic cloves, finely chopped
- 2 cups cherry tomatoes, halved
- 2 boiled eggs
- 4 tbsp extra virgin olive oil
- 1 tbsp tomato purée
- 3 tbsp apple cider vinegar
- 2 tsp smoked paprika
- Dash of Worcestershire sauce
- Juice of ½ lemon
- 100ml filtered water
- Sea salt and black pepper

Method
1. Boil the eggs, peel, and halve them.
2. In a pan, sauté garlic in olive oil over low heat for 1 minute.
3. Add tomatoes and cook for 5 minutes.
4. Add vinegar and cook for an additional 2 minutes.
5. Stir in tomato purée and water. Mash lightly.
6. Add paprika, beans, Worcestershire sauce, lemon juice, salt, and pepper.
7. Simmer for 10–12 minutes.
8. Serve topped with egg halves.

Scrambled Eggs with Creamy Mushrooms
Serves: 2

Ingredients
- 4 large eggs
- 1 tsp natural yoghurt
- 8 chestnut mushrooms, halved
- 1 tbsp coconut oil
- 1 handful fresh rocket leaves
- 1 avocado, mashed
- 1 tsp olive oil
- 1 tsp lemon juice
- 1 tbsp apple cider vinegar
- 3 tbsp filtered water
- Sea salt and black pepper

Method
1. Whisk eggs with water, salt, and pepper.
2. Heat half the coconut oil in each of two pans.
3. In one, cook mushrooms for 2-3 minutes, then stir in yoghurt.
4. In the other, cook the eggs gently for 2-3 minutes, stirring occasionally.
5. Mash avocado with olive oil, lemon, vinegar, salt, and pepper.
6. Serve eggs, mushrooms, avocado, and rocket together.

Breakfast: Turmeric Quinoa and Oat Porridge
Serves: 2

Ingredients
- 1 small cup of quinoa, rinsed
- 1 small cup of whole oats
- 300 ml coconut milk
- 1 mug (approx. 250 ml) oat milk (e.g., Plenish organic)
- 1 tbsp honey or stevia (to taste)
- ½ tsp ground turmeric
- 2 tbsp dried cranberries
- 2 tbsp coconut flakes
- 1 organic apple, grated (skin on, core and seeds removed)

Method
1. In a small saucepan, combine quinoa and oat milk. Bring to a boil, then reduce the heat and simmer with the lid on for 10 minutes, or until the quinoa is tender.
2. Turn off the heat and leave the dish covered for 5 minutes to absorb the remaining liquid.
3. In another medium saucepan, combine the cooked quinoa, oats, turmeric, and coconut milk. Simmer gently for 10 minutes until the oats are tender and the porridge is loose and creamy.
4. Divide between two bowls and top with cranberries, coconut flakes, grated apple, and a drizzle of pure honey (optional).

Breakfast: Overnight Chocolate Chia Seed Pudding
Serves: 2

Ingredients
- 40 g chia seeds
- 200 ml milk or plant milk
- 1 tbsp kefir (coconut or dairy)
- 1 tbsp mixed seeds (e.g., flax, sunflower, pumpkin)
- 1 tsp dark cacao powder
- 1 tbsp desiccated coconut
- 1 tsp stevia (optional)
- A handful of berries (for topping)

Method
1. Combine all ingredients in a large jar with a lid or in a bowl.
2. Shake vigorously (or stir well) for 2-3 minutes to prevent clumping.
3. Refrigerate overnight or for at least 4 hours until set.
4. Serve topped with berries.

Breakfast: Whole Food Loaf
Makes: 10-12 slices

Ingredients
- 200 g gluten-free rolled oats
- 150 g golden linseeds (flaxseeds)
- 60 g sunflower seeds
- 60 g pumpkin seeds
- 100 g raw cashew nuts, crushed
- 40 g chia seeds
- 60 ml extra virgin olive oil

- 500 ml filtered water
- ¼ tsp sea salt

Method

1. In a large bowl, mix all dry ingredients. Stir in the water and olive oil until well combined.
2. Pour into a parchment-lined 1 lb loaf tin. Let soak for 3–4 hours.
3. Preheat oven to 200°C (fan 180°C).
4. Bake in the tin for 40 minutes.
5. Remove the loaf from the tin, discard the paper, and return it to the baking tray upside down. Bake for another 20 minutes.
6. Cool before slicing. Serve with butter and a poached egg.

Breakfast: Zingy Mashed Avocado with Poached Eggs
Serves: 2

Ingredients

- 1 large ripe avocado
- ½ red bell pepper, finely diced
- 2 tbsp apple cider vinegar
- 1 tbsp chopped chives or 1 spring onion
- Juice of ½ lemon
- Sea salt and black pepper, to taste
- 2 organic free-range eggs
- Optional: smoked wild salmon and sourdough toast

Method

1. Scoop the avocado into a bowl and mash until smooth.
2. Mix in the diced pepper, chives, vinegar, lemon juice, salt, and pepper.
3. Poach the eggs to your preference.
4. Serve avocado mash on plates with poached eggs.
5. Add salmon and toast if desired.

Breakfast: Walnut Almond Energy Balls
Makes: 12 medium balls

Ingredients
- 50 g dates or dried figs (pitted)
- 50 g dried apricots (pitted)
- 50 g ground almond flour
- 60 g walnuts
- 2 tbsp coconut oil
- 3 tsp dark cacao powder
- A handful of coconut flakes
- Filtered water, as needed (1 tsp at a time)
- For coating: coconut flakes or cacao powder

Method
1. Soak dates and apricots in warm water for 15 minutes.
2. In a food processor, blend all the ingredients until you have a smooth, sticky dough. Add water as needed to reach the desired texture.
3. Roll mixture into 12 even-sized balls.
4. Coat each ball in coconut flakes or cacao powder.
5. Chill in the fridge for 30 minutes before serving.

Oven-Baked Spinach Falafels
Makes 15 falafels (Freezer-friendly)

Ingredients
- 4 tbsp extra virgin olive oil
- 800g dried chickpeas (soaked overnight in water)
- 1 handful fresh spinach
- 6 garlic cloves, peeled and grated
- 1 brown onion, finely chopped
- 1 small handful chopped parsley
- 1 small handful chopped coriander
- ½ tsp baking powder
- 1 tsp ground cumin
- ¼ tsp ground coriander
- 2 tbsp sesame seeds
- ¼ tsp sea salt

Tahini Dip (serves 2)
- 2 tbsp tahini
- Juice of ½ lemon
- 1 garlic clove, grated

Mix all dip ingredients in a small bowl.

Method
1. Soak chickpeas overnight in water (2 inches above the level of the chickpeas). Drain and rinse well.
2. Preheat oven to 200°C (180°C fan). Line a baking tray with parchment paper and brush it with 1 tbsp olive oil.
3. In a food processor, combine all ingredients except the olive oil. Pulse until thick and whipped. Scrape sides as needed.
4. Form the mixture into 15 balls using a tablespoon. Flatten into patties (~6 cm wide).

5. Place patties on the tray. Brush tops with olive oil and sprinkle with sesame seeds.
6. Bake for 30 minutes or until golden brown.
7. Serve with tahini dip, tzatziki, and roasted peppers.

Freeze uncooked patties in a container for up to 3 months.

Aubergine Salad

Ingredients:
- 1 aubergine (whole or sliced)
- 1 red pepper, chopped
- 2 garlic cloves, crushed
- 1 small bunch parsley, chopped
- 1 tomato, diced
- Juice of 1 lemon
- 1 tsp vinegar
- 1 tbsp olive oil
- Pomegranate seeds (optional)
- Himalayan salt, to taste

Method:
1. Roast or air-fry the aubergine until soft.
2. In a bowl, combine the aubergine with chopped red pepper, tomato, parsley, and garlic.
3. Drizzle with lemon juice, vinegar, and olive oil.
4. Season with salt and top with pomegranate seeds. Mix well and serve.

Lunch and dinner recipes

Vegetable Soup

Ingredients:
- 3 tbsp olive oil or coconut oil (or a mix)
- 3 onions, finely chopped
- 4 garlic cloves, crushed
- 1 courgette, chopped
- 3 carrots, chopped
- 2 tomatoes, chopped
- 2 celery sticks, chopped
- 1 sweet potato, peeled and chopped
- 1 tsp ground cumin
- Sea salt, to taste
- Water (enough to cover the vegetables)

Method:
1. Heat the oil in a medium pot over medium heat. Add the onions and garlic, and sauté until they are soft and fragrant.
2. Add all the vegetables, stir well, and let them cook together for 5 minutes to absorb the flavours.
3. Add enough water to just cover the vegetables. Stir in cumin and salt.
4. Simmer until the vegetables are soft (about 20–25 minutes).
5. Blend the soup with a hand blender until smooth. Serve warm.

Butternut Squash Soup

Ingredients:

- 3 tbsp olive oil or coconut oil
- 3 onions, finely chopped
- 5 garlic cloves, crushed
- 1 medium butternut squash, peeled and chopped
- 4 carrots, chopped
- 1 tsp ground cumin
- Himalayan salt, to taste
- Water (enough to cover)

Method:

1. In a large pot, heat the oil over medium heat. Add onions and garlic, and sauté until soft.
2. Add squash and carrots. Stir and cook for 5 minutes to absorb the flavour.
3. Add enough water to cover, then season with cumin and salt.
4. Simmer until the vegetables are tender (20-25 minutes).
5. Blend until smooth. Serve hot.

Broccoli Soup

Ingredients:

- 3 tbsp olive oil or coconut oil
- 3 onions, finely chopped
- 5 garlic cloves, crushed
- 1 medium head of broccoli, chopped
- 1 tsp ground cumin
- Himalayan salt, to taste
- Water (enough to cover)

Method:

1. Heat oil in a pot. Add onions and garlic; sauté for 5 minutes.
1. Add the broccoli and cook for 3 minutes, stirring occasionally.
2. Pour in enough water to cover the vegetables.
3. Season with cumin and salt, then simmer until broccoli is tender.
4. Blend until smooth and serve.

Red Lentil Soup

Ingredients:

- 3 tbsp olive oil or coconut oil
- 3 onions, finely chopped
- 4 garlic cloves, crushed
- 1 mug red lentils (rinsed)
- 2 celery sticks, chopped
- 2 tomatoes, chopped
- 2 carrots, chopped
- 1 tsp ground coriander
- Himalayan salt, to taste
- Water (to cover)

Method:

1. In a medium pot, heat the oil and sauté the onions and garlic until they are soft.
2. Add carrots, celery, and tomatoes. Stir and cook for 3–5 minutes.
3. Add lentils, stir briefly, then pour in water to cover.
4. Cook until the lentils and vegetables are tender and soft (about 20 minutes).
5. Season with coriander and salt, blend, and serve.

Steamed Vegetables

Ingredients:
- Mixed vegetables (e.g., carrots, cauliflower, broccoli, green beans)
- Olive oil
- Salt and black pepper, to taste
- Optional: minced garlic and fresh ginger

Method:
1. Toss the vegetables with olive oil, salt, pepper, garlic, and ginger before steaming.
2. Place them in a steamer and steam for about 5 minutes until tender but still vibrant.
3. Avoid overcooking. Serve immediately.

Miso-Roasted Aubergine
Serves 2

Ingredients
- 1 aubergine, sliced into strips
- 3 tbsp extra virgin olive oil
- 2 garlic cloves, grated
- 3 tbsp brown rice miso paste
- 2 tbsp rice vinegar
- ½ of a medium avocado
- 1 small handful of sunflower seeds
- 1 small handful of pine nuts
- 4 tbsp chopped chives
- 2 tbsp natural yoghurt
- 1 bag of rocket salad

Method

1. Preheat oven to 200°C (180°C fan). Line a baking tray with parchment paper.
2. Mix the miso, olive oil, rice vinegar, garlic, and avocado to form a paste.
3. Rub paste over aubergine slices. Lay on a tray and roast for 20–25 minutes until golden and soft.
4. Toast pine nuts and sunflower seeds in a dry pan over medium heat for 3 minutes, stirring occasionally.
5. Assemble the rocket on the plates. Add aubergine, sprinkle with toasted seeds and chives.
6. Serve with a spoonful of yoghurt.

Minced Turkey Lettuce Cups
Serves 2

Ingredients

- 1 tbsp coconut oil
- 200g lean minced turkey
- 6 baby gem lettuce leaves
- 1 medium brown onion, finely chopped
- ½ tsp ground turmeric
- ½ tsp paprika
- ½ tsp cumin seeds
- 2 tbsp tahini
- 2 tbsp chopped coriander
- 1 lime, cut into wedges
- 100ml filtered water
- ¼ tsp sea salt

Method
1. Heat the coconut oil in a pan. Sauté onion until golden, then add cumin seeds and fry for 30 seconds.
2. Add turkey mince and cook for 10 mins, stirring. Add turmeric and paprika.
3. Add water and simmer for 10 minutes, until the moisture is absorbed; then season with salt.
4. Spoon turkey into lettuce leaves. Top with tahini and coriander. Serve with lime wedges.

Leftover Chicken Bone Broth Soup
Serves 2

Ingredients
- 1 roast chicken carcass
- Leftover cooked chicken
- Leftover vegetables (e.g., Brussels sprouts, leeks, roast potatoes)
- 3 garlic cloves, chopped
- 1 carrot, chopped
- 1 bag of spinach
- 2 pints of filtered water
- 1 chicken stock cube
- 1 rosemary sprig

Method
1. After your roast, remove the leftover chicken and refrigerate it.
2. Add the carcass to a saucepan, cover with water, and bring to a boil. Add garlic and rosemary. Simmer with lid for 2 hours.

3. Cool and refrigerate. The next day, skim the fat and remove the bones.
4. Add stock cube, carrot, water, chicken, and vegetables. Simmer 5 mins.
5. Add spinach until wilted. Serve hot.

Egg Truffle on Sourdough
Serves 2

Ingredients
- 2 large eggs
- 1 egg yolk
- 1 tsp lemon juice
- 1 tsp Dijon mustard
- 150ml avocado or olive oil
- 1 tbsp truffle oil
- ¼ tsp white vinegar
- 1 spring onion, finely chopped
- 1 tbsp chopped chives
- Sea salt and black pepper
- Mixed salad leaves
- 2 slices seeded sourdough bread

Method
1. Combine truffle and avocado oils. In a bowl, whisk egg yolk, lemon juice, vinegar, and mustard. Gradually whisk in oils until thick.
2. Boil eggs for 6 minutes, then cool, peel, and mash them in a bowl. Then mix with the thick cream and spring onion and season with sea salt and black pepper.
3. Spread the egg mixture on the sourdough. Top with chives. Serve with salad leaves.

Crunchy Waldorf Salad
Serves 2

Ingredients
- 50g walnuts, chopped
- 1 green apple, thinly sliced
- 75g red grapes, halved
- 1 baby gem lettuce
- ½ celery stick, chopped
- 50g Stilton cheese, crumbled

Dressing
- 1 tbsp extra virgin olive oil
- 2 tbsp grass-fed butter
- 2 tbsp Greek yoghurt
- Juice of ½ lemon
- ½ tsp Dijon mustard
- Salt and pepper

Method

Toast the walnuts in a dry pan until they are brown. Let cool.

Scatter lettuce on a platter.

Toss apple, celery, grapes, Stilton, and walnuts with dressing.

Spoon over lettuce and serve.

Crispy Tofu Poke Bowl
Serves 2

Ingredients
- 280–300g firm tofu
- 2 tbsp extra virgin olive oil + extra for drizzling
- 1 small cup of quinoa
- 200ml hot stock (chicken or veg)

- 1 avocado, sliced
- ½ cucumber, diced
- 1 small red onion, diced
- 1 red bell pepper, chopped
- 4 radishes, sliced

Dressing

- 5 tbsp olive oil
- 2 tbsp tahini
- 1 tbsp apple cider vinegar
- ½ tsp Dijon mustard
- Juice of 1 lime or ½ lemon
- 1 tbsp pure honey

Whisk all ingredients together.

Method

1. Cook quinoa in stock for 10 mins, then cover and steam.
2. Dry tofu, cut into chunks, and pan-fry in olive oil for 10 mins, turning to brown all sides.
3. Fluff quinoa and add to bowls. Arrange the tofu and vegetables side by side.
4. Drizzle with dressing and serve.

Creamy Mushroom Soup
Serves 4

Ingredients

- 2 tbsp coconut oil
- 300g button mushrooms, quartered
- 300g chestnut mushrooms, quartered
- 1 brown onion, chopped
- 6 garlic cloves, chopped
- 1 small potato, peeled and quartered

- 2 sprigs thyme, leaves only
- 1.5 pints of hot filtered water
- 1 mushroom stock cube
- 1 tbsp butter
- ½ tsp sea salt
- Black pepper

Method

1. Sauté onion in coconut oil for 3 minutes. Add garlic, cook until golden.
2. Add mushrooms, raise the heat, and cook 5–7 minutes.
3. Add half the water and the stock cube. Stir in potatoes, salt, and thyme. Simmer 10 mins.
4. Let cool, then blend until smooth. Return the pot to the stove, add the remaining water to achieve the desired consistency.
5. Add butter and black pepper. Serve with parmesan on top.

Pea, Broccoli & Leek Soup
Serves 4

Ingredients

- 2 tbsp olive oil + extra to drizzle
- 4 garlic cloves, chopped
- 2 cups broccoli florets
- 2 leeks, chopped
- 1 small potato, chopped
- 100g frozen peas
- 1 L chicken or vegetable stock
- ½ cup pine nuts
- 2 tbsp pumpkin seeds

- Chopped chives (garnish)
- ¼ tsp sea salt
- Black pepper

Method

1. In a large pan, heat olive oil. Sauté garlic and leeks for 8–10 minutes.
2. Add stock, broccoli, peas and potatoes. Simmer 10 mins.
3. Blend until smooth. Season with salt and pepper.
4. Toast pine nuts and pumpkin seeds in a skillet.
5. Serve soup in bowls topped with seeds, chives, and a drizzle of oil.

Vegetable Quinoa with Halloumi Salad
Serves: 2

Ingredients

- 100g halloumi, cut into 4 slices
- 2 tbsp extra virgin olive oil
- 120g cooked quinoa
- 1 tsp dried peri seasoning
- ⅓ cucumber, chopped
- 1 small red onion, chopped
- 5 cherry tomatoes, chopped
- ½ red bell pepper, chopped
- 1 medium beetroot, chopped
- 10 black olives
- ¼ tsp sea salt
- Dressing
- Juice of ½ lemon
- 1 tbsp tahini
- 2 tbsp extra virgin olive oil

- ½ tbsp apple cider vinegar
- ½ tsp Dijon mustard
- Sea salt and black pepper, to taste

Whisk all dressing ingredients together in a small bowl.

Method

1. Heat olive oil in a skillet and fry halloumi for 2 minutes on each side until golden.
2. In a bowl, combine quinoa, salad vegetables, peri seasoning, sea salt, and dressing.
3. Mix well, divide between plates, and top with halloumi.
4. Serve at room temperature.

Spicy Chickpea Croutons
Serves: 2

Ingredients

- 400g chickpeas (cooked or jarred, drained and rinsed)
- 2 tbsp extra virgin olive oil
- 1 tsp smoked paprika
- ½ tsp cayenne pepper
- ½ tsp cumin seeds
- Pinch of sea salt flakes
- Ground black pepper, to taste

Method

1. Preheat oven to 200°C (180°C fan).
2. Pat the chickpeas dry and place them in a baking tin.
3. Add oil and spices; toss to coat.
4. Roast for 20 minutes, stirring occasionally, until golden and crispy.
5. Cool slightly and enjoy as a snack or topping with tahini or as a salad accompaniment.

Sardines & Sundried Tomato Pâté
Serves: 2

Ingredients
- 150g cooked sardine fillets
- 1 tbsp extra virgin olive oil
- 2 tbsp natural plain yoghurt
- 2 spring onions, finely chopped
- 5 sundried tomatoes, finely chopped
- 1 tbsp fresh parsley, chopped
- Pinch of sea salt

Method
1. Mash sardines and yoghurt in a bowl.
2. Stir in remaining ingredients.
3. Serve with seeded crackers or sourdough and a rocket salad.
4. Store in the fridge in an airtight container for up to 2 days.

Salmon Fishcakes with Yoghurt Dip
Serves: 2

Ingredients
- 3 tbsp extra virgin olive oil
- 1 small onion, finely chopped
- 100g steamed baby spinach
- 2 cooked wild salmon steaks
- 1 medium egg
- 1 tbsp ground flaxseeds
- 1 tbsp capers
- 1 tbsp chopped fresh chives
- ¼ tsp sea salt
- Ground black pepper

Yogurt Dip
- ¼ cup Greek yogurt or kefir
- Zest of 1 lemon
- 1 tbsp chopped fresh dill

Mix dip ingredients in a bowl and set aside.

Method
1. Heat 1 tbsp olive oil and sauté the onion until golden.
2. In a bowl, mix crumbled salmon, spinach, onion, egg, flaxseeds, capers, chives, salt, and pepper.
3. Heat the remaining oil and cook the patties (3–4 at a time) for 2 minutes per side, until golden.
4. Serve with yoghurt dip.

Roasted Red Pepper & Bean Soup
Serves: 4

Ingredients
- 2 red bell peppers, chopped
- 150g cherry tomatoes, halved
- 2 shallots, halved
- 3 tbsp extra virgin olive oil
- 1 tsp dried oregano
- 400g butter beans, drained
- 500ml bone broth
- 1 vegetable or chicken stock cube
- 4 tbsp kefir yoghurt
- 10 fresh basil leaves
- Sea salt and black pepper

Method
1. Preheat oven to 200°C (180°C fan).
2. Place peppers, tomatoes, and shallots on a tray; toss with

oil and oregano.
3. Roast for 15 minutes.
4. Add two-thirds of the butter beans and roast for an additional 10 minutes.
5. Transfer to a pot, add broth and stock cube, and blend until smooth. Season with sea salt and pepper to taste.
6. Add remaining beans and heat through.
7. Serve topped with kefir and basil.

Rainbow Slaw with Mango & Feta
Serves: 4

Ingredients
- 200g feta cheese
- ½ small white cabbage, shredded
- ½ small red cabbage, shredded
- 2 celery sticks, finely sliced
- 2 carrots, grated
- 2 tbsp parsley, chopped
- 3 spring onions, chopped
- 4 tbsp mango, diced

Dressing
- 100g natural yoghurt
- 6 tbsp hummus
- 2 tbsp Dijon mustard
- 1 tbsp apple cider vinegar
- ½ off a medium avocado
- ½ tsp sea salt
- Ground black pepper

Whisk dressing ingredients together.

Method
1. Mix all the vegetables and mango in a large bowl.
2. Pour over dressing and combine thoroughly.
3. Top with crumbled feta and serve.

Pomegranate Citrus Salad
Serves: 2

Ingredients
- 2 handfuls mixed salad leaves
- 2 tbsp pomegranate seeds
- 1 orange, peeled and segmented
- 1 medium red onion, finely sliced
- Zest of ½ lemon
- 2 matchbox-sized pieces of feta cheese
- 6 walnuts, crushed

Dressing
- 2 tbsp extra virgin olive oil
- Juice of ½ lemon
- ¼ tsp Dijon mustard
- 1 tbsp orange juice
- ¼ tsp sea salt
- Ground black pepper

Whisk all dressing ingredients together.

Method
1. Arrange salad leaves on plates.
2. Add orange, onion, lemon zest, pomegranate, feta, and walnuts.
3. Drizzle with dressing and serve.
4. Optional: Add brown rice and grilled chicken or fish for a heartier meal.

Poached Salmon & Watercress Niçoise
Serves: 2

Ingredients
- 100g watercress
- 2 boiled eggs
- 120g green beans
- 8 asparagus spears
- 10 green olives
- 4 spring onions, chopped
- 2 poached salmon fillets, flaked

Dressing
- Juice of ½ lemon
- ½ tsp Dijon mustard
- ½ tsp apple cider vinegar
- 2 tbsp extra virgin olive oil

Whisk dressing ingredients together.

Method
1. Boil eggs for 8 minutes, cool, peel, and halve.
2. Steam green beans and asparagus for 5 minutes; rinse with cold water.
3. Steam the salmon for 10 minutes and flake it.
4. Arrange watercress on plates, add salmon, eggs, vegetables, and olives.
5. Drizzle with dressing and serve.

Pesto Seabass with Green Beans
Serves: 2

Ingredients
- 4 tbsp extra virgin olive oil

- 5 garlic cloves
- 1 handful fresh basil
- 2 heaped tbsp grated parmesan
- 3 tbsp pine nuts
- ½ green chilli, finely chopped (optional)
- 150g green beans, trimmed
- Juice of ½ lemon
- 2 seabass fillets
- Sea salt

Method
1. Preheat oven to 200°C (180°C fan).
2. Line a tray with parchment and place the seabass on it.
3. In a pan, heat 1 tbsp oil, garlic, and pine nuts until golden, then transfer them to a blender.
4. Add basil, parmesan, remaining oil, chilli, and salt. Blend into a paste.
5. Spread pesto over the seabass and bake for 10 minutes.
6. Steam green beans for 6-8 minutes. Toss with lemon juice, oil, and seasoning.
7. Serve fish with beans.

Wheat-Free Seeded Crackers
Serves: 4

Ingredients
- 3 tbsp pumpkin seeds
- 3 tbsp flaxseeds
- 3 tbsp chia seeds
- 3 tbsp sunflower seeds
- 3 tbsp sesame seeds
- ½ tsp smoked paprika

- ½ tsp peri peri flakes
- ¼ tsp sea salt
- 100ml filtered water

Method

1. Preheat oven to 200°C (180°C fan).
2. Mix seeds and salt in a bowl. Stir in water and let sit for 5 minutes.
3. Spread mixture thinly on parchment-lined tray.
4. Sprinkle with paprika and peri peri flakes.
5. Bake for 15–18 minutes until golden. Cool for 10 minutes.
6. Serving Suggestion: Break into pieces and enjoy with hummus or pâté. Store leftovers in an airtight container.

Monkfish Coconut Curry
Serves 2

Ingredients:

- 1 tbsp coconut oil
- 1 large onion, finely diced
- 3 garlic cloves, finely chopped
- 1 thumb-sized piece fresh ginger, peeled and grated
- 1 fresh red chilli, finely sliced (with seeds)
- 1 tbsp curry powder
- 1 heaped tsp ground turmeric
- 1 tsp ground coriander
- 2 medium tomatoes, diced
- 1 medium sweet potato, peeled and chopped into 2 cm chunks
- 400 ml fresh fish stock
- 400 g monkfish fillets, cut into 4 cm chunks
- 100 g green beans, trimmed and halved

- 100 ml organic tinned coconut milk
- 2 tbsp chopped fresh coriander leaves
- Sea salt and black pepper, to taste

Method:

1. Heat coconut oil in a large skillet over medium-high heat. Add the onion and sauté for 5 minutes until softened and lightly browned.
2. Add garlic and cook for 1 minute. Stir in the ginger and chilli, cooking for an additional 3 minutes.
3. Add curry powder, turmeric, and coriander. Stir for 1 minute until fragrant.
4. Add tomatoes and fish stock. Bring to a boil, then reduce the heat and simmer for 12–15 minutes, or until the mixture has thickened.
5. Add monkfish, sweet potato, and coconut milk. Simmer gently for 2 to 3 minutes.
6. Add the green beans and cook for an additional 3-4 minutes, until tender.
7. Season to taste, stir in fresh coriander, and serve warm in bowls.

Middle Eastern-Spiced Kidney Beans
Serves 4

Ingredients:

- 800 g cooked kidney beans (2 cans), drained
- 3 tbsp olive oil
- 1 onion, finely sliced
- 4 garlic cloves, finely sliced
- 1 red chilli pepper, chopped
- 1 tbsp curry powder

- 1 tbsp paprika
- 1 tin chopped tomatoes
- 1 celery stick, chopped
- 1 carrot, chopped into 1 cm chunks
- ½ cup water
- 150 g Parmesan cheese shavings
- Sea salt and black pepper, to taste
- Thyme, for garnish

Method:

1. Heat olive oil in a large pot over medium heat. Sauté the onion and garlic until they are golden and soft.
2. Add chilli, curry powder, and paprika. Stir and cook for 1 minute.
3. Add kidney beans, chopped tomatoes, and water. Stir and simmer for 15 minutes.
4. Add carrots and celery. Simmer for an additional 10–15 minutes, until the vegetables are softened.
5. Adjust the consistency with water if needed, then season with salt and pepper.
6. Serve topped with Parmesan shavings and a sprinkle of thyme.

Mediterranean Chicken Fillets with Quinoa Salad
Serves 2

Ingredients:

- 2 small chicken breasts
- ½ tsp oregano
- ½ tsp cumin seeds
- 1 garlic clove, grated
- 2 tbsp extra virgin olive oil
- 120 g cooked quinoa

Salad:

- ⅓ cucumber, finely chopped
- 1 small red onion, finely sliced
- 5 cherry tomatoes, chopped
- ½ red bell pepper, chopped
- 10 black olives, halved

Dressing:

- Juice of ½ lemon
- Pinch of cayenne pepper
- 2 tbsp extra virgin olive oil
- ½ tbsp apple cider vinegar
- ½ tsp Dijon mustard
- Sea salt and black pepper, to taste

Method:

1. Flatten chicken breasts between parchment sheets. Season with salt and pepper, then rub with garlic, oregano, and cumin seeds.
2. Heat olive oil in a pan over medium heat. Cook chicken for 3–4 minutes on each side until golden and cooked through. Let rest, then slice.
3. Combine quinoa and salad ingredients in a bowl. Mix dressing separately, then toss with the salad.
4. Divide the salad onto plates and top with chicken slices.

Lamb & Beef Ragu with Courgette Spaghetti
Serves 3–4

Ragu Ingredients:

- 3 tbsp extra virgin olive oil
- 250 g lean beef mince
- 250 g lean lamb mince

- 2 tbsp tomato purée
- 1 large onion, finely sliced
- 8 garlic cloves, chopped
- 1 tin chopped plum tomatoes
- 1 tsp dried oregano
- 1 beef stock cube
- 1 litre of filtered water
- Handful of chopped parsley
- Sea salt and black pepper

Courgette Spaghetti:

- 3 medium courgettes, spiralized
- ¼ tsp sea salt
- 1 litre boiling water

Method:

1. Heat olive oil in a skillet. Cook the onion for 3 minutes, then add the garlic, dry oregano and cook until golden.
2. Add the minced meat and cook for 10 minutes, breaking it up as needed. Add the stock cube.
3. Add chopped tomatoes and tomato purée. Simmer for 10 minutes.
4. Add half the water, cover, and simmer for 30 minutes. Add the remaining water and simmer for an additional 30 minutes. Let it sit for 10 minutes.
5. Boil water with sea salt. Add spiralized courgettes and cook for 3 minutes. Drain.
6. Serve ragu over courgette spaghetti. Top with parsley.

Hearty Vegetable Tray Bake
Serves 2

Ingredients:
- 1 aubergine, diced
- 1 courgette, chopped
- 1 red pepper, chopped
- 1 red onion, halved
- 1 yellow onion, halved
- 1 garlic bulb, halved
- 1 cup mushrooms, halved
- 4 parboiled new potatoes
- 50 ml extra virgin olive oil
- 1 cup cooked chickpeas
- 1 tbsp dried oregano
- Sea salt and black pepper
- 2 tbsp natural yoghurt, to serve

Method:
1. Preheat oven to 220°C (fan 200°C).
2. Spread vegetables on a baking tray. Drizzle with oil, sprinkle with oregano, salt, and pepper. Mix by hand.
3. Roast for 15 minutes. Add the chickpeas and roast for an additional 10 minutes, until they are cooked through.
4. Serve with a dollop of natural yoghurt.

Chicken Pot with Mushrooms, Spinach & Chickpeas
Serves 4

Ingredients:
- 3 tbsp extra virgin olive oil
- 4 chicken thighs or breasts

- 400 g cooked chickpeas
- 2 cups chicken bone broth
- 1 chicken stock cube
- 1 cup button mushrooms, sliced
- 1 cup chestnut mushrooms
- 1 large onion, finely sliced
- 6 garlic cloves, chopped
- ½ tsp thyme
- 2 tbsp apple cider vinegar
- 1 pack of baby spinach
- 2 tbsp chopped fresh parsley

Method:
1. Heat olive oil in a cast-iron pan. Sauté the onion for 3 minutes, then add the garlic and cook for 1 minute.
2. Add chicken and cook for 8–10 minutes, turning once.
3. Add mushrooms and cook 1 minute. Pour in broth, crumble in a stock cube, and add vinegar and thyme. Simmer for 20 minutes.
4. Stir in the chickpeas and simmer for an additional 10 minutes.
5. Add spinach, cover, and cook for 2–3 minutes to wilt.
6. Sprinkle with parsley and serve warm.

Cannellini Bean & Leek Stew
Serves 2

Ingredients:
- 3 tbsp extra virgin olive oil
- 1 medium onion, sliced
- 4 garlic cloves, crushed
- 2 leeks, cut into chunks

- 400 g chopped tomatoes (tinned)
- 1 cup chicken bone broth
- 1 chicken stock cube
- 400 g cooked cannellini beans
- 1 tbsp natural yoghurt
- Juice of 1 lemon
- ½ tsp dried thyme
- Sea salt and black pepper
- Chopped parsley, to serve

Method:

1. Heat oil in a saucepan over low heat. Sauté the onion for 5 minutes. Add garlic and leeks, cook 1 more minute.
2. Stir in tomatoes, broth, and stock cube. Season and simmer for 20 minutes.
3. Add beans and yoghurt. Simmer for 5 minutes.
4. Adjust the seasoning, then stir in the lemon juice and parsley.
5. Serve with crushed new potatoes, skins on.

Black Dal Makhani
Serves 4

Ingredients

Dal Preparation

- 200g (1 cup) urad lentils
- 2.5L hot filtered water
- 1 tbsp sea salt or pink salt
- 1 tbsp fresh ginger, finely grated

Paste

- 30g coconut oil
- 1 tbsp fresh ginger, finely grated

- 1 tsp cumin seeds
- 5 large garlic cloves, grated
- 3 tbsp tomato purée
- 1 tbsp dried fenugreek leaves
- 200ml coconut cream
- 1 tsp chilli powder (optional)
- 2 tbsp garam masala
- 1 tbsp ground coriander

Topping

- 3 garlic cloves, thinly sliced
- 1 tsp cumin seeds
- 3 tbsp extra virgin olive oil

Method

1. Soak the urad lentils overnight in cold water. Drain and rinse thoroughly.
2. In a deep saucepan, combine the lentils with 2 L of hot water, salt, and grated ginger. Bring to a boil, then reduce the heat, cover, and simmer for about 2 hours, or until the vegetables are tender.
3. Meanwhile, prepare the paste by heating the coconut oil in a pan over medium heat. Add cumin seeds and sauté for 30 seconds. Add ginger, garlic, tomato purée, fenugreek leaves, and coconut cream. Stir well.
4. Cook for 2–3 minutes. Add chilli powder, garam masala, coriander, and a pinch of salt. Stir for another minute.
5. Once the lentils are cooked, stir in the paste and an additional 500ml of hot water. Cover and simmer for a further 30 minutes, until the sauce has thickened and become creamy.
6. For the topping: Warm olive oil in a small pan, add garlic, and sauté over low heat for 30 seconds. Add the cumin

seeds and cook for an additional 30 seconds.
7. Drizzle the garlic-cumin oil over the dal. Serve hot with basmati rice or flatbread and a green salad.

Beef-Stuffed Aubergine
Serves 2

Ingredients
- 2 aubergines
- 2 tbsp olive oil
- 1 tbsp coconut oil
- 1 brown onion, diced
- 4 garlic cloves, finely chopped
- ½ tsp cumin seeds
- ½ tsp ground turmeric
- ½ tsp chilli powder
- ½ tsp ground coriander
- 400g beef mince
- 100g button mushrooms, chopped
- 1 beef stock cube
- ¼ tsp sea salt
- Black pepper, to taste
- 40g green olives, pitted and chopped
- 200ml filtered water
- Rocket salad leaves
- Balsamic vinegar and olive oil, to serve

Method
1. Preheat oven to 200°C (180°C fan).
2. Halve aubergines lengthwise and scoop out the flesh, leaving a thin shell. Chop the flesh and set aside.
3. Place aubergine shells on a baking tray, drizzle with olive

oil, and roast for 15 minutes.

4. Meanwhile, heat the coconut oil in a frying pan. Sauté onion for 3 minutes, add garlic, and cook 1 more minute.
5. Add spices and stir. Increase the heat, add beef mince, and cook for 8 minutes until browned.
6. Stir in mushrooms and chopped aubergine flesh. Lower the heat and add a stock cube, water, salt, and pepper. Cover and simmer for 10 minutes.
7. Stir in chopped olives and remove from the heat.
8. Fill roasted aubergines with the beef mixture.
9. Serve with rocket leaves, a drizzle of balsamic vinegar, olive oil, and a squeeze of lemon juice.

Nourishing Fish Stew
Serves 2

Ingredients

- 300g mixed fish fillets (cod, haddock, salmon)
- 6 whole king prawns (optional)
- 200g canned chopped tomatoes
- 3 tbsp extra virgin olive oil
- 1 small onion, finely chopped
- ½ stick celery, finely chopped
- 5 new potatoes, halved
- 1 courgette, cut into chunks
- 2 garlic cloves, chopped
- 1 tbsp dried rosemary
- 1 sprig thyme
- 1 bay leaf
- ½ tsp ground cumin
- ½ tsp paprika

- 1 tbsp tomato purée
- 100ml fish stock
- A handful of fresh coriander or parsley
- Juice of ½ lemon

Method
1. Remove the skin and bones from the fish, then cut it into chunks.
2. Heat olive oil in a casserole dish. Sauté onion and celery on low heat.
3. Add the courgette and garlic and cook until the onion is golden.
4. Stir in herbs, spices, chopped tomatoes, tomato purée, and potatoes. Simmer briefly.
5. Add fish stock and simmer for 15 minutes.
6. Add fish and prawns. Simmer gently for 10–15 minutes until cooked.
7. Serve in bowls with fresh coriander or parsley and garnish with lemon juice.

Vegetable Stir-Fry with Cauliflower Rice
Serves 4

Ingredients
- 1 head of cauliflower, chopped
- 4 tsp extra virgin olive oil
- 3 tbsp soy sauce
- 5 garlic cloves, minced
- ¼ cup water
- Pinch sea salt
- 1 red onion, sliced
- 1 tbsp grated fresh ginger

- 8 broccoli florets
- 1 cup carrots, peeled and sliced
- 1 cup shiitake mushrooms, chopped
- 1 handful of snap peas
- 400g cooked chickpeas
- Juice of ½ lemon
- Fresh coriander, chopped, to garnish

Method:

Cauliflower Rice

1. Pulse the cauliflower and carrots in a food processor until it reaches a rice-sized consistency, or finely chop it by hand.
2. Heat 2 tsp olive oil in a large skillet over medium heat. Add 1 tsp garlic and sauté for 2 minutes.
3. Add cauliflower, water, and salt. Cover and steam for 2 minutes. Set aside.

Stir-Fry

1. In the same pan, heat the remaining olive oil over medium-high heat.
2. Add the remaining garlic and onion, and cook for 4 minutes, until softened.
3. Add broccoli, mushrooms, snap peas, and ginger. Stir-fry for about 6 minutes.
4. Stir in soy sauce and chickpeas. Remove from heat, add lemon juice.
5. Serve over cauliflower rice, garnished with coriander.

Turmeric and Lemon Chicken
Serves 2

Ingredients
- 100g cooked chickpeas
- 3 tbsp extra virgin olive oil
- ½ tsp turmeric
- 1 medium onion, finely chopped
- 2 organic skinless chicken thighs
- 500ml chicken stock
- Juice of ½ lemon
- 3 garlic cloves, crushed
- 1 tbsp fresh rosemary, chopped
- 1 tsp fresh thyme
- ½ tbsp Dijon mustard
- Sea salt and black pepper, to taste

Method
1. Heat olive oil in a saucepan. Sauté the onion on low heat until golden.
2. Add garlic and cook for 1 minute.
3. Add chicken and brown both sides. Add turmeric, rosemary, and thyme, and cook for 1 minute.
4. Add stock, bring to a boil, cover, and simmer on low for 30 minutes.
5. Add chickpeas, lemon juice, and mustard. Simmer for an additional 10 minutes, until the sauce has reduced.
6. Serve with wholegrain rice and steamed vegetables.

Tofu Thai Green Curry
Serves 2

Ingredients

Curry Paste
- 2 lemongrass stalks, trimmed
- 2 green chillies, chopped
- 1 thumb-sized piece of ginger, grated
- Juice of ½ lime
- 4 garlic cloves, chopped
- 1 medium onion
- 1 tsp ground cumin
- A handful of fresh coriander

Curry
- 200g firm tofu, cubed
- 1 tbsp olive oil
- 1 medium onion, sliced
- 1L vegetable stock
- 200ml coconut milk
- 1 thumb-sized piece ginger, grated
- 1 red bell pepper, thinly sliced
- 4 broccoli florets
- 1 cup button mushrooms
- Sea salt and pepper
- 1 cup cooked wholegrain rice
- Fresh coriander and lime wedges, to serve

Method

Paste

1. Blend all paste ingredients in a food processor. Marinate tofu in half the paste for 3 hours.

Curry

1. Heat oil in a deep pan. Sauté onion for 3-4 minutes.
2. Add tofu and remaining paste, cook for 3 minutes per side. Remove tofu and set aside.
3. Add stock and half the coconut milk. Bring to a boil, then simmer for 30 minutes.
4. Add ginger, remaining coconut milk, tofu, and vegetables. Simmer for 5 minutes.
5. Season with salt and pepper. Serve with rice, coriander, and lime wedges.

Spiced Lamb Rack with Thyme New Potatoes
Serves 2

Ingredients

- 1 small rack of lamb (6-8 chops), fat removed
- 3 tbsp extra virgin olive oil
- 3 garlic cloves, grated
- ¼ tsp each: turmeric, paprika, peri
- 1 tbsp apple cider vinegar
- 1 thumb-sized piece fresh ginger, peeled and grated
- Sea salt and black pepper, to taste
- ½ tsp dried thyme
- 8 medium new potatoes
- 250g steamed vegetables (e.g., cauliflower, broccoli, green beans)
- 1 to 2 tbsp mint sauce

Method

1. Preheat oven to 220°C (200°C fan).
2. Place the lamb in a baking tray. Rub with garlic, spices, vinegar, 1 tbsp olive oil, ginger, salt, and pepper.

3. Roast for 18 minutes for pink or 22 minutes for well done. Rest for 7 minutes before slicing.
4. Meanwhile, boil the potatoes until they are just soft. Drain, then toss with thyme, 2 tbsp olive oil, salt, and pepper.
5. Serve lamb with potatoes, steamed vegetables, and mint sauce.

Smoked Paprika Ratatouille
Serves 2

Ingredients

- 100ml olive oil
- 1 aubergine, chopped into 3cm chunks
- 1 red onion, finely sliced
- 3 courgettes, chopped
- 2 red bell peppers, chopped
- 500g ripe tomatoes, chopped
- 8 garlic cloves, finely chopped
- 4–5 sprigs fresh thyme (leaves only)
- 1 tbsp smoked paprika
- 1 vegetable stock cube
- A handful of fresh basil
- 1 fresh red chilli, chopped
- 1 cup filtered water
- ¼ tsp sea salt
- Black pepper, to taste

Method

- Heat olive oil in a large casserole dish. Fry an aubergine for 10–12 minutes until tender. Set aside.
- Add onion, courgette, and peppers. Cook for 10 minutes until soft.

- Return the aubergine to the pan with tomato, garlic, thyme, chilli, paprika, stock cubes, salt, pepper, and water.
- Simmer covered for 20–25 mins.
- Serve topped with fresh basil.

Slow-Cooked Roast Lamb
Serves 4

Ingredients

- ½ leg organic lamb
- 2 tbsp olive oil
- ¼ tsp sea salt
- 1 sprig each: rosemary, thyme
- 3 garlic cloves, quartered
- 1 tbsp Dijon mustard
- 1 lamb stock cube
- ½ pint filtered water
- Parchment paper + foil

Method

1. Preheat oven to 180°C (160°C fan).
2. Insert garlic into small cuts all over the lamb.
3. Rub with herbs and mustard, season with salt, and drizzle with olive oil.
4. Place in a baking dish with water. Cover with parchment, then foil.
5. Roast for 2.5–3 hours, basting every 30 minutes.
6. Rest for 15 minutes before slicing.
7. Serve with new potatoes and vegetables.

Meat Juice Gravy
- Add 1 cup boiling water and a lamb stock cube to the pan juices. Stir and heat on the stove to make gravy.

Red Lentil Dahl

Serves 4

Ingredients
- 200g split red lentils
- 4 tbsp extra virgin olive oil
- 1 large onion, finely chopped
- 8 garlic cloves, chopped
- 1 tsp cumin seeds
- 1 cinnamon stick
- 1 tsp each: turmeric, coriander, garam masala
- 1 litre of filtered water
- ½ tsp sea salt
- Black pepper, to taste
- Fresh coriander, to serve

Method
1. Rinse lentils under cold water. Place the ingredients in a pot with water, including turmeric, coriander, garam masala, cinnamon, salt, and pepper.
2. Bring to a boil, then reduce the heat and simmer for 30 minutes, or until the mixture has thickened.
3. In a separate pan, heat 2 tbsp oil. Sauté onion and garlic until soft, then add cumin seeds.
4. Stir onion mixture into lentils. Let it sit for 5 minutes.
5. Serve with basmati rice and salad.

Pan-Fried Turkey & Pepper Koftas
Serves 2

Ingredients
- 1 pack minced turkey or chicken
- 1 small egg
- 1 tbsp chickpea flour
- 3 tbsp olive oil
- 1 small onion, finely chopped
- 1 red bell pepper, finely chopped
- ½ orange bell pepper, finely chopped
- 1 red chilli (optional), finely chopped
- 1 tbsp chopped fresh coriander
- 3 garlic cloves, grated
- ¼ tsp sea salt
- 1 tbsp peri peri flakes
- 1 tsp black pepper
- 1 tbsp onion powder
- 1 tbsp tomato paste

Method
1. Combine all ingredients (except oil) in a bowl and mix well.
2. Shape into 4 round burger-sized patties.
3. Heat oil in a large pan. Fry koftas for 4-5 minutes on each side or until cooked through.
4. Serve with a side salad.

Oven-Baked Salmon with Dill & Mustard + Red Slaw
Serves 2

Ingredients
- 2 Alaskan wild salmon fillets
- 1 tbsp olive oil
- 2 tbsp wholegrain mustard
- ½ of a medium avocado
- 100g Greek yoghurt
- Small handful of fresh dill
- 1 beetroot, peeled & grated
- ½ red cabbage, finely sliced
- 1 red onion, finely sliced
- ½ lemon, cut into wedges
- Steamed green beans, to serve
- Salt & pepper, to taste

Method
1. Preheat oven to 200°C (180°C fan).
2. Line a baking tray. Place the salmon skin-side down.
3. Mix the oil, mustard, most of the dill, salt, and pepper. Spread over the salmon.
4. Bake for 10-12 minutes until slightly pink in the centre.

Red Slaw
1. Mix avocado, 2 tbsp yoghurt, beetroot, cabbage, and onion in a bowl.
2. Serve salmon with slaw, green beans, lemon wedges, and remaining yoghurt.
3. Optional: add new potatoes.

Wholesome Beef Stew with Vegetables
Serves 2

Ingredients
- 2 tbsp coconut oil
- 300g sirloin steak, cubed
- 1 onion, finely sliced
- 4 garlic cloves, sliced
- 1 carrot, chopped
- 1 celery stalk, chopped
- 1 small butternut squash, cubed
- 4 new potatoes, halved
- ½ litre beef bone broth
- ½ litre filtered water
- 1 beef stock cube
- 1 bay leaf
- 1 sprig rosemary
- ½ tsp dried oregano
- 1 tbsp curry powder
- ¼ tsp sea salt
- Black pepper, to taste

Method
1. Heat 2 tbsp coconut oil in a skillet. Cook the onion for 3 minutes, then add the garlic and cook for an additional minute.
2. Add another tbsp of oil, then sear the beef on all sides for 3 mins.
3. Add stock cube, herbs, and spices. Stir for 1 min.
4. Add bone broth and simmer for 30 minutes.
5. Add water and vegetables. Bring to a boil, then simmer, covered, for 20 minutes or until the mixture has thickened.
6. Serve in bowls.

Coconut Bread

Ingredients (makes 6-8 small rounds):
- 2 cups coconut flour (sifted)
- 2 tbsp psyllium husk (not powder)
- 1 tbsp olive oil
- 1 tbsp coconut oil (melted)
- 1 tsp sesame seeds (optional, for texture)
- 1 tsp black onion seeds (nigella seeds)
- 1/2 tsp Himalayan pink salt
- 1 to 1 cups warm water (as needed)

Optional Add-ins (for variety):
- ½ tsp baking powder (for a lighter texture)
- ½ tsp garlic powder or cumin (for flavour)

Method:
1. Preheat oven to 200°C (180°C fan). Line a baking tray with parchment paper.
2. Mix dry ingredients (coconut flour, psyllium husk, seeds, salt, and optional spices and baking powder) in a large mixing bowl.
3. Add oils and mix slightly to coat the dry ingredients.
4. Slowly pour in warm water, stirring continuously until a soft, pliable dough forms. Start with 1 cup and add more if needed. Dough should be moist but not sticky.
5. Rest the dough for 10-15 minutes to allow the psyllium to absorb moisture and firm up.
6. Shape the dough: Roll out between two sheets of parchment to ~5mm thickness, then cut into circles or desired shapes.
7. Bake for 30-40 minutes or until golden, firm, and slightly crisp at the edges. Flip halfway if needed for even baking.

8. Cool on a rack for 10 minutes before serving. Best served warm with dips or spreads.

Storage:

Store in an airtight container in the fridge for up to 5 days or freeze for up to 2 months. Reheat in a toaster or oven for the best texture.

Additional reading

Chapter 1
UCLA Health. (2009, January 12). *Most heart attack patients' cholesterol levels did not indicate cardiac risk*. https://www.uclahealth.org/news/release/most-heart-attack-patients-cholesterol-levels-did-not-indicate-cardiac-risk#:~:text=A%20new%20national%20study%20has,on%20current%20national%20cholesterol%20guidelines

Xu, J., Zhang, L., Wu, Q., Zhou, Y., Jin, Z., Li, Z., & Zhu, Y. (2021). Body roundness index is a superior indicator to associate with the cardio-metabolic risk: Evidence from a cross-sectional study with 17,000 Eastern-China adults. *BMC Cardiovascular Disorders, 21*(1), 97. https://doi.org/10.1186/s12872-021-01905-x

Chapter 2
AquaVitae. (n.d.). *Your metabolism and your body composition*. https://aquavitality.com/metabolism-body-composition/

Fisher, P. (n.d.). *What is your metabolic type?* https://liveleanrx.com/what-is-your-metabolic-type/

Ianev, S. (n.d.). *Understanding the four metabolic types*. https://enterprisefitnessacademy.com/blog/2019/04/03/the-4-metabolic-types/

Nunez, K., & Bhagwat, R. (2024, December 23). *Four signs of a healthy metabolism, according to health experts*. https://www.realsimple.com/what-is-healthy-metabolism-7966890

Chapter 3
Haigh, R. (2017, November 17). *Insulin response: It comes from eating protein too.* https://thestrongkitchen.com/blog/post/insulin-response-it-comes-from-eating-protein-too#:~:text=But%20still%2C%20research%20has%20shown,about%2015%20minutes%20after%20ingestion

Chapter 4

Bazire, P. (2020, April 7). *Body fat distribution.* https://drbazire.uk/blog/body-fat-distribution/

Cubeddu, L. X., & Hoffmann, I. S. (2012). Metabolic syndrome: An all or none or a continuum load of risk? *Metabolic Syndrome and Related Disorders, 10*(1), 14–19. https://doi.org/10.1089/met.2011.0058

DiGiacinto, J., & Roland, J. (2021, September 8). *Fatty liver: What it is, and how to get rid of it.* https://www.healthline.com/nutrition/fatty-liver#TOC_TITLE_HDR_7

Fitzgerald, K. (n.d.). *Non-alcoholic fatty liver disease: Dr Robert Rountree shares.* https://www.drkarafitzgerald.com/2019/01/03/non-alcoholic-fatty-liver-disease-dr-robert-rountree/

Medline Plus. (n.d.). *Congenital leptin deficiency.* https://medlineplus.gov/genetics/condition/congenital-leptin-deficiency/#:~:text=LEP%20gene%20mutations%20that%20cause,gain%20associated%20with%20this%20disorder

National Health Service Inform. (n.d.). *Non-alcoholic fatty liver disease.* https://www.nhsinform.scot/illnesses-and-conditions/stomach-liver-and-gastrointestinal-tract/non-alcoholic-fatty-liver-disease-nafld#stages

Ristic, A. (2019, September 9). *Genetic factors for fatty liver.* https://selfdecode.com/blog/article/fatty-liver-pemt-40/

Sheridan, P. A., Paich, H. A., Handy, J., Karlsson, E. A., Hudgens, M. G., Sammon, A. B., Holland, L. A., Weir, S., Noah, T. L., & Beck, M. A. (2012). Obesity is associated with impaired immune response to influenza vaccination in humans. *International Journal of Obesity, 36*(8), 1072–1077. https://doi.org/10.1038/ijo.2011.208

Takahashi, M., Hori, M., Ishigamori, R., Mutoh, M., Imai, T., & Nakagama, H. (2018). Fatty pancreas: A possible risk factor for pancreatic cancer in animals and humans. *Cancer Science, 109*(10), 3013–3023. https://doi.org/10.1111/cas.13766

Walker, B. B., Shashank, A., Gasevic, D., Schuurman, N., Poirier, P., Teo, K., Rangarajan, S., Yusuf, S., & Lear, S. A. (2020). The local food environment and obesity: Evidence from three cities. *Obesity, 28*(1), 40–45. https://doi.org/10.1002/oby.22614

[8] Alqarni, A. A., Aldhahir, A. M., Siraj, R. A., Alqahtani, J. S., Alshehri, H. H., Alshamrani, A. M., Namnqani, A. A., Alsaidalani, L. N., Tawhari, M. N., Badr, O. I., & Alwafi, H. (2023). Prevalence of overweight and obesity and their impact on spirometry parameters in patients with asthma: A multicentre, retrospective study. *Journal of Clinical Medicine, 12*(5), 1843. https://doi.org/10.3390/jcm12051843

[9] Bagnato, C. B., Bianco, A., Bonfiglio, C., Franco, I., Verrelli, N., Carella, N., Shahini, E., Zappimbulso, M., Giannuzzi, V., Pesole, P. L., Ancona, A., & Giannelli, G. (2024). Healthy lifestyle changes improve cortisol levels and liver steatosis in MASLD patients: Results from a randomized clinical trial. *Nutrients, 16*(23), 4225. https://doi.

org/10.3390/nu16234225; Ryan, M. C., Itsiopoulos, C., Thodis, T., Ward, G., Trost, N., Hofferberth, S., O'Dea, K., Desmond, P. V., Johnson, N. A., & Wilson, A. M. (2013). The Mediterranean diet improves hepatic steatosis and insulin sensitivity in individuals with non-alcoholic fatty liver disease. *Journal of Hepatology, 59*(1), 138–143. https://doi.org/10.1016/j.jhep.2013.02.012

[10] Yan, H. M., Xia, M. F., Wang, Y., Chang, X. X., Yao, X. Z., Rao, S. X., Zeng, M. S., Tu, Y. F., Feng, R., Jia, W. P., Liu, J., Deng, W., Jiang, J. D., & Gao, X. (2015). Efficacy of berberine in patients with non-alcoholic fatty liver disease. *PLOS One, 10*(8), e0134172. https://doi.org/10.1371/journal.pone.0134172

[11] Vell, M. S., Creasy, K. T., Scorletti, E., Seeling, K. S., Hehl, L., Rendel, M. D., Schneider, K. M., & Schneider, C. V. (2023). Omega-3 intake is associated with liver disease protection. *Frontiers in Public Health, 11*, 1192099. https://doi.org/10.3389/fpubh.2023.1192099

[12] Rocha, R., Cotrim, H. P., Siqueira, A. C., & Floriano, S. (2007). Fibras solúveis no tratamento da doença hepática gordurosa não-alcoólica: estudo piloto [Non-alcoholic fatty liver disease: treatment with soluble fibres]. *Arquivos de Gastroenterologia, 44*(4), 350–352. https://doi.org/10.1590/s0004-28032007000400013

Chapter 6

Barnardo, A. (2020, March 17). *What is glycation, and how can it age your skin?* https://yora.com/blogs/journal/glycation

International Diabetes Federation. (2006). The IDF consensus worldwide definition of metabolic syndrome. https://idf.org/media/uploads/2023/05/attachments-30.pdf

Johnson, J. (2023, May 16). *What causes food cravings?* https://www.medicalnewstoday.com/articles/318441

Kobo, O., Leiba, R., Avizohar, O., & Karban, A. (2019). Normal body mass index (BMI) can rule out metabolic syndrome: An Israeli cohort study. *Medicine, 98*(9), e14712. https://doi.org/10.1097/MD.0000000000014712

The Vitality Clinic. (2021, May 3). *Blog: All about metabolic flexibility.* https://thevitalityclinic.co.uk/is-this-the-fountain-of-youth/

The Vitality Clinic. (2021, October 15). *Blog: Blood sugar control the key to metabolic health.* https://thevitalityclinic.co.uk/blood-sugar-control-the-key-to-metabolic-health/

Xue, F. (2024, April 16). *Cravings sugar? Your body is probably lacking this nutrient.* https://www.byrdie.com/what-do-sugar-cravings-mean

Chapter 9

Bonsignore, M. R., Borel, A. L., Machan, E., & Grunstein, R. (2013). Sleep apnoea and metabolic dysfunction. *European Respiratory Review, 22*(129), 353-364. https://doi.org/10.1183/09059180.00003413

Piotrowski, B. (2021, April 30). *The link between sleep apnea and gum disease.* https://www.periodonticsnaples.com/the-link-between-sleep-apnea-and-gum-disease#:~:text=People%20with%20sleep%20apnea%20tend,or%20gum%20disease%20to%20develop

British Snoring and Sleep Apnoea Association. (n.d.). *What is sleep apnoea? (sleep apnea)?* https://britishsnoring.co.uk/snoring_&_sleep_apnoea/what_is_sleep_apnoea.php

Castaneda, A., Jauregui-Maldonado, E., Ratnani, I., Varon, J., & Surani, S. (2018). Correlation between metabolic syndrome and sleep apnea. *World Journal of Diabetes, 9*(4), 66-71. https://doi.org/10.4239/wjd.v9.i4.66

ENTUK. (n.d.). *Snoring and obstructive sleep apnoea in adults.* https://www.entuk.org/patients/conditions/34/snoring_and_obstructive_sleep_apnoea_in_adults/

Framnes, S. N., & Arble, D. M. (2018). The bidirectional relationship between obstructive sleep apnea and metabolic disease. *Frontiers in Endocrinology, 9*, 440. https://doi.org/10.3389/fendo.2018.00440

Georgoulis, M., Yiannakouris, N., Kechribari, I., Lamprou, K., Perraki, E., Vagiakis, E., & Kontogianni, M. D. (2021). The effectiveness of a weight-loss Mediterranean diet/lifestyle intervention in the management of obstructive sleep apnea: Results of the "MIMOSA" randomised clinical trial. *Clinical Nutrition, 40*(3), 850-859. https://doi.org/10.1016/j.clnu.2020.08.037

Kostoglou-Athanassiou, I., & Athanassiou, P. (2008). Metabolic syndrome and sleep apnea. *Hippokratia, 12*(2), 81-86.

Weichselbaum, E. (2013, August). *Dietary patterns and the heart.* https://assets.heartfoundation.org.nz/documents/shop/submissions/dietary-patterns-evidence-paper.pdf

Chapter 10

Harvard Health Publishing. (2021, February 15). *Gum disease and heart disease that common thread.* https://www.health.harvard.edu/heart-health/gum-disease-and-heart-disease-the-common-thread

Lamster, I. B., & Pagan, M. (2017). Periodontal disease and the metabolic syndrome. *International Dental Journal, 67*(2), 67-77. https://doi.org/10.1111/idj.12264

Srivastava, M. C., Srivastava, R., Verma, P. K., & Gautam, A. (2019). Metabolic syndrome and periodontal disease: An overview for physicians. *Journal of Family Medicine and Primary Care, 8*(11), 3492–3495. https://doi.org/10.4103/jfmpc.jfmpc_866_19

Chapter 11

Abdollah, F., Briganti, A., Suardi, N., Castiglione, F., Gallina, A., Capitanio, U., & Montorsi, F. (2011). Metabolic syndrome and benign prostatic hyperplasia: Evidence of a potential relationship, hypothesised etiology, and prevention. *Korean Journal of Urology, 52*(8), 507–516. https://doi.org/10.4111/kju.2011.52.8.507

Banerjee, P. P., Banerjee, S., Brown, T. R., & Zirkin, B. R. (2018). Androgen action in prostate function and disease. *American Journal of Clinical and Experimental Urology, 6*(2), 62–77.

Corona, G., Vignozzi, L., Rastrelli, G., Lotti, F., Cipriani, S., & Maggi, M. (2014). Benign prostatic hyperplasia: A new metabolic disease of the aging male and its correlation with sexual dysfunctions. *International Journal of Endocrinology, 2014,* 329456. https://doi.org/10.1155/2014/329456

Ngai, H. Y., Yuen, K. S., Ng, C. M., Cheng, C. H., & Chu, S. P. (2017). Metabolic syndrome and benign prostatic hyperplasia: An update. *Asian Journal of Urology, 4*(3), 164–173. https://doi.org/10.1016/j.ajur.2017.05.001

Chapter 12

Dong, J., & Rees, D. A. (2023). Polycystic ovary syndrome: Pathophysiology and therapeutic opportunities. *BMJ Medicine, 2*(1), e000548. https://doi.org/10.1136/bmjmed-2023-000548

Hajam, Y. A., Rather, H. A., Neelam, N., Kumar, R., Basheer, M., & Reshi, M. S. (2024). A review on critical appraisal and pathogenesis of polycystic ovarian syndrome. *Endocrine and Metabolic Science, 14,* 100162. https://doi.org/10.1016/j.endmts.2024.100162

Sadeghi, H. M., Adeli, I., Calina, D., Docea, A. O., Mousavi, T., Daniali, M., Nikfar, S., Tsatsakis, A., & Abdollahi, M. (2022). Polycystic ovary syndrome: A comprehensive review of pathogenesis, management, and drug repurposing. *International Journal of Molecular Sciences, 23*(2), 583. https://doi.org/10.3390/ijms23020583

Singh, S., Pal, N., Shubham, S., Sarma, D. K., Verma, V., Marotta, F., & Kumar, M. (2023). Polycystic ovary syndrome: Etiology, current management, and future therapeutics. *Journal of Clinical Medicine, 12*(4), 1454. https://doi.org/10.3390/jcm12041454

Chapter 13

Aberdeen Orthopaedic Network. (2021, July 27). *Hip osteoarthritis: The four stages.* https://www.aberdeenorthopaedics.com/hip-osteoarthritis-the-four-stages/

Li, H., George, D. M., Jaarsma, R. L., & Mao, X. (2016). Metabolic syndrome and components exacerbate osteoarthritis symptoms of pain, depression and reduced knee function. *Annals of Translational Medicine, 4*(7), 133. https://doi.org/10.21037/atm.2016.03.48

ProHealth Clinic. (2024, April 19). *How to regenerate knee cartilage naturally.*

https://prohealthclinic.co.uk/blog/how-to-regenerate-knee-cartilage-naturally/#:~:text=Natural%20strategies%20for%20cartilage%20regeneration,supplements%20like%20glucosamine%20and%20chondroitin

Zheng, L., Zhang, Z., Sheng, P., & Mobasheri, A. (2021). The role of metabolism in chondrocyte dysfunction and the progression of osteoarthritis. *Ageing Research Reviews, 66*, 101249. https://doi.org/10.1016/j.arr.2020.101249

Chapter 14

Antani, M. R., & Dattilo, J. B. (2023, August 8). Varicose veins. In *StatPearls*. StatPearls Publishing. https://www.ncbi.nlm.nih.gov/books/NBK470194/

Bradbury, A. W. (2011). Pathophysiology and principles of management of varicose veins. In R. Fitridge (Ed.), *Mechanisms of vascular disease: A reference book for vascular specialists* (pp. 451-458). University of Adelaide Press. https://www.ncbi.nlm.nih.gov/books/NBK534256/

Lim, C. S., & Davies, A. H. (2009). Pathogenesis of primary varicose veins. *The British Journal of Surgery, 96*(11), 1231-1242. https://doi.org/10.1002/bjs.6798

LiverDoctor. (n.d.). *A sluggish liver can cause varicose veins.* https://www.liverdoctor.com/a-sluggish-liver-can-cause-varicose-veins/

Chapter 16

Altomare, R., Cacciabaudo, F., Damiano, G., Palumbo, V. D., Gioviale, M. C., Bellavia, M., Tomasello, G., & Lo Monte, A. I. (2013). The Mediterranean diet: A history of health. *Iranian Journal of Public Health, 42*(5), 449-457.

Brehm, B. J., Seeley, R. J., Daniels, S. R., & D'Alessio, D. A. (2003). A randomised trial comparing a very low carbohydrate diet and a calorie-restricted low fat diet on body weight and cardiovascular risk factors in healthy women. *The Journal of Clinical Endocrinology and Metabolism, 88*(4), 1617-1623. https://doi.org/10.1210/jc.2002-021480

Marrone, G., Guerriero, C., Palazzetti, D., Lido, P., Marolla, A., Di Daniele, F., & Noce, A. (2021). Vegan diet health benefits in metabolic syndrome. *Nutrients, 13*(3), 817. https://doi.org/10.3390/nu13030817

Mawer, R. (2020, November 9). *A ketogenic diet to lose weight and fight metabolic disease.* https://www.healthline.com/nutrition/ketogenic-diet-and-weight-loss

Chapter 17
Science Learning Hub. (2022, November 18). *Energy requirements of the body.* https://www.sciencelearn.org.nz/resources/1835-energy-requirements-of-the-body

Chapter 18
Morselli, L. L., Guyon, A., & Spiegel, K. (2012). Sleep and metabolic function. *Pflugers Archiv: European Journal of Physiology, 463*(1), 139-160. https://doi.org/10.1007/s00424-011-1053-z

Newsom, R., & Truong, K. (2024, April 11). *Sleep and weight loss.* https://www.sleepfoundation.org/physical-health/weight-loss-and-sleep

Sleep Doctor. (n.d.). *Four things to know about how sleep affects metabolism.* https://thesleepdoctor.com/physical-health/sleep-and-weight-loss/#:~:text=Sleep%20also%20affects%20individual%20metabolism,diseases%20associated%20with%20weight%20gain

Suni, E., & Rehman, A. (2023, December 8). *How do you determine poor sleep quality.* https://www.sleepfoundation.org/sleep-hygiene/how-to-determine-poor-quality-sleep

The Vitality Clinic. (2021, November 26). *Sleep: It's a vital part of our physical, mental, and emotional well-being.* https://thevitalityclinic.co.uk/sleep-its-a-vital-part-of-our-physical-mental-and-emotional-well-being/

Chapter 19
Bergmann, N., Gyntelberg, F., & Faber, J. (2014). The appraisal of chronic stress and the development of the metabolic syndrome: A systematic review of prospective cohort studies. *Endocrine Connections, 3*(2), R55–R80. https://doi.org/10.1530/EC-14-0031

Chandola, T., Brunner, E., & Marmot, M. (2006). Chronic stress at work and the metabolic syndrome: Prospective study. *BMJ (Clinical Research Ed.), 332*(7540), 521-525. https://doi.org/10.1136/bmj.38693.435301.80

Hjemdahl P. (2002). Stress and the metabolic syndrome: An interesting but enigmatic association. *Circulation, 106*(21), 2634-2636. https://doi.org/10.1161/01.cir.0000041502.43564.79

Janczura, M., Bochenek, G., Nowobilski, R., Dropinski, J., Kotula-Horowitz, K., Laskowicz, B., Stanisz, A., Lelakowski, J., & Domagala, T. (2015). The relationship of metabolic syndrome with stress, coronary heart disease and pulmonary function--An occupational cohort-based study. *PLOS One, 10*(8), e0133750. https://doi.org/10.1371/journal.pone.0133750

Pyykkönen, A. J., Räikkönen, K., Tuomi, T., Eriksson, J. G., Groop, L., & Isomaa, B. (2010). Stressful life events and the metabolic syndrome: The prevalence, prediction and prevention of diabetes (PPP)-Botnia Study. *Diabetes Care, 33*(2), 378–384. https://doi.org/10.2337/dc09-1027

Rosmond, R. (2005). Role of stress in the pathogenesis of the metabolic syndrome. *Psychoneuroendocrinology, 30*(1), 1–10. https://doi.org/10.1016/j.psyneuen.2004.05.007

Wallace, J. (2020, September 8). *Six types of stress and how to manage them effectively.* https://www.psychreg.org/types-of-stress/

Chapter 20

Blue Zones. (n.d.). *Food guidelines.* https://www.bluezones.com/recipes/food-guidelines/

Erynn. (2020, March 15). *How the aging baby boomers are going to change 2020.* https://seniorshelpingseniorsnh.com/elderly-home-caregivers/how-the-aging-baby-boomers-are-going-to-change-2020

Marks, G. (2014, February 12). *This is why the baby boomers are the worst generation ever.* https://www.huffpost.com/entry/this-is-why-the-baby-boom_b_4441735

Medical Research Council. (2012, September 21). *The baby boomers under the doctor at retirement.* https://medicalxpress.com/news/2012-09-baby-boomers-doctor.html

Money and Markets Staff. (2020, February 6). *Why boomers and Gen X have more in common than either group realise.* https://moneyandmarkets.com/baby-boomers-generation-z-more-in-common/

Park, A. (2013, February 5). *Baby boomers: Not the healthiest generation.* https://healthland.time.com/2013/02/05/baby-boomers-not-the-healthiest-generation/

Robertson, R. (2024, December 3). *Why people in blue zones live longer than the rest of the world.* https://www.healthline.com/nutrition/blue-zones

Scripps. (2025, March 6). *10 top health concerns of baby boomers.* https://www.scripps.org/news_items/5475-top-health-concerns-of-baby-boomers

University College London. (2020, July 14). *Middle-aged face more years of ill health than baby boomers.* https://www.ucl.ac.uk/news/2020/jul/middle-aged-face-more-years-ill-health-baby-boomers

End notes

Introduction
[1] Lorenzo, C., Williams, K., Hunt, K. J., & Haffner, S. M. (2007). The National Cholesterol Education Program - Adult Treatment Panel III, International Diabetes Federation, and World Health Organization definitions of the metabolic syndrome as predictors of incident cardiovascular disease and diabetes. *Diabetes Care*, 30(1), 8–13. https://doi.org/10.2337/dc06-1414

[2] de la Monte, S. M., & Wands, J. R. (2008). Alzheimer's disease is type 3 diabetes - Evidence reviewed. *Journal of Diabetes Science and Technology*, 2(6), 1101–1113. https://doi.org/10.1177/193229680800200619

[3] Hamer, M., Sharma, N., & Batty, G. D. (2019). Association of objectively measured physical activity with brain structure: UK Biobank study. Journal of Epidemiology & Community Health, 73(11), 970–976. https://doi.org/10.1136/jech-2019-212233

[4] Office for National Statistics. (2022). *Health state life expectancies, UK: 2018 to 2020*. https://www.ons.gov.uk/peoplepopulationandcommunity/healthandsocialcare/healthandlifeexpectancies

The History of Metabolic Syndrome
[1] Joslin, E. P. (1923). *The treatment of diabetes mellitus: With observations based upon three thousand cases*. Lea & Febiger.

[2] Kylin, E. (1923). Studien über das Hypertonie-Hyperglykämie-Hyperurikämiesyndrom. *Zentralblatt für Innere Medizin*, 44, 105–127.

[3] Mandal, A. (2023, July 3). *History of metabolic syndrome*. https://www.news-medical.net/health/History-of-Metabolic-Syndrome.aspx; Vague, J. (1956). The degree of masculine differentiation of obesities: A factor determining predisposition to diabetes, atherosclerosis, gout, and uric calculous disease. *The American Journal of Clinical Nutrition*, 4(1), 20–34. https://doi.org/10.1093/ajcn/4.1.20

[4] Avogaro, P., Crepaldi, G., Enzi, G., & Tiengo, A. (1967). Associazione di iperlipemia, diabete mellito e obesità di medio grado. *Acta Diabetologica Latina*, *4*(1), 572–590. https://doi.org/10.1007/BF01544100

[5] Singer, P. (1977). Diagnosis of primary hyperlipoproteinemias. *Zeitschrift für die Gesamte Innere Medizin und Ihre Grenzgebiete*, *32*(8), 129–133.

[6] Haller, H. (1977). Epidemiology and associated risk factors of hyperlipoproteinemia. *Zeitschrift für die gesamte innere Medizin und ihre Grenzgebiete*, *32*(8), 124–128.

[7] Phillips, G. B. (1978). Sex hormones, risk factors and cardiovascular disease. *The American Journal of Medicine*, *65*(1), 7–11. https://doi.org/10.1016/0002-9343(78)90685-x

[8] Reaven, G. M. (1988). Banting Lecture 1988. Role of insulin resistance in human disease. *Diabetes*, *37*(12), 1595–1607. https://doi.org/10.2337/diab.37.12.1595

[9] Reaven G. (2001). Syndrome X. *Current Treatment Options in Cardiovascular Medicine*, *3*(4), 323–332. https://doi.org/10.1007/s11936-001-0094-6

[10] Alberti, K. G. M. M., Zimmet, P., & Shaw, J. (2005). The metabolic syndrome—A new worldwide definition. *The Lancet*, *366*(9491), 1059–1062. https://doi.org/10.1016/S0140-6736(05)67402-8; Alberti, K. G. M. M., Zimmet, P., Shaw, J., & Grundy, S. M. (2006). The IDF consensus worldwide definition of the metabolic syndrome. *Diabetes & Vascular Disease Research*, *3*(3), 160–163.

[11] de Luca, C., & Olefsky, J. M. (2008). Inflammation and insulin resistance. *FEBS Letters*, *582*(1), 97–105. https://doi.org/10.1016/j.febslet.2007.11.057

[12] Alberti, K. G., Eckel, R. H., Grundy, S. M., Zimmet, P. Z., Cleeman, J. I., Donato, K. A., Fruchart, J. C., James, W. P., Loria, C. M., Smith, S. C., Jr, International Diabetes Federation Task Force on Epidemiology and Prevention, National Heart, Lung, and Blood Institute, American Heart Association, World Heart Federation, International Atherosclerosis Society, & International Association for the Study of Obesity. (2009). Harmonizing the metabolic syndrome: A joint interim statement of the International Diabetes Federation Task Force on Epidemiology and Prevention; National Heart, Lung, and Blood Institute; American Heart Association; World Heart Federation; International Atherosclerosis Society; and International Association for the Study of Obesity. *Circulation*, *120*(16), 1640–1645. https://doi.org/10.1161/CIRCULATIONAHA.109.192644

[13] World Health Organization. (2010). *Definition and diagnosis of diabetes mellitus and intermediate hyperglycemia: Report of a WHO/IDF consultation*. https://iris.who.int/handle/10665/43588

[14] Lim, E. L., Hollingsworth, K. G., Aribisala, B. S., Chen, M. J., Mathers, J. C., & Taylor, R. (2011). Reversal of type 2 diabetes: Normalisation of beta cell function in association with decreased pancreas and liver triacylglycerol. *Diabetologia*, *54*(10), 2506–2514. https://doi.org/10.1007/s00125-011-2204-7

[15] Fryar, C. D., Carroll, M. D., & Ogden, C. L. (2020). *Prevalence of overweight, obesity, and severe obesity among adults aged 20 and over: United States, 1960–1962 through 2017–2018.* https://www.cdc.gov/nchs/products/databriefs/db360.htm

[16] Bray, G. A., Nielsen, S. J., & Popkin, B. M. (2004). Consumption of high-fructose corn syrup in beverages may play a role in the epidemic of obesity. *The American Journal of Clinical Nutrition, 79*(4), 537–543. https://doi.org/10.1093/ajcn/79.4.537

[17] Robinson, E., Boyland, E., Chisholm, A., Harrold, J., Maloney, N. G., Marty, L., Mead, B. R., Noonan, R., & Hardman, C. A. (2021). Obesity, eating behavior and physical activity during COVID-19 lockdown: A study of UK adults. *Appetite, 156*, 104853. https://doi.org/10.1016/j.appet.2020.104853

[18] Sidor, A., & Rzymski, P. (2020). Dietary choices and habits during COVID-19 lockdown: Experience from Poland. *Nutrients, 12*(6), 1657. https://doi.org/10.3390/nu12061657

Chapter 1

[1] National Institute for Health and Care Excellence. (2022, April 8). *Keep the size of your waist to less than half of your height, NICE recommends.* https://www.nice.org.uk/news/articles/keep-the-size-of-your-waist-to-less-than-half-of-your-height-nice--recommends

Chapter 2

[1] Araújo, J., Cai, J., & Stevens, J. (2019). Prevalence of optimal metabolic health in american adults: National Health and Nutrition Examination Survey 2009-2016. *Metabolic Syndrome and Related Disorders, 17*(1), 46–52. https://doi.org/10.1089/met.2018.0105

[2] Office for National Statistics. (2015). *How has life expectancy changed over time?* https://www.ons.gov.uk/peoplepopulationandcommunity/birthsdeathsandmarriages/lifeexpectancies/articles/howhaslifeexpectancychangedovertime/2015-09-09

[3] For a global overview of these shifts, see Monteiro, C. A., Cannon, G., Levy, R. B., Moubarac, J. C., Louzada, M. L. C., Rauber, F., & Jaime, P. C. (2020). Ultra-processed foods: A global perspective on public health and policy. *Nutrients, 12*(7), 1958.

[4] Franco, M., Bilal, U., Orduñez, P., Benet, M., Morejón, A., Caballero, B., Kennelly, J. F., & Cooper, R. S. (2013). Population-wide weight loss and regain in relation to diabetes burden and cardiovascular mortality in Cuba 1980-2010: Repeated cross sectional surveys and ecological comparison of secular trends. *BMJ (Clinical Research Ed.), 346*, f1515. https://doi.org/10.1136/bmj.f1515

[5] Stanhope, K. L. (2016). Sugar consumption, metabolic disease and obesity: The state of the controversy. *Critical Reviews in Clinical Laboratory Sciences, 53*(1), 52–67. https://doi.org/10.3109/10408363.2015.1084990

[6] Mayo Clinic Staff. (n.d.). *Metabolism and weight loss: How you burn calories.* https://www.mayoclinic.org/healthy-lifestyle/weight-loss/in-depth/metabolism/art-20046508

[7] Health.com. (2024, December 15). *What your body type means for your health.* https://www.health.com/body-type-8699069

Chapter 3

[1] Frankenberg, A. D. V., Reis, A. F., & Gerchman, F. (2017). Relationships between adiponectin levels, the metabolic syndrome, and type 2 diabetes: A literature review. *Archives of Endocrinology and Metabolism, 61*(6), 614–622. https://doi.org/10.1590/2359-3997000000316; Yanai, H., & Yoshida, H. (2019). Beneficial effects of adiponectin on glucose and lipid metabolism and atherosclerotic progression: Mechanisms and perspectives. *International Journal of Molecular Sciences, 20*(5), 1190. https://doi.org/10.3390/ijms20051190

[2] Frankenberg, A. D. V., Reis, A. F., & Gerchman, F. (2017). Relationships between adiponectin levels, the metabolic syndrome, and type 2 diabetes: A literature review. *Archives of Endocrinology and Metabolism, 61*(6), 614–622. https://doi.org/10.1590/2359-3997000000316; Yanai, H., & Yoshida, H. (2019). Beneficial effects of adiponectin on glucose and lipid metabolism and atherosclerotic progression: Mechanisms and perspectives. *International Journal of Molecular Sciences, 20*(5), 1190. https://doi.org/10.3390/ijms20051190

[3] Dicken, S. J., & Batterham, R. L. (2024). Ultra-processed food and obesity: What Is the evidence? *Current Nutrition Reports, 13*(1), 23–38. https://doi.org/10.1007/s13668-024-00517-z

[4] Zupo, R., Donghia, R., Castellana, F., Bortone, I., De Nucci, S., Sila, A., Tatoli, R., Lampignano, L., Sborgia, G., Panza, F., Lozupone, M., Colacicco, G., Clodoveo, M. L., & Sardone, R. (2023). Ultra-processed food consumption and nutritional frailty in older age. *GeroScience, 45*(4), 2229–2243. https://doi.org/10.1007/s11357-023-00753-1

[5] Azemati, B., Rajaram, S., Jaceldo-Siegl, K., Sabate, J., Shavlik, D., Fraser, G. E., & Haddad, E. H. (2017). Animal-protein intake is associated with insulin resistance in Adventist Health Study 2 (AHS-2) Calibration substudy participants: A cross-sectional analysis. *Current Developments in Nutrition, 1*(4), e000299. https://doi.org/10.3945/cdn.116.000299

[6] Turner, K. M., Keogh J. B., Clifton P. M. (2015). Red meat, dairy, and insulin sensitivity: A randomized crossover intervention study. *The American Journal of Clinical Nutrition, 101*(6), 1173–1179. https://doi.org/10.3945/ajcn.114.104976.

[7] Vanhaecke T., Perrier E. T., & Melander O. (2021). A journey through the early evidence linking hydration to metabolic health. *Annals of Nutrition and Metabolism, 9,* 4–9. https://doi.org/10.1159/000515021

[8] Rodak, K., Kokot, I., & Kratz, E. M. (2021). Caffeine as a factor influencing the functioning of the human body—Friend or foe? *Nutrients, 13*(9), 3088. https://doi.org/10.3390/nu13093088

[9] Maddatu, J., Anderson-Baucum, E., & Evans-Molina, C. (2017). Smoking and the risk of type 2 diabetes. *Translational Research, 184*, 101–107. https://doi.org/10.1016/j.trsl.2017.02.004

[10] Luo, J., Rossouw, J., Tong, E., Giovino, G. A., Lee, C. C., Chen, C., Ockene, J. K., Qi, L., & Margolis, K. L. (2013). Smoking and diabetes: Does the increased risk ever go away? *American Journal of Epidemiology, 178*(6), 937–945. https://doi.org/10.1093/aje/kwt071

[11] Kosmas, C. E., Rodriguez Polanco, S., Bousvarou, M. D., Papakonstantinou, E. J., Peña Genao, E., Guzman, E., & Kostara, C. E. (2023). The triglyceride/high-density lipoprotein cholesterol (TG/HDL-C) ratio as a risk marker for metabolic syndrome and cardiovascular disease. *Diagnostics, 13*(5), 929. https://doi.org/10.3390/diagnostics13050929

[12] Lazris, A., Roth, A. R., Haskell, H., & James, J. (2021). Prediabetes Diagnosis: Helpful or harmful? *American Family Physician, 104*(6), 649–651.

Chapter 4

[1] Morland, K., Diez Roux, A. V., & Wing, S. (2006). Supermarkets, other food stores, and obesity: The Atherosclerosis Risk in Communities Study. *American Journal of Preventive Medicine, 30*(4), 333–339. https://doi.org/10.1016/j.amepre.2005.11.003

[2] Walker, B. B., Shashank, A., Gasevic, D., Schuurman, N., Poirier, P., Teo, K., Rangarajan, S., Yusuf, S., & Lear, S. A. (2020). The local food environment and obesity: Evidence from three cities. *Obesity, 28*(1), 40–45. https://doi.org/10.1002/oby.22614

[3] Kohli, P., & Greenland, P. (2006). Role of the metabolic syndrome in risk assessment for coronary heart disease. *JAMA, 295*(7), 819–821.

[4] Alqarni, A. A., Aldhahir, A. M., Siraj, R. A., Alqahtani, J. S., Alshehri, H. H., Alshamrani, A. M., Namnqani, A. A., Alsaidalani, L. N., Tawhari, M. N., Badr, O. I., & Alwafi, H. (2023). Prevalence of overweight and obesity and their impact on spirometry parameters in patients with asthma: A multicentre, retrospective study. *Journal of Clinical Medicine, 12* (5), 1843. https://doi.org/10.3390/jcm12051843

Chapter 5

[1] Office for National Statistics. (n.d.). *Leading causes of death, UK*. Retrieved January 29, 2025, from https://www.ons.gov.uk/peoplepopulationandcommunity/healthandsocialcare/causesofdeath/articles/leadingcausesofdeathuk/latest

[2] Primatesta, P., & Poulter, N. R. (2006). Improvement in hypertension management in England: Results from the Health Survey for England 2003. *Journal of Hypertension, 24*(6), 1187–1192. https://doi.org/10.1097/01.hjh.0000226211.58026.f8

[3] Gupta, P., Perkovic, V., & Huxley, R. (2016). Burden of hypertension among normal weight adults: A population-based study. *Journal of Hypertension, 34*(4), 597–603.

https://doi.org/10.1097/HJH.0000000000000851

[4] American Heart Association. (n.d.). *Home blood pressure monitoring.* https://www.heart.org/en/health-topics/high-blood-pressure/understanding-blood-pressure-readings/monitoring-your-blood-pressure-at-home

[5] Cohen, J. B., Cohen, D. L., Herman, L. J., & Townsend, R. R. (2019). Cardiovascular events and mortality in white-coat hypertension: A systematic review and meta-analysis. *Annals of Internal Medicine, 170*(12), 853–862. https://doi.org/10.7326/M19-0223

[6] Tinetti, M. E., Han, L., Lee, D. S. H., McAvay, G. J., Peduzzi, P., Gross, C. P., Zhou, B., & Lin, H. (2014). Antihypertensive medications and serious fall injuries in a nationally representative sample of older adults. *JAMA Internal Medicine, 174*(4), 588–595. https://doi.org/10.1001/jamainternmed.2013.14764

[7] LeBlanc, E. S., Hillier, T. A., Pedula, K. L., & Rizzo, J. H. (2011). Hip fracture and increased short-term but not long-term mortality in healthy older women. *Archives of Internal Medicine, 171*(20), 1831–1837. https://doi.org/10.1001/archinternmed.2011.447

[8] Intersalt Cooperative Research Group. (1988). Intersalt: an international study of electrolyte excretion and blood pressure. *British Medical Journal, 297*(6644), 319–328.

[9] Bell, L. L., & Taylor, M. C. (2022). *The impact of pet ownership on human health: A systematic review. PMC, 17*(4), 25-30. https://pmc.ncbi.nlm.nih.gov/articles/PMC9356927

Chapter 6

[1] Lenoir, M., Serre, F., Cantin, L., & Ahmed, S. H. (2007). Intense sweetness surpasses cocaine reward. *PLOS One, 2* (8), e698. https://doi.org/10.1371/journal.pone.0000698

Chapter 7

[1] Khera, A. V., & Kathiresan, S. (2017). Genetics of coronary artery disease: Discovery, biology and clinical translation. *Nature Reviews Genetics, 18*(6), 331–344. https://doi.org/10.1038/nrg.2016.160

[2] Sachdeva, A., Cannon, C. P., Deedwania, P. C., Labresh, K. A., Smith, S. C., Jr, Dai, D., Hernandez, A., & Fonarow, G. C. (2009). Lipid levels in patients hospitalized with coronary artery disease: An analysis of 136,905 hospitalizations in Get With The Guidelines. *American Heart Journal, 157*(1), 111–117.e2. https://doi.org/10.1016/j.ahj.2008.08.010

[3] Gordon, D. J., Probstfield, J. L., Garrison, R. J., Neaton, J. D., Castelli, W. P., Knoke, J. D., Jacobs, D. R., Bangdiwala, S., & Tyroler, H. A. (1989). High-density lipoprotein cholesterol and cardiovascular disease: Four prospective American studies. *Circulation, 79*(1), 8–15. https://doi.org/10.1161/01.CIR.79.1.8

[4] Siri, P. W., & Krauss, R. M. (2005). Influence of dietary carbohydrate and fat on LDL and HDL particle distributions. *Current Atherosclerosis Reports*, 7(6), 455–459. https://doi.org/10.1007/s11883-005-0062-9

[5] Howard, B. V., Van Horn, L., Hsia, J., Manson, J. E., Stefanick, M. L., Wassertheil-Smoller, S., Kuller, L. H., LaCroix, A. Z., Langer, R. D., Lasser, N. L., Lewis, C. E., Limacher, M. C., Margolis, K. L., Mysiw, W. J., Ockene, J. K., Parker, L. M., Perri, M. G., Phillips, L., Prentice, R. L., ... & Brunner, R. L. (2006). Low-fat dietary pattern and risk of cardiovascular disease: The Women's Health Initiative Randomized Controlled Dietary Modification Trial. *JAMA*, 295(6), 655–666. https://doi.org/10.1001/jama.295.6.655

Chapter 8

[1] For more information, see British Liver Trust. (n.d.). *Key facts and statistics*. https://britishlivertrust.org.uk/information-and-support/statistics/

[2] Nayagam, S., Williams, J., & Thursz, M. (2021). Disease burden and economic impact of diagnosed non-alcoholic steatohepatitis (NASH) in the United Kingdom. *Frontline Gastroenterology*, 12(4), 322–332. https://doi.org/10.1136/flgastro-2020-101538

[3] Song, J., da Costa, K. A., Fischer, L. M., Kohlmeier, M., Kwock, L., Wang, S., & Zeisel, S. H. (2005). Polymorphism of the PEMT gene and susceptibility to nonalcoholic fatty liver disease (NAFLD). *FASEB Journal*, 19(10), 1266–1271. https://doi.org/10.1096/fj.04-3580com

[4] Ou, H. Y., Wang, C. Y., Yang, Y. C., Chen, M. F., & Chang, C. J. (2013). The association between nonalcoholic fatty pancreas disease and diabetes. *PLOS One*, 8(5), e62561. https://doi.org/10.1371/journal.pone.0062561; Yu, T. Y., & Wang, C. Y. (2017). Impact of non-alcoholic fatty pancreas disease on glucose metabolism. *Journal of Diabetes Investigation*, 8(6), 735–747. https://doi.org/10.1111/jdi.12665

[5] For more information, see Lambert, J. E., Ramos-Roman, M. A., Browning, J. D., & Parks, E. J. (2014). The influence of dietary fat on liver fat accumulation in humans. *Proceedings of the Nutrition Society*, 73(1), 80–85. https://doi.org/10.1017/S0029665113003904

[6] Taylor, R., Al-Mrabeh, A., Zhyzhneuskaya, S., Peters, C., Barnes, A. C., Aribisala, B. S., Hollingsworth, K. G., Mathers, J. C., Sattar, N., & Lean, M. E. J. (2018). Remission of human type 2 diabetes requires decrease in liver and pancreas fat content but is dependent upon capacity for β cell recovery. *Cell Metabolism*, 28(4), 547–556.e3. https://doi.org/10.1016/j.cmet.2018.07.003

[7] Hallsworth, K., Fattakhova, G., Hollingsworth, K. G., Thoma, C., Moore, S., Taylor, R., Day, C. P., & Trenell, M. I. (2011). Resistance exercise reduces liver fat and its mediators in non-alcoholic fatty liver disease independent of weight loss. *Gut*, 60(9), 1278–1283. https://doi.org/10.1136/gut.2011.242073

[8] Yan, H.-M., Xia, M.-F., Wang, Y., Chang, X.-X., Yao, X.-Z., Rao, S.-X., Zeng, M.-S., & Li, X.-M. (2015). Efficacy of berberine in patients with non-alcoholic fatty liver disease.

PLOS ONE, 10(8), e0134172. https://doi.org/10.1371/journal.pone.0134172

[9] Guo, X., Yang, B., Tan, J., Jiang, J., Li, H., & Wang, X. (2020). Effects of omega-3 polyunsaturated fatty acid supplementation on non-alcoholic fatty liver disease: A meta-analysis. *Nutrition Reviews*, 78(9), 737-746. https://doi.org/10.1093/nutrit/nuz103

Chapter 9

[1] Young, T., Finn, L., Peppard, P. E., Szklo-Coxe, M., Austin, D., Nieto, F. J., Stubbs, R., & Hla, K. M. (2008). Sleep disordered breathing and mortality: Eighteen-year follow-up of the Wisconsin sleep cohort. *Sleep*, 31(8), 1071-1078.

[2] Doumit, J., & Prasad, B. (2016). Sleep apnea in type 2 diabetes. *Diabetes Spectrum*, 29(1), 14-19. https://doi.org/10.2337/diaspect.29.1.14

[3] Stegman, S. S., Burroughs, J. M., & Henthorn, R. W. (1996). Asymptomatic bradyarrhythmias as a marker for sleep apnea: Appropriate recognition and treatment may reduce the need for pacemaker therapy. *Pacing and Clinical Electrophysiology*, 19(6), 899-904. https://doi.org/10.1111/j.1540-8159.1996.tb03385.x

[4] Georgoulis, M., Yiannakouris, N., Kechribari, I., Lamprou, K., Perraki, E., Vagiakis, E., & Kontogianni, M. D. (2020). The effectiveness of a weight-loss Mediterranean diet/lifestyle intervention in the management of obstructive sleep apnea: Results of the MIMOSA randomized clinical trial. *Clinical Nutrition*, 39(8), 2371-2379. https://doi.org/10.1016/j.clnu.2020.09.003

[5] Vasta, C. (2024, April 29). *Exercises to reduce sleep apnoea*. https://www.sleepcareonline.com/articles/exercises-to-reduce-sleep-apnea/

Chapter 10

42% of the adult increases the risk of obesity and suffering a heart attack twofold.
[1] Centers for Disease Control and Prevention. (2022, May 17). *Gum disease facts*. https://www.cdc.gov/oral-health/data-research/facts-stats/fast-facts-gum-disease.html

Gum D diabetes, non-alcoholic liver disease, dementia, and colorectal cancer.
[2] Medical News Today. (2019, March 11). *Gum disease increases the risk of heart attacks and strokes*. https://www.medicalnewstoday.com/articles/gum-disease-increases-the-risk-of-heart-attacks-and-strokes

Association between metabolic syndrome and periodontal disease.
[3] D'Aiuto, F., Nibali, L., Parkar, M., Suvan, J., & Tonetti, M. S. (2010). Oxidative stress, systemic inflammation, and severe periodontitis. *Journal of Dental Research*, 89(11), 1241-1246. https://doi.org/10.1177/0022034510375830

Number of metabolic syndrome components present in an individual.

[4] Kuo, L. C., Polson, A. M., & Kang, T. (2008). Associations between periodontal

diseases and metabolic syndrome: A systematic review and meta-analysis. *Journal of Clinical Periodontology, 35*(5), 347–365. https://doi.org/10.1111/j.1600-051X.2008.01218.x

Oral care can also reduce inflammatory markers.

[5] D'Aiuto, F., Orlandi, M., & Gunsolley, J. C. (2019). Evidence that periodontal treatment improves biomarkers and CVD outcomes. *Journal of Clinical Periodontology, 46*(Suppl 21), 92–105. https://doi.org/10.1111/jcpe.13052

Link between periodontal disease and benign prostatic hyperplasia (BPH).

[6] See, for example, Baek, S.-H., Han, S. J., Park, S. C., & Choi, H. G. (2022). A cross-sectional study for association between periodontitis and benign prostatic hyperplasia. *Coatings, 12*(2), 265. https://doi.org/10.3390/coatings12020265

Bacteria infecting the gum plaques in the mouth isolated from prostate fluids.

[7] Estemalik, J., Demko, C., Bonomo, R. A., Wadhwa, P., Sim, C., & Novak, M. J. (2017). Simultaneous detection of oral pathogens in subgingival plaque and prostatic fluid of men with periodontal and prostatic diseases: A pilot study. *Journal of Periodontology, 88*(8), 778–787. https://doi.org/10.1902/jop.2017.160477

Chapter 11

[1] Parsons, J. K., & Kashefi, C. (2008). Physical activity, benign prostatic hyperplasia, and lower urinary tract symptoms. *European Urology, 53*(6), 1228–1235. https://doi.org/10.1016/j.eururo.2008.01.077

[2] Kim, J. W., Oh, M. M., Yoon, C. Y., Lee, J. G., Bae, J. H., Hong, S. K., & Kim, J. J. (2012). Association between metabolic syndrome and lower urinary tract symptoms in Korean men. *International Neurourology Journal, 16*(1), 23–29. https://doi.org/10.5213/inj.2012.16.1.23

[3] Smith, D. P., et. al. (2014). Relationship between lifestyle and lower urinary tract symptoms: A longitudinal study of 45 and Up Study participants. *The Journal of Urology, 191*(1), 174–181. https://doi.org/10.1016/j.juro.2013.06.088

[4] Liu, Z. M., Wong, C. K., & Chen, Y. M. (2016). Fruit and vegetable intake in relation to lower urinary tract symptoms and erectile dysfunction among Southern Chinese elderly men: A 4-year prospective study of Mr OS Hong Kong. *Medicine, 95*(2), e2555. https://doi.org/10.1097/MD.0000000000002555

[5] Kristal, A. R., Arnold, K. B., Schenk, J. M., Neuhouser, M. L., Goodman, P., Penson, D. F., Thompson, I. M., & Lin, D. W. (2008). Race/ethnicity, obesity, health-related behaviors and the risk of symptomatic benign prostatic hyperplasia: Results from the Prostate Cancer Prevention Trial. *The Journal of Urology, 180*(2), 474–479. https://doi.org/10.1016/j.juro.2008.04.029

[6] Lu, Z., Wu, C., Zhang, J., Ye, Y., Zhang, Z., Liao, M., Huang, L., Tian, J., Tan, A., & Mo, Z. (2019). Drinking frequency but not years may be associated with lower urinary

tract symptoms: Result from a large cross-sectional survey in Chinese men. *Risk Management and Healthcare Policy*, *12*, 633-642. https://doi.org/10.2147/RMHP.S238012

[7] Zhang, L., Li, H., & Xu, L. (2019). Statin use and the risk of benign prostatic hyperplasia: A systematic review and meta-analysis. *European Journal of Clinical Pharmacology*, *75*(5), 619-626. https://doi.org/10.1007/s00228-019-02691-4

[8] Choi, H. S., Lee, S. H., Lee, S. H., Lee, S. H., Lee, S. H., Lee, S. H., ... & Lee, S. H. (2015). The effects of statins on benign prostatic hyperplasia in elderly men. *The Journal of Urology*, *193*(5), 1712-1717. https://doi.org/10.1016/j.juro.2014.12.086

[9] Zhao, J., Zhang, L., Zhang, Y., & Zhang, X. (2013). Impact of type 2 diabetes on lower urinary tract symptoms in men. *BMC Urology*, *13*(1), 12. https://doi.org/10.1186/1471-2490-13-12

Chapter 12

[1] Liu, Y., Zhang, H., Zhang, L., Yuan, Z., Guo, X., & Jiang, H. (2022). Gut microbiota dysbiosis in polycystic ovary syndrome (PCOS): An updated review. *Scientific Reports*, *12*, 25041. https://doi.org/10.1038/s41598-022-25041-4.

[2] Kandaraki, E. A., Kolibianakis, E. M., Chatzianastasiou, K., Koutsou, A., Tarlatzis, B. C., & Papanikolaou, E. G. (2011). Elevated serum bisphenol A levels in women with polycystic ovary syndrome: A case-control study. *Human Reproduction*, *26*(6), 1525-1530. https://doi.org/10.1093/humrep/der102.

[3] Kandaraki, E. A., Papanikolaou, E. G., & Tarlatzis, B. C. (2012). Bisphenol A impacts the hormonal profile in patients with polycystic ovary syndrome, but not in healthy women. *Gynecological Endocrinology*, *28*(5), 424-428. https://doi.org/10.3109/09513590.2011.627066.

[4] Kandaraki, E. A., Papanikolaou, E. G., & Tarlatzis, B. C. (2021). Changes in ghrelin and glucagon following a low glycemic load diet in women with polycystic ovary syndrome. *Journal of Clinical Endocrinology & Metabolism*, *106*(3), e1061-e1070. https://doi.org/10.1210/clinem/dgaa907

[5] Zhang, Y., Zhang, L., Zhang, H., & Zhang, Y. (2021). The effect of low glycemic index diet on the reproductive and clinical features of polycystic ovary syndrome: A systematic review and meta-analysis. *Frontiers in Endocrinology*, *12*, 688. https://doi.org/10.3389/fendo.2021.688

[6] Stepto, N. K., Cassar, S., Joham, A. E., Harrison, C. L., Moran, L. J., & Teede, H. J. (2019). Exercise interventions in polycystic ovary syndrome: A systematic review and meta-analysis. *Human Reproduction Update*, *25*(5), 576-593. https://doi.org/10.1093/humupd/dmz022

[7] Karamali, M., Mirmiran, P., Moghadam, S. K., & Azizi, F. (2019). Changes in hormonal profile and body mass index in women with polycystic ovary syndrome after probiotic

intake: A 12-week placebo-controlled and randomized clinical study. *Nutrients, 11*(3), 405. https://doi.org/10.3390/nu11030405

[8] Hoeger, K. M., Kochman, L., Wixom, N., Craig, K., Miller, R. K., & Guzick, D. S. (2004). A randomized, 48-week, placebo-controlled trial of intensive lifestyle modification and/or metformin therapy in overweight women with polycystic ovary syndrome: A pilot study. *Fertility and Sterility, 82*(2), 421–429. https://doi.org/10.1016/j.fertnstert.2004.02.104

[9] Panidis, D., Farmakiotis, D., Rousso, D., Kourtis, A., Katsikis, I., & Krassas, G. (2008). Obesity, weight loss, and the polycystic ovary syndrome: Effect of treatment with diet and orlistat for 24 weeks on insulin resistance and androgen levels. *Fertility and Sterility, 89*(4), 899–906. https://doi.org/10.1016/j.fertnstert.2007.04.043

Chapter 13

[1] Zagaria, M. A. E. (2004). Osteoarthritis in seniors. *U.S. Pharmacist, 1*, 20–24. https://www.uspharmacist.com/article/osteoarthritis-in-seniors

[2] Ponzio, D. Y., Syed, U. A. M., Purcell, K., Cooper, A. M., Maltenfort, M., Shaner, J., & Chen, A. F. (2018). Low prevalence of hip and knee arthritis in active marathon runners. *The Journal of Bone and Joint Surgery, 100*(2), 131–137. https://doi.org/10.2106/JBJS.16.01071

[3] Zhuo, Q., Yang, W., Chen, J., Wang, Y., & Zhang, Y. (2012). Metabolic syndrome meets osteoarthritis. *Nature Reviews Rheumatology, 8*(12), 729–737. https://doi.org/10.1038/nrrheum.2012.135

[4] Veronese, N., & Reginster, J. Y. (2019). The effects of metabolic syndrome on osteoarthritis: Evidence from epidemiological and clinical studies. *Aging Clinical and Experimental Research, 31*(5), 543–548. https://doi.org/10.1007/s40520-018-1062-8

[5] Niu, J., Clancy, M., Aliabadi, P., & Felson, D. T. (2017). Metabolic syndrome and progression of knee osteoarthritis: The Framingham Osteoarthritis Study. *Arthritis Care & Research, 69*(2), 176–182. https://doi.org/10.1002/acr.23045

Chapter 14

[1] Hirai, H. (1990). Prevalence and risk factors of varicose veins in Japanese women. *Angiology, 41*(3), 228–232.

[2] Lee, A. J., Robertson, L. A., Boghossian, S. M., Allan, P. L., Ruckley, C. V., Fowkes, F. G., & Evans, C. J. (2015). Progression of varicose veins and chronic venous insufficiency in the general population in the Edinburgh Vein Study. *Journal of Vascular Surgery: Venous and Lymphatic Disorders, 3*(1), 18–26.

Chapter 16

[1] USA Facts. (2021). *Obesity rate nearly triples in the United States over the last 50 years.* https://usafacts.org/articles/obesity-rate-nearly-triples-united-states-over-last-50-years

[2] United Nations Conference on Trade and Development. (1999). *Jamaica: Economic liberalization policies in the 1990s.* https://unctad.org/system/files/official-document/poedmm176.en.pdf

[3] Boume, P. A., & McGrowder, D. A. (2009). Health status of patients with self-reported chronic diseases in Jamaica. *North American Journal of Medical Sciences, 1*(7), 356–364. https://doi.org/10.4297/najms.2009.7356

[4] Unwin, D. (2021). *A lower carb diet sheet for type 2 diabetes.* Public Health Collaboration. https://phcuk.org/wp-content/uploads/A_5_page_low_carb_diet_leaflet_Unwin_2021-converted.pdf

[5] Taylor, R., Al-Mrabeh, A., Zhyzhneuskaya, S., Peters, C., Barnes, A. C., Aribisala, B. S., Hollingsworth, K. G., Mathers, J. C., Sattar, N., & Lean, M. E. J. (2018). Remission of human type 2 diabetes requires decrease in liver and pancreas fat content but is dependent upon capacity for β cell recovery. *Cell Metabolism, 28*(4), 547–556.e3. https://doi.org/10.1016/j.cmet.2018.07.003

[6] Huang, R. Y., Huang, C. C., Hu, F. B., & Chavarro, J. E. (2016). Vegetarian diets and weight reduction: A meta-analysis of randomized controlled trials. *Journal of General Internal Medicine, 31*(1), 109–116. https://doi.org/10.1007/s11606-015-3390-7

[7] Elorinne, A. L., Alfthan, G., Erlund, I., Kivimäki, H., Paju, A., Salminen, I., Turpeinen, U., & Voutilainen, S. (2016). Food and nutrient intake and nutritional status of Finnish vegans and non-vegetarians. *PLOS One, 11*(2), e0148235. https://doi.org/10.1371/journal.pone.0148235

[8] Shenoy, S. F., Poston, W. S., Reeves, R. S., Kazaks, A. G., & Foreyt, J. P. (2010). Weight loss in individuals with metabolic syndrome given DASH diet counseling when provided a low sodium vegetable juice: A randomized controlled trial. *Nutrition Journal, 9*, 8. https://doi.org/10.1186/1475-2891-9-8

[9] Zhang, L., Zhang, Y., Zhang, X., Zhang, Y., Zhang, Y., & Zhang, Y. (2018). Antibiotic exposure in early life increases risk of childhood obesity: A systematic review and meta-analysis. *Scientific Reports, 8*(1), 15018. https://doi.org/10.1038/s41598-018-33475-3

Chapter 17

[1] Booth, F. W., Roberts, C. K., & Laye, M. J. (2017). Lack of exercise is a major cause of chronic diseases. Comprehensive Physiology, 2(2), 1143–1211. https://doi.org/10.1002/cphy.c110025; Warburton, D. E., Nicol, C. W., & Bredin, S. S. (2006). Health benefits of physical activity: The evidence. *CMAJ: Canadian Medical Association Journal, 174*(6), 801–809. https://doi.org/10.1503/cmaj.051351

[2] McGuire, D. K., Levine, B. D., Williamson, J. W., Snell, P. G., Blomqvist, C. G., Saltin, B., & Mitchell, J. H. (2001). A 30-year follow-up of the Dallas Bed Rest and Training Study: I. Effect of age on the cardiovascular response to exercise. *Circulation, 104*(12), 1350–1357. https://doi.org/10.1161/circ.104.12.1350

[3] Trapp, E. G., Chisholm, D. J., Freund, J., & Boutcher, S. H. (2008). The effects of high-

intensity intermittent exercise training on fat loss and fasting insulin levels of young women. *International Journal of Obesity, 32*(4), 684–691. https://doi.org/10.1038/sj.ijo.0803781

[4] Tseng, B. Y., Uh, J., Rossetti, H. C., Cullum, C. M., Diaz-Arrastia, R. F., Levine, B. D., Lu, H., & Zhang, R. (2013). Masters athletes exhibit larger regional brain volume and better cognitive performance than sedentary older adults. *Journal of Magnetic Resonance Imaging, 38*(5), 1169–1176

[5] Fiatarone, M. A., Marks, E. C., Ryan, N. D., Meredith, C. N., Lipsitz, L. A., & Evans, W. J. (1990). High-intensity strength training in nonagenarians. *JAMA, 263*(22), 3029–3034.

[6] Hamer, M., Batty, G. D., & Singh-Manoux, A. (2015). Association of body mass index and waist-to-hip ratio with brain structure: UK Biobank study. *Neurology, 84*(6), 625–632. https://doi.org/10.1212/WNL.0000000000001239

[7] Estruch, R., Ros, E., Salas-Salvadó, J., Covas, M. I., Corella, D., Arós, F., Gómez-Gracia, E., Ruiz-Gutiérrez, V., Fiol, M., Lapetra, J., Lamuela-Raventós, R. M., Serra-Majem, L., Pintó, X., Basora, J., Muñoz, M. A., Sorlí, J. V., Martínez, J. A., & Martínez-González, M. A. (2018). Primary prevention of cardiovascular disease with a Mediterranean diet supplemented with extra-virgin olive oil or nuts. *New England Journal of Medicine, 378*(25), e34. https://doi.org/10.1056/NEJMoa1800389

Chapter 18

[1] Antunes, L. C., Levandovski, R., Dantas, G., Caumo, W., & Hidalgo, M. P. (2010). Obesity and shift work: Chronobiological aspects. *Nutrition Research Reviews, 23*(1), 155–168. https://doi.org/10.1017/S0954422410000016; Sooriyaarachchi, P., Jayawardena, R., Pavey, T., & King, N. (2021). Shift work and body composition: A systematic review and meta-analysis. *Minerva Endocrinology, 46*(2), 201–213. https://doi.org/10.23736/S2724-6507.21.03534-X

[2] Foster, G. D., Sanders, M. H., Millman, R., Zammit, G., Borradaile, K. E., Newman, A. B., Wadden, T. A., Kelley, D., Wing, R. R., & Pi-Sunyer, F. X. (2009). Obstructive sleep apnea among obese patients with type 2 diabetes. *Diabetes Care, 32*(6), 1017–1019. https://doi.org/10.2337/dc08-1776; Kendzerska, T., Gershon, A. S., Hawker, G., Leung, R. S., & Tomlinson, G. (2014). Obstructive sleep apnea and incident diabetes. A historical cohort study. *American Journal of Respiratory and Critical Care Medicine, 190*(2), 218–225. https://doi.org/10.1164/rccm.201312-2209OC

[3] Herth, J., Sievi, N. A., Schmidt, F., & Kohler, M. (2023). Effects of continuous positive airway pressure therapy on glucose metabolism in patients with obstructive sleep apnoea and type 2 diabetes: A systematic review and meta-analysis. *European Respiratory Review, 32*(169), 230083. https://doi.org/10.1183/16000617.0083-2023; Martínez-Cerón, E., Barquiel, B., Bezos, A. M., Casitas, R., Galera, R., García-Benito, C.,

Ramos, A., Fernández-Navarro, I., & Alonso-Álvarez, M. L. (2016). Effect of continuous positive airway pressure on glycemic control in patients with obstructive sleep apnea and type 2 diabetes: A randomized clinical trial. *American Journal of Respiratory and Critical Care Medicine, 194*(4), 476–485. https://doi.org/10.1164/rccm.201510-1942OC

[4] Van Cauter, E., Leproult, R., & Plat, L. (2000). Age-related changes in slow-wave sleep and REM sleep and relationship with growth hormone and cortisol levels in healthy men. *JAMA, 284*(7), 861–868. https://doi.org/10.1001/jama.284.7.861

[5] Spiegel, K., Leproult, R., & Van Cauter, E. (1999). Impact of sleep debt on metabolic and endocrine function. *The Lancet, 354*(9188), 1435–1439. https://doi.org/10.1016/S0140-6736(99)01376-8

[6] American Society for Biochemistry and Molecular Biology. (2019, September 16). *Lack of sleep affects fat metabolism.* https://www.sciencedaily.com/releases/2019/09/190916114020.htm

[7] Jurado-Fasoli, L., Mochon-Benguigui, S., Castillo, M. J., & Amaro-Gahete, F. J. (2020). Association between sleep quality and time with energy metabolism in sedentary adults. *Scientific Reports, 10*(1), 4598. https://doi.org/10.1038/s41598-020-61493-2

[8] St-Onge, M. P., Mikic, A., & Pietrolungo, C. E. (2016). Effects of diet on sleep quality. *Advances in Nutrition, 7*(5), 938–949. https://doi.org/10.3945/an.116.012336

Chapter 19

[1] Brand, A. (2024, September 20) Most stressful jobs in the UK revealed. https://hrreview.co.uk/hr-news/wellbeing-news/most-stressful-jobs-in-the-uk-revealed/

[2] Chandola, T., Brunner, E., & Marmot, M. (2006). Chronic stress at work and the metabolic syndrome: Prospective study. *BMJ (Clinical Research Ed.), 332*(7540), 521–525. https://doi.org/10.1136/bmj.38693.435301.80

[3] Troxel, W. M., Matthews, K. A., Gallo, L. C., & Kuller, L. H. (2005). Marital quality and occurrence of the metabolic syndrome in women. *Archives of Internal Medicine, 165*(9), 1022–1027. https://doi.org/10.1001/archinte.165.9.1022

[4] Block, J. P., He, Y., Zaslavsky, A. M., Ding, L., & Ayanian, J. Z. (2009). Psychosocial stress and change in weight among US adults. *American Journal of Epidemiology, 170*(2), 181–192. https://doi.org/10.1093/aje/kwp104

[5] Krolow, R., Noschang, C., Arcego, D. M., Huffell, A., Pettenuzzo, L. F., Dalmaz, C., & Gelain, D. P. (2019). Divergent metabolic effects of acute versus chronic repeated forced swim stress in rats. *Obesity, 27*(5), 773–779. https://doi.org/10.1002/oby.22390

[6] Jackson, S. E., Kirschbaum, C., & Steptoe, A. (2017). Hair cortisol and adiposity in a population-based sample of 2,527 men and women aged 54 to 87 years. Obesity, 25(3), 539–544. https://doi.org/10.1002/oby.21733

[7] Farrell, K., & Antoni, M. H. (2010). Insulin resistance, obesity, inflammation, and depression in polycystic ovary syndrome: Biobehavioral mechanisms and interventions. *Fertility and Sterility, 94*(5), 1565–1574. https://doi.org/10.1016/j.fertnstert.2010.03.081

[8] Hansen, A. L., Thomsen, R. W., Brøns, C., Svane, H. M. L., Jensen, R. T., Andersen, M. K., Hansen, T., Nielsen, J. S., Vestergaard, P., Højlund, K., Jessen, N., Olsen, M. H., Sørensen, H. T., & Vaag, A. A. (2023). Birthweight is associated with clinical characteristics in people with recently diagnosed type 2 diabetes. *Diabetologia, 66*(9), 1680–1692. https://doi.org/10.1007/s00125-023-05936-1; Mu., M., Wang, S. F., Sheng, J., Zhao, Y., Li, H. Z., Hu, C. L., & Tao, F. B. (2012). Birth weight and subsequent blood pressure: A meta-analysis. *Archives of Cardiovascular Diseases, 105*(2), 99–113. https://doi.org/10.1016/j.acvd.2011.10.006; Wibaek, R., Andersen, G. S., Linneberg, A., Hansen, T., Grarup, N., Thuesen, A. C. B., Jensen, R. T., Wells, J. C. K., Pilgaard, K. A., Brøns, C., Vistisen, D., & Vaag, A. A. (2023). Low birthweight is associated with a higher incidence of type 2 diabetes over two decades independent of adult BMI and genetic predisposition. *Diabetologia, 66*(9), 1669–1679. https://doi.org/10.1007/s00125-023-05937-0

[9] Curhan, G. C., Willett, W. C., Rimm, E. B., Spiegelman, D., Ascherio, A. L., & Stampfer, M. J. (1996). Birth weight and adult hypertension, diabetes mellitus, and obesity in US men. *Circulation, 94*(12), 3246–3250. https://doi.org/10.1161/01.CIR.94.12.3246; Sadrzadeh, S., Hui, E. V. H., Schoonmade, L. J., Painter, R. C., & Lambalk, C. B. (2017). Birthweight and PCOS: Systematic review and meta-analysis. *Human Reproduction Open, 2017*(2), hox010. https://doi.org/10.1093/hropen/hox010; Zhang, N., Liu, X., & Li, J. (2021). Birth weight and adult obesity index in relation to the risk of hypertension: A dose-response meta-analysis of prospective cohort studies. *Frontiers in Cardiovascular Medicine, 8*, 624914. https://doi.org/10.3389/fcvm.2021.624914

[10] Palmisano, G. L., Innamorati, M., & Vanderlinden, J. (2021). Life adverse experiences in relation with obesity and binge eating disorder: A systematic review. *Journal of Behavioral Addictions, 10*(1), 1–20. https://doi.org/10.1556/2006.2021.00002; Schmeer, K. K., & Tarrence, J. (2020). Childhood socioeconomic hardship, family conflict, and young adult hypertension. *Social Science & Medicine, 255*, 112982. https://doi.org/10.1016/j.socscimed.2020.112982

[11] Kiecolt-Glaser, J. K., Newton, T. L., Cacioppo, J. T., MacCallum, R. C., Glaser, R., & Malarkey, W. B. (2001). Marital conflict and endocrine function: Are men really more physiologically affected than women? *Journal of Consulting and Clinical Psychology, 69*(1), 46–59. https://doi.org/10.1037/0022-006X.69.1.46

[12] Ishizaki, M., Nakagawa, H., Morikawa, Y., Honda, R., Yamada, Y., & Kawakami, N. (2008). Influence of job strain on changes in body mass index and waist circumference—6-year longitudinal study. *Scandinavian Journal of Work, Environment & Health, 34*(4), 288–296.

[13] Cleveland Clinic. (2016). *High cholesterol: Causes, symptoms and how it affects the body*. https://my.clevelandclinic.org/health/articles/11918-cholesterol-high-cholesterol-diseases

[14] Powell, L. H., Shahabi, L., & Thoresen, C. E. (2003). Religion and spirituality:

Linkages to physical health. *American Psychologist, 58*(1), 36–52. https://doi.org/10.1037/0003-066x.58.1.36

[15]Hansen, A. L., Olson, G., Dahl, L., Thornton, D., Grung, B., Graff, I. E., Frøyland, L., & Thayer, J. F. (2014). Reduced anxiety in forensic inpatients after a long-term intervention with Atlantic salmon. *Nutrients, 6*(12), 5405–5418. https://doi.org/10.3390/nu6125405

[16] Banel, D. K., & Hu, F. B. (2009). Effects of walnut consumption on blood lipids and blood pressure: A meta-analysis and systematic review. *American Journal of Clinical Nutrition, 90*(1), 56-63. https://doi.org/10.3945/ajcn.2009.27457

Chapter 20

[1] Gimeno, L., Goisis, A., Dowd, J. B., & Ploubidis, G. B. (2024). Cohort differences in physical health and disability in the United States and Europe. *The Journals of Gerontology. Series B, Psychological Sciences and Social Sciences, 79*(8), gbae113. https://doi.org/10.1093/geronb/gbae113

[2] Pierce, M. B., Silverwood, R. J., Nitsch, D., Adams, J. E., Stephen, A. M., Nip, W., Macfarlane, P., Wong, A., Richards, M., Hardy, R., Kuh, D., & NSHD Scientific and Data Collection Teams (2012). Clinical disorders in a post war British cohort reaching retirement: Evidence from the First National Birth Cohort study. *PLOS One, 7*(9), e44857. https://doi.org/10.1371/journal.pone.0044857

[3] Miyawaki, C. E., Bouldin, E. D., Taylor, C. A., & McGuire, L. C. (2020). Baby boomers as caregivers: Results from the Behavioral Risk Factor Surveillance System in 44 states, the District of Columbia, and Puerto Rico, 2015-2017. *Preventing Chronic Disease, 17*, E80. https://doi.org/10.5888/pcd17.200010

[4] King, D. E., Matheson, E., Chirina, S., Shankar, A., & Broman-Fulks, J. (2013). The status of baby boomers' health in the United States: The healthiest generation? *JAMA Internal Medicine, 173*(5), 385–386. https://doi.org/10.1001/jamainternmed.2013.2006

[5] Zhang, T., Song, J., Shen, Z., Yin, K., Yang, F., Yang, H., Ma, Z., Chen, L., Lu, Y., & Xia, Y. (2024). Associations between different coffee types, neurodegenerative diseases, and related mortality: Findings from a large prospective cohort study. *The American Journal of Clinical Nutrition, 120*(4), 918–926. https://doi.org/10.1016/j.ajcnut.2024.08.012

[6] Abe, S. K., & Inoue, M. (2021). Green tea and cancer and cardiometabolic diseases: A review of the current epidemiological evidence. *European Journal of Clinical Nutrition, 75*(6), 865–876. https://doi.org/10.1038/s41430-020-00710-7; Zamani, M., Kelishadi, M. R., Ashtary-Larky, D., Amirani, N., Goudarzi, K., Torki, I. A., Bagheri, R., Ghanavati, M., & Asbaghi, O. (2023). The effects of green tea supplementation on cardiovascular risk factors: A systematic review and meta-analysis. *Frontiers in*

nutrition, 9, 1084455. https://doi.org/10.3389/fnut.2022.1084455

[7] Buettner, D. (n.d.). *Blue Zones Diet: Food Secrets of the World's Longest-Lived People.* https://www.bluezones.com/2020/07/blue-zones-diet-food-secrets-of-the-worlds-longest-lived-people/

[8] MedlinePlus. (n.d.). *Lactose intolerance.* https://medlineplus.gov/genetics/condition/lactose-intolerance/

[9] Orlich, M. J., Singh, P. N., Sabaté, J., Jaceldo-Siegl, K., Fan, J., Knutsen, S., Beeson, W. L., & Fraser, G. E. (2013). Vegetarian dietary patterns and mortality in Adventist Health Study 2. *JAMA Internal Medicine, 173*(13), 1230–1238. https://doi.org/10.1001/jamainternmed.2013.6473

[10] Colman, R. J., Beasley, T. M., Kemnitz, J. W., Johnson, S. C., Weindruch, R., & Anderson, R. M. (2014). Caloric restriction reduces age-related and all-cause mortality in rhesus monkeys. *Nature Communications, 5,* 3557. https://doi.org/10.1038/ncomms4557

[11] Spritzler, F. (2019, June 18). *Does eating slowly help you lose weight?* https://www.healthline.com/nutrition/eating-slowly-and-weight-loss

[12] Solan, M. (2023, August 1). *The (almost) last word on alcohol and health.* https://www.health.harvard.edu/staying-healthy/the-almost-last-word-on-alcohol-and-health

[13] Aubrey, A. (2024, April 29). *Elevator or stairs? Your choice could boost longevity, study finds.* https://www.npr.org/sections/health-shots/2024/04/29/1247532191/longevity-stairs-climbing-exercise-heart-disease; Paddock, S. (2024, April 25–27). Evaluating the cardiovascular benefits of stair climbing: a systematic review and meta-analysis [Conference presentation]. ESC Preventive Cardiology, Athens, Greece. https://esc365.escardio.org/presentation/279143

[14] Lee, D. H., Rezende, L. F. M., Joh, H. K., Keum, N., Ferrari, G., Rey-Lopez, J. P., Rimm, E. B., Tabung, F. K., & Giovannucci, E. L. (2022). Long-term leisure-time physical activity intensity and all-cause and cause-specific mortality: A prospective cohort of US adults. *Circulation, 146*(7), 523–534. https://doi.org/10.1161/CIRCULATIONAHA.121.058162

[15] Shen, X., Wu, Y., & Zhang, D. (2016). Nighttime sleep duration, 24-hour sleep duration and risk of all-cause mortality among adults: A meta-analysis of prospective cohort studies. *Scientific Reports, 6,* 21480. https://doi.org/10.1038/srep21480

Index

A

Abdominal fat, 96, 104
Acanthosis nigricans, 88, 140
Adipose tissue. See also Central obesity
Adrenal gland, 137
Alcohol, 98, 101
Antioxidants, 176, 291
Arteries
    atherosclerosis, 115, 153
    stiffness, 115
Arthritis. See Osteoarthritis

B

Baby Boomers, 332
Beans, 175, 77, 338
Behaviour change. *See also* Health goal setting
    barriers, 71, 176
    habits, 272
Benign Prostatic Hyperplasia (BPH), 214
Blood glucose
    high, 38, 138

monitoring, 142, 293
regulation, 150
Blood pressure
high, 112
lifestyle management, 126
Blue Zoners, 332
dietary patterns, 337
longevity, 332
Body mass index BMR, 30, 98
Bone health, 244

C

Carbohydrates
refined, 48, 50
whole-food sources, 50, 276
Cardiovascular health, 199
Central obesity, 94
Cholesterol
dietary, 155
HDL ("good"), 154
LDL ("bad"), 87, 91
particle size, 158, 173
management strategies, 175
Circulation, 115, 164
Cooking methods, healthy, 349
Congenital disorders. *See also* Genetic
Continuous glucose monitoring, 142, 197
Cortisol, 103, 141
Cuba, 51, 277
Cysts, 67, 85

D

Dairy products, 76

Diet
 DASH plan, 126
 Dehydration, 80, 292
 Metabolic diet prescription, 275
 Mediterranean, 284
 Western diet, 50, 114, 276
 Paleo diet, 278
 plant-based, 280
 low-carbohydrate, 278
 fasting, 92, 145, 290

Diabetes, 38, 92, 129

Dinner recipes, 370

E

Eisenhower, Dwight D., 153

Energy balance, 279

Environmental risk factors, 104, 231

Ethnicity, 31, 205

Exercise
 Metabolic exercise prescription, 294
 aerobic activity, 300, 305
 resistance training, 234, 300, 305
 HIIT, 234, 300
 Walking, 299

F

Familial hypercholesteraemia, 161

Fasting, 92, 290

Fatty liver disease, 180

Fats
- saturated, 282
- unsaturated, 281
- trans fats, 76, 174

Fatigue, 137
Fibre, dietary, 71
Fish, 56, 277
Fructose, 74, 132, 133
Fruits, 74, 277
Functional medicine, 16

G

Genetics, 103, 161
Gestational diabetes, 86, 138
Glucose metabolism, 10, 69, 71
Glycaemic index & load, 72, 145
Glycated haemoglobin, 88, 134
Glycogen, 61
Gout, 73
Gut microbiome, 77

H

Habits. *See also* Behaviour change
Health goal setting, 264
Heart
- Attack, 4, 26
- Disease, 26, 115
- Failure, 117, 118

Heavy metals, 56
Hormones
- insulin, 69

cortisol, 137

Hypertension. *See* Blood pressure, high

High blood sugar. *See* Blood glucose

High-density lipoprotein HDL, 154

High Fructose Corn Syrup HFCS, 73

History of metabolic syndrome, 18

Hormones. *See* insulin & cortisol

Hyperinsulinaemia, 69

Hypoglycaemia, 13

I

Immune system, 85

Inactivity *See* Sedentary life

Inflammation, 75

Infertility, 87, 226

Insulin resistance, 66

Intermittent fasting. *See also* Diet, fasting

J

Joints, 237

K

Kidney disease, 9, 117, 235

L

Lifestyle medicine, 15–18, 405, 410

Lipids. *See* Cholesterol

Low-density lipoprotein LDL, 89

Liver. *See* Fatty liver disease, 189

Lunch recipes, 370

M

Maradonna, Diego, 43

Menopause, 58

Mental health conditions, 136

Metabolic health screening, 26

Metabolic syndrome

    causes, 21, 76, 84

    complications, 85

    reversal, 106

Metabolism: the engine of life, 43

Mindset, 264

N

Nixon, Richard, 48

Nutrients

    micronutrients, 74

    Carbohydrates, 71

    Protein, 79

    Fat, 153

    Minerals, 52, 55

    Vitamins, 52

O

Obesity. *See* Central obesity, 94

Obstructive sleep apnoea OSA, 191

Omega 3, 107, 126, 176, 258

Organic food, 288

Osteoarthritis, 237

Ovarian health. *See* Polycystic ovary syndrome, 226

Oxygen, 54

P

Pelé, 43

Periodontal disease, 204

Physical activity. *See* also Exercise, 294

Polycystic Ovary Syndrome (PCOS), 226

Post-meal glucose level, 37

Pre-diabetes, 37

Processed food, 22, 77, 102

Psychological well-being, 136

R

Recipes
    breakfasts, 349
    lunches, 370
    dinners, 370
    snacks and sides, 349

Relationship, 317

Risk factors, metabolic, 28

S

Screening, 26

Sedentary life, 29, 86, 295

Sleep
    Apnoea, 191
    Metabolic sleep prescription, 307

Silver fillings. *Also* amalgum fillings, 56

Skin tags, 88, 140

Stress
    Management, 325
    Metabolic stress and relationship prescription, 317

Stroke, 2

Sugar
  added, 73, 102
  cravings, 148
Symptoms of metabolic syndrome, 6, 28

T
Tests - blood, 26, 141
Thyroid dysfunction, 51
Trans fats, 76, 174
Triglycerides, 38, 156, 219

U
Ultra-processed food UPF, 77

V
Varicose veins, 251
Vegetables, 277, 286
Vision problems, 116, 35
Vitamin D, 235

W
Waist circumference, 31, 8
Weight loss, 92, 125, 291
Whole grains, 72
Wild fish, 57, 277

X
Xanthelasma, 162

AVAILABLE FORMATS

Your Metabolic Shift ebook, Paperback, and Hardcover

COMING SOON

Your Metabolic Shift Audiobook, Whole Food Cookbook, and Digital Book.

To help you put the principles of Your Metabolic Shift into daily practice, you now have access to the **Your Metabolic Shift: 12-Week Reset Program**—a practical, step-by-step guide designed to help you reboot your metabolism, build powerful new habits, and create lasting change. Download Your 12-week Metabolic Reset Program Here: **www.drshariefibrahim.com**

Your Metabolic Shift starts here.

www.ingramcontent.com/pod-product-compliance
Lightning Source LLC
LaVergne TN
LVHW041616060526
838200LV00040B/1309